OXFORD MEDICAL PUBLICATIONS

Cancer Pain Management

Cancer pain management:
a comprehensive approach

Edited by

KAREN H. SIMPSON
Consultant in Pain Management,
Pain Management Service,
St James's University Hospital,
and Senior Clinical Lecturer,
University of Leeds, UK

KEITH BUDD
Consultant in Pain Management,
The Mornington Clinic, Cottingley Manor,
Bingley, West Yorkshire, UK

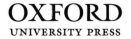

OXFORD
UNIVERSITY PRESS

OXFORD
UNIVERSITY PRESS

Great Clarendon Street, Oxford OX2 6DP
Oxford University Press is a department of the University of Oxford.
It furthers the University's objective of excellence in research, scholarship,
and education by publishing worldwide in

Oxford New York

Athens Auckland Bangkok Bogotá Buenos Aires Calcutta
Cape Town Chennai Dar es Salaam Delhi Florence Hong Kong Istanbul
Karachi Kuala Lumpur Madrid Melbourne Mexico City Mumbai
Nairobi Paris São Paulo Singapore Taipei Tokyo Toronto Warsaw

with associated companies in
Berlin Ibadan

Oxford is a registered trade mark of Oxford University Press
in the UK and in certain other countries

Published in the United States
by Oxford University Press, Inc., New York

A catalogue record for this title is available from the British Library

Library of Congress Cataloging in Publication Data

Cancer pain management : associated therapy to common practice / edited
by Karen H. Simpson, Keith Budd.
Includes bibliographical references and index.
1. Cancer pain.   I. Simpson, Karen H.   II. Budd, Keith.
[DNLM: 1. Neoplasms–therapy.   2. Pain–prevention & control.   3. Palliative Care. QZ
266 C21625 2000]
RC262 .C2911915 2000   616.99'406–dc21   00-032389

ISBN 0–19–262877–1 (alk. paper)

1 3 5 7 9 10 8 6 4 2

Typeset in Sabon by
Jayvee, Trivandrum, India
Printed in Great Britain
on acid-free paper by
Biddles Ltd.,
Guildford & King's Lynn

Contents

Contributors

Dawn L. Alison, *Macmillan Senior Lecturer in Oncology and Palliative Medicine, University of Leeds and St James's University Hospital, Leeds, UK*

Harald Breivik, *Professor and Chairman, Department of Anaesthesiology, The National Hospital, Oslo, Norway*

Meredith Dickens, *Anderson Cancer Centre, Texas USA*

Geoffrey Dunn, *Hospice Director, Great Lakes Hospice, Erie USA*

Ann Elfred, *Deputy Superintendent Physiotherapist, St Christopher's Hospice, London, UK*

Jacqueline Filshie, *Consultant in Anaesthetics and Pain Management, The Royal Marsden Hospital, Surrey and London, UK*

Lorna Foyle, *Independent Lecturer Practitioner/Lecturer, Dove House Hospice, Hull, UK*

Samuel J. Hassenbusch, *Anderson Cancer Centre, Texas USA*

Elliott S. Krames, *Pacific Pain Treatment Centre, San Francisco, USA*

Wendy P. Makin, *Macmillan Consultant in Palliative Care and Oncology, Christie Hospital and Holt Radium Institute, Manchester, UK*

Betty O'Gorman, *Superintendent Physiotherapist, St Christopher's Hospice, London, UK*

P. Poulain, *Assistant Professor, Institute Gustave Roussy, France*

Sunil K. Rohira, *Consultant in Pain Management and Anesthesiology. The Specialists Orthopedic Medical Corporation Fairfield. California, USA*

Lynne Russon, *Senior Registrar in Palliative Medicine, St James's University Hospital Leeds, UK*

Suzanne M. Skevington, *Professor of Health Psychology, University of Bath, UK*

David Stoter, *Manager, Chaplaincy Department and Bereavement Centre, Queen's Medical Centre, Nottingham, UK*

Elizabeth A. Thompson, *Senior Registrar in Palliative Medicine, Beatson Oncology Centre and Glasgow Homeopathic Hospital, UK*

John W. Thompson, *Emeritus Professor of Pharmacology, University of Newcastle upon Tyne and Emeritus Consultant Clinical Pharmacologist. Newcastle Health Authority, UK*

M. Vieyra, *Institute Gustave Roussy, France*

J. C. D. Wells, *Consultant in Pain Management, Liverpool, UK*

Stephen Wilkinson, *Lecturer in Medical Ethics, Department of Philosophy, Keele University, UK*

C. Wood, *Institute Gustave Roussy, France*

Preface

The world-wide incidence of cancer has increased and, in spite of major therapeutic advances, many tumours remain incurable. Cancer pain is a significant problem for millions of people and their physicians. Adequate control of this pain can improve quality of life and is an essential part of palliation. The oral or parenteral administration of primary and secondary analgesics drugs is the mainstay of pain management for most patients with cancer.

There are many publications that cover the pharmacology and therapeutics of the analgesic drugs. This book is about other aspects of pain control. It starts by recognizing those ethical issues that should underpin all management decisions. What follows emphasizes aspects of treatment and care that can sometimes be given a low priority or forgotten. The use of any analgesic drug or pain relieving technique should always be in the context of the care of the whole patient, including the psychological, spiritual, and nursing context. In addition, special considerations may be needed for children with cancer pain.

Physical methods of treatment such as physiotherapy and peripheral neural stimulation (transcutaneous electrical nerve stimulation or acupuncture) can be of great value and are discussed. This is also true of palliative surgery, radiotherapy, and chemotherapy that can be vital for cancer pain management.

Specialized management techniques such as simple or complex nerve blocks, spinal cord stimulation, percutaneous cordotomy, or neurosurgery may be needed for selected patients with pain that is difficult to control. Each of these different topics warrants a chapter so that they can be addressed and explained such that their value can be fully explored.

We have brought together experts from a variety of differing clinical areas, all with specific interest and expertise in cancer pain management, to focus on these strategies. Appropriate pain control involves so much more than the provision of medication. It must encompass the total care of the patient and often needs a multi-professional team to deliver this service.

We believe that this book provides a comprehensive review of the different analgesic modalities which, when used appropriately, will provide optimal pain control for patients with cancer-related pain. However, it must be understood that this goal also encompasses those who care and those who just wait.

Leeds	K.H.S.
Bingley	K.B.
August 2000	

ONE

Philosophy of cancer pain management

KAREN H. SIMPSON

Pain relief for patients with cancer should be part of a more comprehensive management plan to address the many factors affecting their quality of life (Ventifredda 1989). Pain control should encompass the concept of 'total pain', appreciating that pain has sensory, emotional, socioeconomic, and spiritual components. The World Health Organization developed its Analgesic Ladder to allow information on simple methods of pain control to be widely disseminated. This had a huge global impact. However, strong opioids are still not available to some of the world's population. Education and legislation to improve this situation is essential.

Pain in cancer is not just a medical issue and pain management should not be seen in isolation, but as part of a continuum of care delivered by a group of professionals (Levy 1991). Patients with cancer often present with a variety of symptoms of which pain is only one. A study of 1635 patients with cancer pain presenting to a pain clinic found that the average patient had 3.3 other symptoms. The most common were insomnia (59%), anorexia (48%), constipation (33%), sweating (28%), and nausea (27%) (Grond et al. 1994). It may, therefore, be necessary to treat patients with cancer pain using several different strategies. A multi-disciplinary approach by a co-ordinated team is needed so that pain management can be tailored to individual requirements and the need for crisis interventions can be reduced.

Failure to recognize and treat cancer pain is still a problem (Von Roenn et al. 1993). Undergraduate education in all aspects of palliative care is often inadequate (Billings and Block 1997) and insufficient continuing education of doctors in cancer pain management is a factor in the poor delivery of pain control worldwide (Elliott and Elliott 1991; Weissman 1996). A study of 81 doctors showed that only 5% could convert a parenteral dose of morphine to an equivalent dose of a controlled release preparation and also that they were unfamiliar with the palliative use of radiation (Mortimer and Bartlett 1997). A study of knowledge about pain assessment and management in 318 nurses showed a lack of knowledge about opioids (Hamilton and Edgar 1992). There is evidence of insufficient knowledge at many different levels and in various settings (Lebovits et al. 1997). Since cancer pain should be managed by a team, it is important to educate multi-professionally. Setting standards for pain management (Bookbinder et al. 1996) and the use of role model programs (Janjan et al. 1996) are possible ways forward.

Research and audit are needed to define best practice and assess whether it is being applied. In addition funding is required to evaluate potential new avenues for pain control and it should be realized that: basic science research forms the foundation on which clinical research can be built; rigorous assessment of the available methods of pain control is required; the benefits of good pain management need to be determined and documented; resources for health care are finite and should therefore be used on the most effective therapies. The ethical problem of resource allocation necessitates support from both research and audit.

The problem of cancer pain

There has been a worldwide increase in the incidence of cancer (Davies *et al.* 1990). Many of the cancers which are becoming commoner, for example lung, are not curable. Cancer cure rates in industrialized countries are 40–50%, but are much less in developing countries. Each year seven million new cancers are diagnosed and five million people die from cancer worldwide. At any one time about fourteen million people in the world are living with cancer. Many cancers occur in the older age group, where pain management may pose particular problems (Portenoy 1992) and this has important socioeconomic implications. Cancer pain in children involves some different issues which are distinct from those seen in adults (Liben 1996; Ljungman *et al.* 1996; see Chapter 7).

The World Health Organization has estimated that four million people in the world have cancer pain. Increased pain occurs as disease progresses, but also depends on the site of the cancer, disease stage, and treatment. Pain may not be a significant problem for patients in the early stages of disease, with fewer than 10% of patients with solid tumours reporting pain that interferes with mood or activity. About one in three patients with metastatic disease report significant pain.

The majority of patients with end stage disease have pain problems (Cleeland 1984). Pain is a significant problem even in ambulatory patients undergoing active treatment (Portenoy *et al.* 1992). More than 50% patients with cancer probably have unrelieved pain and breakthrough pain is often a particular problem (Portenoy and Hagen 1990; Yarbro *et al.* 1997).

Assessment of pain

It is important to try to determine the cause of pain before deciding on possible methods of pain control. Pain intensity, quality, distribution, temporal variation, and aggravating and relieving factors should be considered. Assessment of the patient's mood, sleep, activities of daily living and drug use help to put the pain problem into context. To treat this pain validated, easy to use, and repeatable assessment tools should be used. Pain should be evaluated in terms of the role it plays in the overall suffering of the patient and the carers. The quality of the patient's life should be assessed with the focus on the patient's perceptions (Slevin *et al.* 1988). Under treatment of cancer pain may be due to inadequate assessment of the problem (Gonzalez *et al.* 1991; Grossman *et al.* 1991) and, therefore, previous techniques used for pain control must be considered.

Unproductive efforts should not be repeated, as this may demoralize patients, carers, and other team members. The response of pain to treatment should be carefully and regularly monitored: a sudden increase in pain is most likely to be due to disease progression (Collin 1993). However, occult local tissue infection should also be considered (Coyle and Portenoy 1991). Sometimes pain may resist opioid medication (Fitzgibbon and Galter 1994). Psychosocial and spiritual problems may make the response of the pain to morphine irrelevant (see Chapters 3 and 4).

Pain in patients with cancer comes from a variety of sources, for example, tumour invading bones or viscera, pressing on nerves, or fungating through mucous membranes and skin. Pain may also be due to cancer therapy (surgery, radiation, or chemotherapy). Pain is unrelated to cancer in 3–10% sufferers. Most patients with cancer have multiple pain problems, usually at least three. Consideration of the pathophysiology of the pain can sometimes assist in selecting treatments (Ashby *et al.* 1992). Taking a careful history from the patient may give useful clues about the source of the pain and a careful physical examination is vital.

Appropriate investigation should be performed to elucidate pain mechanisms. Pain may be nociceptive which is usually related to tissue damage. This type of pain is often associated with an identifiable lesion and is commonly well localized. It may be aching or throbbing in quality. Visceral pain in solid organs or hollow organs is usually more diffuse and may be colicy in nature. Nociceptive and visceral pain often responds to opioids and anti-inflammatory drugs; nerve blocks may also be helpful in this type of pain. Neuropathic pain is sustained by aberrant processing in the peripheral and central nervous system. It is often associated with abnormal sensations which do not follow a dermatomal pattern. Pain may be maintained by or independent of the autonomic nervous system. Neuropathic pain is common in the cancer population (Cherny *et al.* 1994) and often partially resists opioid medication (Portenoy *et al.* 1990). However, as opioid responsiveness is not usually predictable, opioids should not be withheld because of assumptions about pain mechanisms. Central neuropathic pain is not usually helped by neurolytic procedures.

Methods of pain control

The basic principles of pain management are to decrease pain and improve quality of life, to do no further harm, to allow patient and carers choices, and to use resources as effectively as possible. Disease modification should always be considered in each patient and, therefore, surgery, radiation, or chemotherapy may be appropriate in some circumstances. Oral analgesic drugs remain the mainstays of cancer pain management: these are effective treatment for 90% patients. However, there are alternatives for patients whose pain resists oral drugs, those in whom medication produces side-effects or those in whom simple drug delivery methods cannot be used. Such alternatives may include neural blockade or spinal drug delivery. Neural blocks may target main divisions of the nervous system and may involve local anaesthetic, steroid, or neurolytic agents. Nerve blocks may be aimed at peripheral nerves, spinal cord, or autonomic ganglia. These techniques have a significant role in about 10% patients with cancer pain (Cleeland *et al.* 1994). Physical treatments such as electrical stimulation or acupuncture may also be appropriate in a significant number of patients. Ideally, a combined approach aimed at several different levels within the nervous system might provide the best pain relief with the fewest adverse effects. Rehabilitation is an extremely important part of pain management. The importance of psychological, social, and spiritual support must not be forgotten. Good communication with patients, carers, and with other professionals is essential for optimum treatment.

References

Ashby, M.A., Fleming, B.G., Brooksbank, M., Rounsefell, B., Runciman, W.B., Jackson, K., Muirden, N., Smith, M. (1992). Description of a mechanistic approach to pain management in advanced cancer. A preliminary report. *Pain*, **51**, 153–61.

Billings, J.A., and Block, S. (1997). Palliative care in undergraduate medical education. Status report and future directions. *Journal of the American Medical Association*, **278**, 733–8.

Bookbinder, M., Coyle, N., Kiss, M., Goldstein, M.L., Horlitz, K., Thaler, H., *et al.* (1996). Implementing national standards for cancer pain management: program model and evaluation. *Journal of Pain and Symptom Management*, **12**, 334–47.

Cherny, N.I., Thaler, H.T., Friedlander,-Klar, H., Lapin, J., Foley, K.M., Houde, R., and Portenoy, R.K. (1994). Opioid responsiveness of cancer pain syndromes caused by neuropathic or nociceptive mechanisms: a combined analysis of controlled single-dose studies. *Neurology*, **44**, 857–61.

Cleeland, C.S. (1984). The impact of pain on the patient with cancer. *Cancer*, **54** (11 Suppl), 2635–41.

Cleeland, C.S., Gonin, R., Hatfield, A.K., Edmondson, J.H., Burn, K.H., Stewart, J.S., and Pandaya, K.J. (1994). Pain and its treatment in patients with metastatic cancer. *New England Journal of Medicine*, **330**, 592–6.

Collin, E., Poulain, P., Gauvain-Piquard, A., Petit, G., and Pichard-Leandri, E. (1993). Is disease progression the major factor in 'morphine tolerance' in cancer pain treatment? *Pain*, **55**, 319–26.

Coyle, N., and Portenoy, R.K. (1991). Infection as a cause of rapidly increasing pain in cancer patients. *Journal of Pain and Symptom Management*, **6**, 266–9.

Davies, D.C., Hoel, D., Fox, J., and Lopez, A. (1990). International trends in cancer mortality. *Lancet*, **336**, 474–81.

Elliott, T.E., and Elliott, B.A. (1991). Physician acquisition of cancer pain management knowledge. *Journal of Pain and Symptom Management*, **6**, 224–9.

Fitzgibbon, D.R., and Galter, B.S. (1994). The efficacy of opioids in cancer pain syndromes. *Pain*, **58**, 429–31.

Gonzalez, G.R., Elliot, K.J., Portenoy, R.K., and Foley, K.M. (1991). The impact of a comprehensive evaluation on the treatment of cancer pain. *Pain*, **47**, 141–4.

Grossman, S.A., Sheidler, V.K., Swedeen, K., Mucenski, J., and Paintadosi, S. (1991).

Correlation of patients and caregivers ratings of cancer pain. *Journal of Pain and Symptom Management*, **6**, 53–7.

Ground, S., Zech, D., Diefenbach, C., and Bischoff, A. (1994). Prevalence and pattern of symptoms in patients with cancer pain: a prospective evaluation of 1635 cancer patients referred to a pain clinic. *Journal of Pain and Symptom Management*, **9**, 372–82.

Hamilton, J., and Edgar, L. (1992). A survey of examining nurses' knowledge of pain control. *Journal of Pain and Symptom Management*, **7**, 18–26.

Janjan, N.A., Martin, C.G., Payne, R., Dahl, J.L., Weissman, D.E., and Hill, C.S. (1996). Teaching cancer pain management: durability of educational effects of a role model program. *Cancer*, **77**, 996–1001.

Lebovits, A.H., Florence, I., Bathina, R., Hunko, V., Fox, M.T., and Bramble, C.Y. (1997). Pain knowledge and attitudes of healthcare providers: practice characteristic differences. *Clinical Journal of Pain*, **13**, 237–43.

Levy, M.H. (1991). Effective integration of pain management into comprehensive cancer care. *Postgraduate Medical Journal*, **67** (Suppl 2), 35–43.

Liben, S. (1996). Pediatric palliative medicine: obstacles to overcome. *Journal of Palliative Care*, **12**, 24–8.

Ljungman, G., Kreuger, A., Gordh, T., Berg, T., Sorensen, S., and Rawal, N. (1996). Treatment of pain in pediatric oncology: a Swedish nationwide survey. *Pain*, **68**, 385–94.

Mortimer, J.E., and Bartlett, N.L. (1997). Assessment of knowledge about cancer pain management by physicians in training. *Journal of Pain and Symptom Management*, **14**, 21–8.

Portenoy, R.K., (1992). Pain management in the older cancer patient. *Oncology*, **6** (Suppl 2), 86–98.

Portenoy, R.K., and Hagen, N.A. (1990). Breakthrough pain: definition, prevalence and characteristics. *Pain*, **41**, 273–81.

Portenoy, R.K., Foley, K.M., and Intrussi, C.E. (1990). The nature of opioid responsiveness and its implications for neuropathic pain: new hypotheses derived from studies of opioid infusions. *Pain*, **43**, 273–86.

Portenoy, R.K., Miransky, J., Thaler, H.T., Hornung, J., Bianchi, C., Cibas-Kong, I., Feldhamer, E., Lewis, F., Matomoros, I., and Sugar, M.Z. (1992). Pain in ambulatory patients with lung or colon cancer: prevalence, characteristics and effect. *Cancer*, **70**, 1616–24.

Slevin, M.L., Plant, H., Lynch, D., Drinkwater, J., and Gregory, N.M. (1988). Who should measure quality of life, the doctor or the patient. *British Journal of Cancer*, **57**, 109–12.

Ventifridda, V. (1989). Continuing care a major issue in cancer pain management. *Pain*, **36**, 137–43.

Von Roenn, J.H., Cleeland, C.S., Gonin, R., Hatfield, A., and Pondaya, K.J. (1993). Physicians' attitudes and practice in cancer pain management. A survey for the Eastern Co-operative Oncology group. *Annals of Internal Medicine*, **119**, 121–6.

Weissman, D.E. (1996). Cancer pain education for physicians in practice: establishing a new paradigm. *Journal of Pain and Symptom Management*, **12**, 364–71.

World Health Organization (1990). *Cancer pain relief and palliative care*. Technical Report Series 804, Geneva, WHO.

Yarbro, J.W., Bornstein, R.S., and Mastrangelo, M.J. (1997). Cancer pain management: update on breakthrough pain. *Seminars in Oncology*, **24** (Suppl 16), S16–42.

TWO

Ethical issues

LYNNE RUSSON AND STEPHEN WILKINSON

Those treating patients with cancer pain are faced with ethical issues daily, even though they may not be recognized as such. However, the difficulties rarely fit into neat philosophical categories. This chapter discusses informed consent, beneficence, non-maleficence, and the doctrine of double effect, and how such issues might influence patient care.

Informed consent

Decisions concerning the management of cancer pain should rest on informed consent by an autonomous patient. Informed consent is defined as:

A voluntary, uncoerced decision made by a sufficiently competent or autonomous person on the basis of adequate information and deliberation, to accept rather than reject some proposed course of action. (Gillon 1986, p. 113)

It is widely accepted that obtaining the patient's consent prior to any medical intervention is a requirement of both ethics and law (Beauchamp and Childress 1994; Gillon 1986; McHale *et al.* 1997). In more serious cases (e.g. surgery) consent should be explicit and, where possible, written. But in more minor cases (e.g. an external examination) oral consent, or even merely implied consent may suffice. Obviously, the consent requirement applies only to cases where the patient is 'competent'. When the patient is not competent (e.g. because they are unconscious or severely cognitively impaired) it may be ethical to proceed with treatment provided that the treatment is in the best interests of the patient.

Why does consent matter?

There are two main reasons for taking consent seriously. First the consent requirement benefits both the individual patient in question and patients in general, by making patients more willing to present themselves for examination or treatment. If patients were fearful that, once they stepped inside a doctor's surgery or hospital, they might be treated against their will, they would be deterred from presenting at all. Respecting patients' rights to choose or refuse treatments also helps to establish relationships of trust between patients and health-care professionals. The relationship between doctor and patient should be one of partnership and collaboration and, clearly, this objective would be hard to achieve if doctors regularly carried out treatment without consent.

The second reason for requiring informed consent relates to respect for patient autonomy. A patient behaves autonomously when they act on those desires that, on reflection, they have decided (without distorting external influences) to endorse. Autonomy is much more than simply desire. It is the capacity to think and decide independently, to act on the basis of that decision and to communicate the decision to others.

Not all patients are fully autonomous; non-competent ones may lack the capacity for self-determination. When patients are autonomous, we should respect their autonomy. This can be done by providing them with sufficient information to make their own rational and informed choices and, where possible, providing treatment in accordance with those choices.

The three elements of valid consent

Consent consists not merely of the patient uttering 'yes' when asked whether they accept a proposed course of treatment. It is a more substantial notion. The following three conditions must be met for consent to be valid.

- It must be fully voluntary and not the result of coercion, of manipulation or of either real or perceived threats.
- The patient must be sufficiently competent.
- The patient must be adequately informed.

The rest of our discussion of consent is devoted to showing how these three elements might be applied in practice, with special reference to the management of cancer pain.

Voluntariness

Fortunately, explicit coercion and threats are rare in everyday practice. Manipulation, however, is much more common. For example, one might choose to say 'this method of pain relief has a 50% chance of giving you complete relief', rather than 'this method of pain relief has a 50% chance of not giving you relief despite the recognized risks', to persuade patients to consent, by making them think positively about the treatment. To avoid manipulation, practitioners should be careful to convey information to patients in a way which is as 'neutral' as possible—expressing the same point in several different ways. Saying, for instance, that there are several ways of viewing the benefits and risks involved. Practitioners should also be aware that even if no real threat exists, patients may sometimes perceive there to be a threat. They may believe for instance that if they don't do what the doctor recommends, they will be labelled as 'uncooperative' or 'non-compliant' and, as a result, receive a lower level of care. Patients in pain and with a terminal illness are an extremely vulnerable group. Practitioners can help to alleviate this problem by making it clear to patients that, whatever choice they make, the team of carers will continue to do their best for the patient (insofar as the patient allows them to do so).

Competence

A patient is competent if they can make reasonable decisions after understanding the information they are given and are able to assess rationally the pros and cons of a particular procedure. It is sometimes impossible to distinguish clearly between competence and non-competence, because the idea of competence is based on notions like 'understanding' and 'reasonableness' which are matters of degree. So there will inevitably be difficult borderline cases.

To be competent an individual should:

- Understand in broad terms and simple language, what the treatment is, its purpose and nature, and why it has been proposed.
- Understand its principal benefits, risks, and alternatives.
- Understand in broad terms the consequences of not receiving the proposed treatment.
- Make a choice, free from undue pressure.
- Retain the information long enough to make an effective decision.

It is impossible to deem a person competent or incompetent by a single test. Competence varies from day to day and procedure to procedure. Practitioners should take care to ensure that they regularly test patients' competence, to avoid incorrect classification. Practitioners should ensure that they do not operate with overly 'substantive' (as opposed to 'procedural') conceptions of reasonableness and understanding. In other words, they should be careful not to deem the patient incompetent for making a decision with which they disagree. For the purposes of competence, what matters, is the patient's ability to go through a recognizable reasoning process. The patient is not necessarily incompetent just because the outcome of that process seems to most of the rest of us to be irrational. The following examples illustrate these differences.

A Jehovah's witness refuses a blood transfusion in a life-threatening situation. If this was the decision reached following a reasoning process when the pros and cons of both treatment and non-treatment were fully understood, although this would seem to many of us to be irrational, the patient would still be competent to make such a decision.

In contrast a patient who suffers from dementia is offered a lumbar plexus block for malignant infiltration of his psoas muscle causing considerable pain. As a result of the dementia he has lost his general reasoning abilities and therefore bases his decision solely on avoiding a painful injection. This patient would be considered incompetent and therefore unable to give informed consent.

Information

In order for a consent to be valid, the patient must be provided with an appropriate level of information. But how much information should be provided? If the patient is not given enough, then consent will not be informed. But it is also possible to give too much complex information, causing the patient to become confused and/or distressed. When prescribing amitriptyline, for example, which of the numerous side-effects should be mentioned? Dry mouth and sedation, or do we include urinary retention, tachycardias, weight gain, and agranulocytosis. Which of the long list of potential complications of all drugs and treatments should we mention? The bioethics literature commonly refers to three standards of disclosure (Beauchamp and Childress 1994).

The first of these is known as the professional practice standard in which the level of disclosure is adequate if it conforms to conventional practice. Perhaps the most attractive feature of this view is that it respects professional autonomy, by allowing practitioners themselves to set the standard. There are, however, serious problems with it. What counts as 'conventional medical practice'? There is likely to be much disagreement within the professions about what level of disclosure is acceptable, so which subgroup of the profession should be taken to determine the standard? Should it be the lowest standard, the highest standard, or some sort of average? The professional practice standard allows no room for criticising whole groups of professionals and no room for the idea that a profession as a whole doesn't have high enough standards.

The second standard—the reasonable person standard—an adequate level of disclosure to enable a hypothetical reasonable person to make an informed decision. This standard does not rely on existing conventions in the way that the professional practice standard does and is, in this respect at least, rather better. However, there are still problems, the most serious of which is that the standard takes no account of the differing needs of individual patients. The amount of information given is based not on individual needs, but rather on a hypothetical reasonable person.

The third level of disclosure is usually called the subjective standard, although a better name for it would be the individual patient standard. According to this view, the level of information is appropriate if it enables the individual patient in question to make an informed choice. This is the most demanding of the standards and can be seen as best practice. It is demanding because it places an obligation on the doctor to assess each individual patient to determine what level of information is appropriate. This may be difficult to do with any accuracy within the time available. The main disadvantages of using the individual patient standard are that it can be expensive (in terms of professionals' time) and professionals may not be in a position to assess individual patients' informational needs accurately.

Conclusion

The consent requirement is important because it promotes patient welfare and respects patient autonomy. For a consent to be valid, practitioners need to ensure that patients are competent, that they are not coerced or manipulated in any way and that an appropriate level of information is provided.

Patient welfare: beneficence, non-maleficence

When discussing the possible types of treatment or intervention available to a particular patient it is important to consider the selection offered in the best interests of the patient and not to forget there is often a price to pay. The price may only be a day in hospital, but for some cancer patients with limited time this may be too high a price.

Beneficence and non-maleficence

These are both welfare-duties, duties that are concerned with patients' health, interests, and well-being. Beneficence means doing good, improving patient welfare, and making patients better than they otherwise would be. Non-maleficence means not harming, not making patients worse. All treatment decisions, including decisions about the treatment of cancer pain, should be based (at least in part) on these two fundamental moral principles. Non-maleficence is commonly thought to be more important than beneficence, i.e. it is thought that harming someone is worse than failing to benefit them.

The whole idea of sound, 'evidence-based' clinical practice can be seen as being based on the thoughts about beneficence and non-maleficence. In other words, what the health services should be providing, where possible, are interventions which have been shown to be maximally beneficent (i.e. those which improve patients' health and/or quality of life as much as possible) and minimally maleficent (i.e. those where the probability of side-effects and suffering are kept to a minimum). Within the context of cancer pain treatment, we need to consider beneficence and non-maleficence together to produce a 'benefits versus risks and burdens' equation. The patient must be allowed to assess for themselves the relative importance of each element in this equation (Randall and Downie 1996).

For example, a patient with intractable pain affecting a lower limb caused by an osteosarcoma may readily accept the potential pain-relieving benefit of an epidural system, despite the risks of life-threatening infection and the burden of increased hospitalization. A young man with pancreatic cancer and upper abdominal pain may feel that the significant risk of impotence outweighs the potential pain relieving effects of a coeliac plexus block.

Professionals have an obligation to provide treatments that have a high benefits: risks ratio, for example, a single fraction of palliative radiotherapy to a painful bony metastasis in prostatic cancer. This treatment often provides the patient with good pain relief with a simple non-invasive procedure and without all the adverse effects of high dose curative radiotherapy regimens. If the balance of benefits to burdens or risks is equally weighted, the treatment is considered optional and the autonomous patient should make the final decision. If, however, the burdens and risks clearly outweigh the likely benefits, some would argue the treatment should not be offered, because to do so would breach the moral principle of non-maleficence.

Patients can only make valid choices on the basis of shared information about diagnosis, prognosis, realistic treatment options, and risks of adverse effects. In-depth knowledge and effective communication by the team caring for the patient are therefore vital.

Conclusion

Health-carers are under a general obligation to maximize benefits and to minimize risks and burdens. Patients' own preferences and values should, where possible, be taken into account when assessing the levels of benefit and burden. The very same side-effect may be relatively easily tolerated by one patient, but regarded as intolerable by another. If a possible treatment is likely overall to benefit the patient, then there is a strong moral reason to provide it. Conversely, if a possible treatment is likely overall to harm the patient, then there is a strong moral reason not to offer it. In both cases, though, these reasons need to be considered alongside the patient's preferences and alongside issues of informed consent.

There are occasions when attempting to relieve the patient's pain may actually cause them considerable harm, such as an intrathecal implantable system which causes meningitis. This is considered to be a recognized risk of the procedure. There are also situations when the beneficial pain-relieving treatment produces its effect by simultaneously causing an adverse effect, this is discussed in the doctrine of double effect.

The doctrine of double-effect

Although often criticised by moral philosophers, the doctrine of double effect (DDE) is widely accepted by health-care practitioners and by various religious groups, most notably the Catholic Church. Some lawyers have argued that it has a role in English Law (Beauchamp and Childress (1994c; Brazier 1992; Gillon 1986; Glover 1977; Harris 1985; McHale *et al.* 1997; Mackie 1977; McMahan 1994; Price 1997). The main idea behind DDE is that, provided certain conditions are met, one is not responsible for all the effects of one's actions, but only for those which are intended. The doctrine of double-effect is, therefore, normally applied to cases in which an action (such as administering a drug) has both a good effect (e.g. pain relief) and a bad effect (e.g. adverse effects, perhaps including hastening death). The doctrine of double-effect states:

Provided that the good effect is what was intended and the bad effect is a merely foreseen but unintended side-effect, then the action is ethically permissible.

In order to render DDE remotely plausible, though, it needs to be formulated in a slightly more detailed way. One such formulation is as follows. An action is ethically permissible provided that all the following conditions are met (Beauchamp and Childress 1994; Price 1997; Sheldon and Wilkinson 1997).

- The action is not intrinsically wrong (i.e. wrong independent of its effects).
- The intended end (i.e. those effects which are aimed at) must be good.
- The bad effects of the action must not be aimed at and must not themselves be means of achieving the good effects.
- The good effects must be sufficiently good to outweigh the bad effects. (This is sometimes referred to as the 'proportionality condition'.)

Why is DDE relevant to the management of cancer pain?

DDE is best illustrated by the use of diamorphine. Take the case of a weak, terminally ill patient who is in pain. A doctor administers diamorphine, which (in this case) causes depressed ventilation and hastens the patient's death. Why isn't this (either morally or legally) a case of murder? The short answer is that the doctor didn't have the relevant intention, since the intention was to relieve the patient's pain, not to kill.

A fuller answer can be provided using the doctrine of double effect. Assuming that the administration of diamorphine is not intrinsically wrong (wrong independently of its effects) we need to ask three questions, corresponding to the last three parts of the doctrine in order to see whether it would classify the action as permissible.

First, was the intended end (pain relief) good? Almost certainly 'yes': relieving pain seems uncontroversially to be a good thing.

Second, was the bad effect (hastened death) aimed at and was it a means of achieving the good effect (pain relief)? Again, almost certainly 'no' (to both parts of the question). The doctor did not intend death (indeed, would probably prefer the patient to survive) and death was not the means of causing pain relief. Rather, death and pain relief were both effects of a common cause, the administration of diamorphine.

Finally, is the good effect (pain relief) sufficiently good to outweigh the bad effect (hastened death)?

This is a much harder question and the answer will vary depending on the details of the case. If the pain was relatively minor and the patient lost 10 years of life, then most would, we suppose, agree that the 'proportionality condition' had not been met. The patient would be better off keeping both the pain and the extra ten years, rather than losing both. But if the pain was intolerable and the patient only lost a few hours of life then most would, we suppose, feel that the patient had benefited overall from the administration of diamorphine.

For this sort of reason, the doctrine of double-effect is more widely applied to 'end of life' situations, than to others. The idea being that it is easier to outweigh the loss of a small quantity of remaining life with other benefits (in terms of quality of life) than to outweigh the loss of a large quantity of remaining life.

It might seem, as if the doctrine of double-effect sanctions some forms of euthanasia, since we talk in terms of patients benefiting from having their lives shortened. However, it must be stressed that it is not supposed to be a way of justifying euthanasia. It is instead an attempt to establish that there is an ethically significant difference between those cases where death is a foreseen but unintended side-effect of an intervention, and those in which death is intended, either as an end in itself, or as a means of achieving pain relief.

Two criticisms are commonly levelled at this doctrine. The first is that, in practice, it is very hard to tell which effects are intended and which are merely foreseen. Sometimes, even the person who is carrying out the action in question might not be sure about this. The second is that, by cleverly redescribing the relevant situations, we can manipulate DDE in order to generate whatever result strikes us as convenient. (Harris 1985.) If correct, this second objection would mean that DDE doesn't really provide any guidance, since we can usually get it to support whatever we do, provided that we describe our actions in a certain way.

Conclusion

If accepted, the doctrine of double-effect means that interventions with harmful side-effects (including, in some cases, hastened death) are acceptable provided that the four conditions outlined are met. However, professionals should remain mindful of the fact that there are both practical and theoretical problems with this doctrine.

References

Beauchamp, T., and Childress, J. (1994). *Principles of biomedical ethics* (4th edn). Oxford University Press, Oxford.

Brazier, M. (1992). *Medicine, patients and the law*, (2nd edn). Penguin, Harmondsworth.

Gillon, R. (1986). *Philosophical medical ethics*. John Wiley & Sons, Chichester.

Glover, J. (1977). *Causing death and saving lives*. Penguin, Harmondsworth.

Harris, J. (1985). *The value of life*. Routledge, London.

Mackie, J. (1977). *Ethics*. Penguin, Harmondsworth.

McHale, J., Fox, M., and Murphy, J. (1997). *Health care law*. Sweet & Maxwell, London.

McMahan, J. (1994). Revising the doctrine of double effect. *Journal of Applied Philosophy*, **11**, 201–12.

Price, D. (1997). Euthanasia, pain relief, and double effect. *Legal Studies*, **17**, 323–42.

Randall, F., and Downie, R.S. (1996). *Palliative care ethics*. Oxford Medical Publications, Oxford.

Sheldon, S., and Wilkinson, S. (1997). Conjoined twins: the legality and ethics of sacrifice. *Medical Law Review*, **5**, 149–71.

THREE

Psychological support

SUZANNE M. SKEVINGTON

Illness is the innately human experience of symptoms and suffering . . . and how the sick person and the members of the family or wider social network perceive, live with and respond to symptoms and disability. (Arthur Kleinman 1988)

Introduction: some theoretical and methodological issues

Melzack and Wall's (1965) classic paper on the Gate Control theory of pain is a prime example of how brilliant theoretical insights can lead to a plethora of therapeutic interventions. Without it, we would not have discovered transcutaneous electrical nerve stimulation (TENS), understood how distraction works as a coping strategy, or made serious strides in the pharmacological targeting of analgesics. It is also exciting because, for the first time, the central psychological mechanisms that contribute to the experience and reporting of pain were made explicit within a theory of pain rather than being seen as incidental. Consequently psychology has become an integral part of multi-disciplinary research into pain and its treatment.

Although the exact nature of the electrochemical messages transmitted to the spinal cord centres (via descending controls) still require fuller neurophysiological elucidation, experimental and clinical evidence no longer leaves room for substantial doubt that psychological factors form in integral part of the mechanism (Melzack and Wall 1982). This enables us to explain relatively common clinical instances where pain is present in the absence of injury, malignancy, or other pathology and, conversely, a spectrum of organic damage in the absence of perceived pain. Such insights challenge the traditional and erroneous notion that pain results solely from damage or pathology. So the dual incorporation of theory into pragmatic research produces progress simultaneously on two fronts; firstly, it satisfies the primary goal of helping to relieve suffering and, secondly, at the same time it advances scientific understanding about how pain mechanisms work.

The accurate assessment of pain is not an easy issue but psychometricians are trained to design, develop, and test instruments to see whether they are reliable, valid, and responsive to changes in the clinical condition. The scores from these instruments are often used in clinical decision-making and hence the goal for users should be to select them with full knowledge of their strengths and weaknesses and to be aware that the interpretation of their results requires both caution and expertise. Without good measures of pain, how can we be confident that care and treatment are appropriately prescribed and when instigated, are providing sufficient relief? Basic research on measurement is an important precursor to the delivery of good health care. Some selected issues surrounding measurement that particularly concern practitioners are addressed here.

Assessments that contain a large number of questions may be burdensome for severely ill cancer patients and the demand from clinicians for short and easy scales is no greater than in this field. However it is wrong to assume that to be useful, all assessments for cancer patients must be short. The amount of pain and distress commonly associated with different cancers is very varied, and within each diagnostic group there is considerable heterogeneity too, so the general term 'cancer' is not helpful to selection here. Many patients who are diagnosed early and treated successfully and those who are ostensibly 'cured', may well be able and willing to cope with more comprehensive assessment of their pain. Indeed, they may welcome it, in the hope that it may improve communications between them and those who care for them. Reluctance to accept more comprehensive instruments of pain and quality of life in this field has tended to lead to a poverty of conceptualization, where the need to reduce the number of items in a scale has overshadowed the desirability of making a holistic assessment of the patient's condition, so raising questions about its adequacy. Astutely, Cleeland *et al.* (1996) comment on the inevitable compromise that must be achieved between asking every possible question and the practical and theoretical demands of establishing a suitable method of pain assessment. But new scales are more often judged in this area by how few items are included rather than whether the instrument is precise and reliable in its measurement, whether its scores change in a sensitive way when there are visible changes in a patient's clinical condition, and whether it is a valid measure of what it purports to measure. With alacrity as the driving priority, the best instruments may be overlooked in favour of the poorer ones, and patients and research may suffer as a consequence.

Several methods have been developed for use in reporting subjective pain (Skevington 1995). If assessing the intensity of pain is the prime goal, then the use of a visual analogue scale (VAS) may be sufficient (Fig. 5.1, p. 53). The VAS is a plain, 100 mm line with labels at the poles (Huskisson 1983). However a comparison of different types of similar scale by Jensen *et al.* (1986) suggests that scales other than the popular VAS may be understood better by a wider range of people and have better predictive validity. In their evaluation, the Numerical Rating Scale (NRS) is judged to be the best, where 100 equal divisions are marked along a 10 cm line (Fig. 5.1, p. 53). However pain is a multidimensional concept consisting of many different qualities and it is arguable that the assessment of pain quantity through pain intensity is only one of many dimensions that might be usefully assessed. These qualities are best demonstrated in a hardy perennial among multidimensional instruments—the McGill Pain Questionnaire (MPQ) (Melzack 1975). In this measure 20 classes of pain are described, each containing several descriptions e.g. tingling, agonizing, burning, aching. The 5-point weightings attributed to each description are accumulated to give both quantitative and qualitative scores. A short form MPQ of 15 items is also available (Melzack 1987) which may be of value in assessing the severely ill. An advantage of this measure is that it examines qualities of pain e.g. sensory and affective dimensions as well as pain intensity, within the same instrument and, in this way, there is much more comprehensive evaluation of pain than in comparable unidimensional measures.

The MPQ is a generic measure that is designed to assess pain in many different medical conditions. But specific measures that directly assess the condition of a particular diagnostic group, for instance melanoma patients, are also attractive because the questions are seen to be more directly relevant to the respondent's condition. However, the use of specific scales precludes comparisons between patients who have other diseases or conditions and so specific measures are less useful than generic ones for resource allocation within the health service. In the end, the choice of measure depends on what the results will be used for, assuming that the psychometric properties of both types of instrument are equally sound. However the specificity of a measure allows for the assessment of features that would not necessarily be relevant to other conditions. For instance, nausea and vomiting are unlikely to be relevant to quality of life assessment in well people or rheumatoid arthritis patients even though they may centrally affect the quality of life of those with a malignancy who are receiving chemotherapy.

Nevertheless, specific measures may enable other types of comparisons to be made. Recently, Cleeland *et al.* (1996) have shown how specific measures like the Brief Pain Inventory (BPI) can be of considerable use in making cross-cultural comparisons between cancer patients in diverse countries, worldwide. In the BPI, patients report their worst, least, and average pain intensity over the past week using a 10-point scale and then show how much pain interferes with various activities. Data from France, China, the Philippines, and USA confirms that pain has two main dimensions; one for activity and another representing emotions. This pattern persists regardless of whether mild, moderate, or severe cancer patients are being assessed. Subsequent samples from Vietnam and India have largely served to support the initial results. The scale promises to be a suitable tool with which to assess whether pain from cancer is being adequately treated.

So theory and measurement inform the practical ways in which psychologists approach the subject of pain in general and cancer pain in particular. In the sections that follow we consider a wide range of psychosocial support and interventions that may be offered to cancer patients and their families. As many cancer patients receive their diagnosis and have their treatment program co-ordinated by their general practitioner, the first sections examine important issues associated with the consultation.

Understanding beliefs about pain and illness

Foundations for the successful management of pain and suffering associated with the diseases of cancer depend upon being able to understand the patient's perspective. As this is achieved, the information enables communications, advice, and choice of treatment to be pitched at an appropriate level and so this knowledge has inherent and practical value. At the same time it instigates the process of developing trust between patient and health professional that is fundamental to the success of almost every therapeutic relationship including the management of cancer and any associated pain.

The range of beliefs and expectations people hold about health and health care are many and varied, even within relatively homogeneous societies and so assumptions about a patient's beliefs and expectations cannot be anticipated accurately. To misunderstand at this early stage may cause unnecessary distress in those who are already trying to adjust to unpleasant news and an uncertain future. It is important that health professionals dealing with cancer patients have the opportunity to develop and practice the skills needed to become comfortable with investigating a patient's network of beliefs and expectations. This investigation should be carried out without delay, as soon as the symptoms presented suggest cancer, as an integral part of psychosocial care.

Making time to review these beliefs and expectations at appropriate intervals is an integral part of this strategy. Beliefs and expectations about pain in particular and illness in general are not static but are dynamically revised as time goes on. In the same way that treatment is reviewed regularly, changes in psychological state should provide milestones to prime further discussion about beliefs and expectations so that the picture is regularly updated and any misunderstandings can be corrected before they cause undue anxiety. Research in psychoneuroimmunology has begun to show how excessive anxiety, with its attendant adrenaline flow, can exacerbate many physical conditions and accelerate a decline in health (Liebskind 1991). Anxiety and depression are also well known factors that accentuate pain, so reviewing beliefs and expectations in order to keep undue anxiety and depression at bay, are vital to the successful management of cancer patients as they can speed or impair recovery.

One of the most important things patients want to know is their diagnosis and whether it is serious. In one study, only a small minority (14%) had any prior convictions about what might be wrong with their health (Reader *et al*. 1957). So how can we find out what patients believe? Reader *et al*. (1957) found that patients do expect to be questioned by their doctors but that not all doctors know how to do this effectively. At the earliest stages of symptom reporting, when diagnosis is uncertain, it is desirable to ask open-ended questions (Weinman and Higgins 1975). Open ended questions usually begin with 'who', 'where', 'how', 'when', 'what' 'tell me about...'. These contrast with closed questions like 'did/didn't', 'have/haven't', 'will/won't which lead the respondent to articulate a simple, unelaborated answer of 'yes' or 'no'. A question such as 'What do **you** think might be the matter with you'? invites patients to express any fears about the possibility of cancer or even to say that they do not think that it is cancer. Asking in a relaxed style serves the dual purpose of enabling patients to open up a discussion about worrying thoughts, and for that anxiety to be defused before it develops into a chronic condition. While this approach might on the face of it sound like an invitation to make one's own diagnosis, it precludes health professionals from trying to make a wild guess about what their patients might be thinking and at the same time seeming to volunteer suggestions about the patients' beliefs which could be misinterpreted by an anxious or hypervigilant patient as a hint about their real condition. The reduction of uncertainty by ruling out the unrealistic, is a sensible aim. When patients are in pain, they are particularly keen to know how long the pain is likely to last (Williams and Thorn 1989) and where this can be reasonably predicted and realistically answered, it is likely to improve well-being by reducing uncertainty.

Another area of psychological concern that may affect well-being surrounds beliefs about being to blame for negative health events (Williams and Thorn 1989). Retrospectively, many patients with a diagnosis of cancer will scrutinize their lifestyle and ask themselves whether something in their environment or past behaviour might have caused the cancer. Irrespective of the veracity of findings from medical research, patients will do better psychologically if carers can encourage them not to blame themselves for their past behaviour. The advice to 'go easy on yourself' seems to be a particularly important message that can be delivered to relieve suffering, within the current social climate that demands that people take responsibility for their own health. Patients with cancer who are perceived by society to have neglected their health are likely to detect disapproval and internalize self-blame, and perceptions of being a victim are not conducive to well-being (Buller and Buller 1987). Health professionals are in a position to dissipate some of this in their role as an authoritative source. This is not to deny that sound medical research findings exist, but to preclude additional suffering from self-blame and feelings of victimization by counselling the comfort of probabilities, individual differences and circumstances. Self-blame is a well known precursor of depression, so action to prevent self-blame affords some protection against the development of chronic negative mood states that in turn can exacerbate the pain. Legitimate explanations about genetics, misfortune, and other factors beyond the patient's control such as particular environmental conditions, are likely to reduce anxiety and be more comforting, where they are known in the health literature.

Patients could also be encouraged to search for a suitable explanation for their illness, as being able to identify a cause can assist the development of well-being, especially in the period immediately following diagnosis and treatment. Research on breast cancer patients by Taylor *et al.* (1984) has shown that those who were able to identify an explanation for their illness in the two years subsequent to a diagnosis of breast cancer showed better adjustment to their illness than those who did not derive a cause. But the picture was not quite so simple, because if patients in this study attributed their cancer to a particular stressor, or if they were inclined to blame others, despite the derivation of an explanation, their psychological state was worse. So it would appear that using certain sorts of explanations about the causes of illness can be very important to the states of well-being during and following treatment for cancer. For many patients, this insight can be an important feature of coming to terms with having a life-threatening illness.

Patients may also have beliefs about bodily sensations other than pain, that raise fears about recurrence during or after treatment has been completed. Ambiguous sensations are the most fear-provoking because they generate anxiety about whether or not to seek further medical help and what consequences that action might bring. From the time of diagnosis, patients should be actively encouraged to visit early if they experience new sensations so that where unfounded, their anxieties can be tackled in the reassuring style that makes no reference to hypochondria. Where anxieties are realistic and founded, then the relabelling of sensations can be encouraged to assist coping. An extensive literature on coping with chronic pain suggests that a rich variety of strategies may be used (Rosensteil and Keefe 1983). To view a sensation as warmth instead of pain for instance, can assist in more positive psychological thinking and better mood.

The use of pleasant and neutral imagery has been found to be helpful (Fernandez and Turk 1989). Other strategies include using coping statements about self, and being able to ignore sensations. Strategies to divert attention are productive, but those where people hope and pray (rather than using an active strategy) are found to be less useful. Lastly, believing with a high degree of confidence that you are able to control events (self-efficacy) and more specifically decreasing the aversiveness of pain, is also a productive pain relieving strategy (Lawson *et al.* 1990). These beliefs about control are closely related to coping (Crisson and Keefe 1988).

Considerable research attention has been focused on beliefs about controlling pain. If people believe they can personally control their pain then this is beneficial to well being. Experimental research by Bowers (1968) underlines the power of these beliefs. The study showed that it is not actually controlling the pain that gives pain relief, but believing that you can control the pain if you want or need to, is much more important and effective. Beliefs about the personal control of pain have been well researched with a number of different methodologies that point to the same conclusion—being in personal control is best. However those in pain may also believe in part or whole, that their pain is controlled by what the doctors can do for them or is even controlled by events beyond anybody's control; by factors such as chance events or misfortune. These beliefs also affect the style and frequency of coping activities. So in short, determining where the locus or site of control is perceived to be, is one step along the road to deciding what plan or pattern of pain control activities is most likely to be effective.

In general, those with acute pain and illness are more likely to have stronger beliefs in their personal ability to control pain than those in chronic pain who rely more on explanations about chance or misfortune. Those in chronic pain also tend to have stronger beliefs that the doctors are in control of the pain. This may be because constant or recurrent pain has an attritional effect on well-being in general and coping beliefs in particular. Using the Beliefs in Pain Control Questionnaire (BPCQ), Skevington (1990) found that ovarian cancer patients with little pain had strong beliefs about the personal control of pain but weak beliefs both about the powers of doctors to control pain and that pain is controlled by chance happenings. In contrast, patients with pains associated with breast cancer and its treatments showed a pattern of beliefs more typical of chronic pain patients, namely weaker beliefs about being able to control the pain personally and strong beliefs both in the powers of doctors to control pain and that pain is controlled by bad luck.

Following an extensive review, Wallston (1989) and others, have concluded that beliefs about personal control are associated with being healthy and beliefs about chance indicate poorer health, in mental and physical terms. This body of knowledge suggests that health professionals would improve and sustain well-being in oncology patients by encouraging beliefs about the personal control of pain, by discouraging unrealistic beliefs in the powers of doctors to control it and by trying to challenge and change explanations that involve chance, bad luck, or misfortune. Explanations that pain is controlled by chance seem to be the most counterproductive of the three types of belief to restoring well-being and are more likely to be associated with helplessness and depressed mood.

Patients might be encouraged to explore whatever psychologically positive and/or medically harmless strategies they know of and like, that may assist in the process of building beliefs in the personal control of pain and health and maintaining them. Chicken soup is the time honoured example in medicine, under the assumption that if it does no good, it will also do no harm. Other coping strategies might include the use of heat, water, exercise, distraction, changing to a healthier diet, relaxation etc. In this way oncologists may harness the benefits of the placebo effect to develop beliefs about greater levels of personal pain control and need not be apologetic about doing this in the interests of creating or sustaining psychological well-being. From this area of study arises a demand for information on how health professionals can access beliefs and expectations successfully. Training in this area could include instruction on how to respond to disclosures in a manner that is conducive to improving psychological well-being in cancer patients. Also methods of how to convert information about different types of beliefs and expectations into productive clinical practice. At the same time, any such training should also include self-reflective consideration of how professionals themselves can sustain these practices without undue distress and eventual burnout.

Suffering and bad news

The way in which a life-threatening diagnosis of cancer is delivered and the management of treatment, affect the ways in which cancer patients adjust to their illness and react to its treatment. Emotional reactions of distress are central in this process, and reducing suffering should be a prime concern at the time of diagnosis, as well as throughout treatment for malignancy. Suffering is defined as an exceptionally unpleasant experience that is commonly and closely associated with pain and distress (Rose and Adams 1989). It occurs when a person perceives their impending destruction and persists either until such time as the threat passes, or until the person can restore their integrity in other ways (Cassel 1982). Contrary to popular thinking, suffering is not confined to the physical symptoms of a disease but is much more broad-ranging. This definition is important because it explains why reducing symptom intensity alone does not necessarily bring significant relief from suffering in all patients. Suffering has a wider remit, covering a range of social, personal, and interpersonal conditions. It may affect or be affected by a person's body image, their social roles such as mother, colleague, dancer, and their identity, as well as their personal relationships with others (Cassel 1982). Indeed an exploratory approach is recommended during consultations as health professionals are often unable to predict what issues patients will identify as an important source of suffering; patients have a range of highly individual beliefs and meanings that they assign to their experiences. Mistaken judgements on the part of health professionals about another person's suffering may themselves cause considerable suffering.

Suffering may be increased by social isolation (Rodin and Salovey 1989); this may be a problem in communities where cancer is still a stigma and for elderly, immobile people. Health professionals need to ascertain whether patients have an appropriate (to them) social support system or whether to establish one rapidly from the formal health-care system, if this appears to be absent. This could be of central importance to the well-being of cancer patients not only at the time that malignancy is diagnosed but throughout the illness until a cure is established or death occurs. The hospice movement has done much to raise awareness on this front but only provides this service in the final stages of the process and to selected individuals.

Society is not always sympathetic to families who are suffering a bereavement. Paradoxically, it may treat harshly those who do not conform to norms about how much suffering a bereaved person is expected to show (Wortman and Silver 1989). These norms and expectations are culturally determined and may not necessarily be apparent to observers outside the immediate social group. But Wortman and Silver (1989) conclude that there is no consensus in the literature about a 'best' way to grieve. For this reason health professionals should keep an open mind and avoid giving prescriptive advice about how best to grieve. They may also be able to play an active role in disseminating attitudes of open-mindedness among relevant others, so that the distress of grieving is not overlaid and prolonged by adding to it social disapproval from others.

The way in which help is given can be affected by the explanations or attributions that are made by the helper about whether the sick person is somehow responsible for their illness or to blame (Ickes and Kidd 1976). If such attributions translate into an attendant loss of support, this may well add to the suffering of those trying to cope with malignancy e.g. a person with lung cancer who smoked 50 cigarettes a day during their adult life. Informal caregivers in the family also face 'a dilemma of caring', because dependency and neediness may be created through the provision of care, love, and support and this may in turn, demotivate potential caregivers and reduce their support (Thompson and Pitts 1992).

Those in pain are invariably 'petitioners for aid' (Sternbach 1983). They usually go to the consultation in search of help and information. Control of the information flow by health professionals seems to be the key to the psychological success of consultations with cancer patients. Breaking bad news is not a pleasant activity for anyone but Donovan (1993) reports that doctor's attitudes towards breaking bad news particularly to those with a malignancy, has improved considerably since the 1960s. In USA, more than 90% of doctors now claim that they are in favour of telling patients their diagnosis and say that they would want to be told themselves, if they had cancer. But in studies where oncologist's behaviour has been observed, there is still found to be a discrepancy between what doctors say and what they actually do. Donovan (1993) found that communications were worst in 'paternalistic' consultations where a diagnosis of cancer had not been disclosed. Her studies underscore the message that most patients do want to know the bad news about themselves, whether it is about cancer, terminal illness, or dying. Studies reviewed by her indicate that when patients have this information, they adjust better, have greater peace of mind, a more positive attitude, and lower uncertainty and anxiety. While disclosure may have a short term negative impact, particularly if the news is delivered abruptly, Donovan shows that the distress from uncertainty is far worse, long-term. The mutual support and trust that disclosure brings promotes good doctor–patient communications throughout the most difficult phases of the illness and in dying.

However Donovan draws back from recommending full disclosure for every patient. A preferable strategy for greater well-being is for individual disclosures that are timed and delivered as the patient needs to know. This way the information flow is regulated by the doctor using her or his knowledge of the medical, psychological, and social history of the patient, combined with their professional judgement and skill about how to deliver the very best advice to that patient. So a partnership for decision-making is the model for best practice (Donovan 1993). Finally, Donovan acknowledges that conveying bad news will always be unpleasant for doctors but if done with care and skill, they will have the satisfaction of knowing it was less unpleasant for their patients. Ray *et al.* (1984) looked closely at the delivery of bad news to women with breast cancer and provide an example of how such work can be done in this context.

Having looked at some aspects of the consultation, it may seem self-evident to state that the consultation is essentially a social process involving two people. But it is easy to forget that much of the research in this area provides a one-sided view of this two-way process as most studies focus on what patients think, do, and say. Considerably less attention has been paid to looking at health professionals and their beliefs, statements, motives, and actions during a consultation. Furthermore, remarkably few studies have investigated the dynamics between patients and health professionals, within the same consultation. In any interaction between two people, a 'chemistry' is generated that could not easily be predicted from looking at them as individuals. This is the subject of social psychology and needs to be applied more readily in the health context. There is an erroneous assumption that health professionals are able to behave in a standard way towards all their patients; they are assumed to be a constant against which patient behaviour can be measured. But health professionals have their varying opinions and bad days like everyone else, and it would demand unreasonable, superhuman skills to expect them to behave in an identical way towards everyone who comes through the surgery door. As a precaution, practitioners should be more sceptical in their interpretation of the results of studies that only present a one-sided view. Despite the ethical problems inherent in carrying out such research, this rich series of interactions needs to be much more thoroughly investigated.

Different approaches to psychological treatment

The contribution of psychological factors to the aetiology and treatment of cancer pain has a long history. Medical psychologists of the 1950s and 60s drew from psychosomatic theories and designed personality tests to explain variations in cancer pain and the patient's response to treatment. The hunt for personality characteristics that would explain these phenomena was extensive, expensive, and prolonged (Skevington 1995). It proved to be disappointing both in practical terms of relieving suffering and intellectually, as a theoretical model. However amongst the many hundreds of traits investigated, one of the most consistent findings is that generalized distress, and in particular, emotions like anxiety, depression, and hostility, are closely associated with the experience and reporting of cancer pain and go some way to predicting response to treatment. For instance, the level of distress reported prior to bone marrow transplant surgery is a good predictor of the intensity of pain from oral mucositis afterwards (Syrjala and Chapko 1995). Some of the many ways of relieving anxiety and depression that have assisted in the better management of cancer pain are discussed below.

Other approaches have also been developed which have challenged the psychosomatic tradition. Arising from an interest in behaviourism came an application to pain based on learning principles—cognitive behaviour therapy (CBT). This has been one of the most successful areas in which psychological processes are used to explain how people with chronic pain behave and to generate a series of skills that can be taught to enable them to manage it (Fordyce 1976). These operant programs do not 'cure' the pain, nor do they aim to do so (Pither 1989) but pain management programs were set up explicitly to reduce disability and to help those with chronic pain lead more normal lives. Many published studies have shown that pain management programs are able to increase a patient's physical activity, reduce their pain behaviours, limit the amount of strong analgesics taken, encourage them to use the health services less, and possibly, return them to work. These programs have been found to be most effective in the management of chronic, painful musculo-skeletal disorders and especially for chronic low back pain (Linton 1986).

Learning is a salient psychological concept that helps us to explain the way people respond to pain in many situations. Different sectors of society express their pain in broadly different styles, depending on learning appropriate to their ethnic group, gender, age group, and so on. Some are more predisposed to visit a doctor than others, even when they suffer from exactly the same symptom or condition and this depends not only on symptom intensity and its inconvenience but also on the norms and expectations in their culture. These social phenomena provide evidence of differential learning about when and where it is appropriate to report pain and some of the best examples are described by medical anthropologists (see Kleinman 1988). The social influence of others also affects this process particularly in situations where symptoms are ambiguous or the presence of illness is unclear. In this void of information we rely on others to legitimate our illness and to provide cues about whether a visit to a doctor is appropriate (Telles and Pollack 1981). Comparisons with others are often used in this decision-making process. The information received from social encounters and the way it is interpreted helps to explain why some people will visit a doctor promptly with rectal bleeding for instance, while others might ignore it for a very long time. Furthermore there may be social, financial, or personal rewards or incentives to adopt the sick role, like much needed attention from loved ones and the provision of sick or disability payments. At the same time these can act as a disincentive to continue working.

Why have cognitive behaviour therapy techniques not been widely used in the relief of chronic cancer pain? The answer in part, comes from the very nature of the pain associated with cancer itself. Cancer pain can arise from tumour growth in bones, nerves, and other organs as disease-related pain. But there may also be pain generated by the treatment, such as that following radiation and chemotherapy and after surgical procedures. In addition, chronic pain may arise as a 'phantom' after the removal of cancerous tissues, as with post-mastectomy pain. Although attention tends to focus on the pain of the cancer itself, a recent review of patients in palliative care with far advanced cancer found that in only half of the cases was the pain caused by the cancer *per se* (Twycross *et al.* 1996). An implication of these findings is that the pain arising from treatments might require the design of a different psychological intervention to that required to combat either the pain of the tumour itself or any phantom pain.

In recent years there has been growing demand for psychological interventions that might be helpful to the terminally ill, yet psychologist's are not commonly seen as an integral member of the palliative care team (see Doyle *et al.* 1993). This may be because there has been some reluctance to use established techniques like cognitive behaviour therapy to relieve malignant pain in the knowledge that cancer pains have organic origins rather than the psychological mechanisms believed to underlie many cases of chronic, intractable low back pain. Consequently, malignant pain may require quite different styles of intervention to non-malignant pain (Wilson and Gil 1996). A second observation concerns the diverging goals of providing pharmacological treatment for those with and without a malignancy. In the case of non-malignant pain, a principal aim of treatment has been to reduce addictive levels of analgesics. This contrasts with the aim of gradually increasing levels of analgesic as necessary, utilizing the principles of the WHO analgesic ladder to relieve cancer and related pains as the disease progresses (WHO 1990). Furthermore, if psychological pressures are brought to bear on the way cancer patients report their pain, alterations to these pain reports might interfere with the delivery of adequate and appropriate analgesia, at the time that it is most needed (Syrjala and Chapko 1995). An aim of pain management programs is to change the way that those with non-malignant illness report their pain, so that pain complaints are actively discouraged. This goal is patently undesirable where malignancy is concerned.

Despite these caveats, some trials have been carried out. For example, Moorey and Greer (1989) selected and modified some techniques from cognitive behaviour therapy in forming a package of treatments called adjuvant psychological therapy. The aim has been to manage depression and anxiety in cancer patients better and by reducing these also to alleviate pain and suffering. A study by Spiegel and Bloom (1983) showed inconclusive results for the use of hypnosis and supportive therapy in the relief of cancer pain. (This is included here because parallels have been drawn between the techniques that induce hypnosis with those used in the relaxation and imagery training that forms part of cognitive behaviour therapy; Syrjala *et al.* 1995). In addition, Turk and Feldman (1992) have argued that several of the psychosocial factors known to affect coping with non-malignant pain are also salient to the management of cancer patients. They point out that beliefs about being in control of the pain and illness (Thompson 1981) and being confident and self-efficacious about being able to perform desired activities are particularly relevant in the cancer pain context. Together this picture begins to suggest that modified cognitive behavioural techniques may have more mileage in relieving suffering connected with cancer than was hitherto anticipated.

But although interest in the roles of relaxation and imagery in the treatment of cancer pain has grown, well controlled trials are still difficult to locate. Reviewing studies published since 1982, Wallace (1997) points out that it is still hard to draw reliable conclusions for a host of methodological reasons. Reliable conclusions from published studies tend to be marred by small numbers in groups, large scale drop out rates during trials and poor or even absent control groups. Many studies also rely on traditional outcome measures such as the amount of medication consumed, rather than using a more sensible combination of biological, psychological, and social methods. Furthermore amount of medication itself is neither an appropriate nor reliable measure in the case of cancer, as demand for opioids does not increase steadily and in a linear fashion as time progresses, but is closely related to stages of treatment and changes in malignant disease.

As psychological variables are only modest predictors of pain, the relationship between analgesic intake, amount of pain experienced, and psychological state remains unclear. In a recent study, 74 patients with oral mucositis pain following bone marrow transplant for cancer were randomly assigned to one of three conditions during the week preceding the bone marrow transplant. Some received active psychotherapy, others had relaxation and imagery training with or without other components of cognitive behaviour therapy, and a third group had treatment as usual. Those who received relaxation and imagery—whether or not it was coupled with cognitive behaviour therapy—reported significantly less pain than patients allocated to the other two groups. However cognitive behaviour therapy was not confirmed to be superior, as expected. Patients who improved tended to affirm the helpfulness of relaxation and imagery in coping with pain and also found it useful in dealing with troublesome nausea and stress (Syrjala *et al.* 1995).

In summary Dalton and Feuerstein (1988) and Syrjala and Chapko (1995) make cautious claims for the success of psychological factors in predicting cancer pain or pathology as it is evident that pain reports alone cannot altogether explain pathology. They conclude that where biological, psychological, and social variables have been assessed together as a biopsychosocial model, they are partially able to predict cancer pain. Furthermore the performance of these combined variables is as good as that of more traditional biomedical models. However biobehavioural models (arising from cognitive behaviour therapy) have not surpassed biomedical models in their ability to predict painful outcomes (see Syrjala and Chapko 1995 for a review). Much more work is needed to establish the efficacy of each of these models.

Health professionals

One focus of research interest has concerned the management of cancer pain by health professionals. Most physicians receive only 3 to 4 hours of training in pain management (Stephenson 1996) despite the large proportion of patients who they see each day who report pain as their most troublesome symptom. In one study, 33 physicians spent 7 minutes interviewing a simulated patient with terminal unresectable rectal cancer and their performance was examined on 12 dimensions (Sloan *et al.* 1996). The factors that discriminated the best interviews from the worst were whether the doctor asked for a description of the pain, inquired about factors that aggravated the pain, elicited a previous pain history, and noted details of other symptoms. Disturbingly, Sloan *et al.* concluded that these doctors were not competent in the assessment and management of severe pain indicating that further training in pain relief is urgently needed on the curriculum. Despite the existence of WHO guidelines for the administration of pain relief to cancer patients, 82% of their sample prescribed on an 'as needed' (p.r.n.) basis rather than 'by the clock', as recommended. They were also inclined to prescribe the same weak opioids to patients that had been prescribed on the previous occasion, even though these drugs had failed to provide adequate pain relief. So the principles of the WHO pain ladder were not being applied. Lastly, they found no differences in the pain management behaviour of junior and senior staff, suggesting that those receiving more recent training did not show any better practice. Although the sample was small, the study shows that medical training needs to be changed substantially to teach pain management to adequate levels. In recent years the International Association for the Study of Pain has published a series of curricula for six health professional groups which currently await implementation in training.

Focusing on the psychosocial aspects of treatment, a recent view has been that therapists may be trained to reduce mood disturbance in patients with cancer, and in so doing, increase their survival time. In a study by Classen *et al.* (1997), 24 therapists who had either been trained in individual psychotherapy or providing social support for patients or in the medical management of breast cancer were chosen from 12 centres to participate in a program that would facilitate positive mood, active coping, and improve support. The results showed that therapists performed these activities better as the training progressed. However, any successes in applying these skills to the treatment of patients and whether it made a difference to the patient's outcomes, has yet to be reported.

Taking action at a national level, the American Pain Society has proposed guidelines for the practical management of cancer pain in order to encourage the development and maintenance of standards in hospitals and Bookbinder *et al.* (1996) report a quality assurance study which has started to assess its impact. These guidelines begin with the recognition of pain and follow with prompt treatment to relieve it. They establish levels to trigger review procedures and incorporate a survey of patient satisfaction; they emphasize the need to make information about analgesic levels and types readily available and the need to promise patients attentive analgesic care. Lastly, they note the necessity of defining explicit policies for the application of advanced technologies, such as the use of infusion devices and the administration of systemic opioids via subcutaneous, intravenous, and epidural routes. To improve awareness levels about good practice, they included a series of interesting techniques such as the viewing of specially designed videotapes, holding focus groups, creating a pain management game, and through pain rounds and nurse liaisons. Although a large proportion of the 696 hospitalized patients interviewed were largely satisfied or very satisfied with the treatment they received, neither levels of pain intensity nor pain relief were significantly reduced following this intervention. Improvements in patient satisfaction may be due to factors such as having to wait less time for pain medication or medication change.

Macrae (1991) has reviewed the main reasons why patients do not get enough pain relief. Even some pharmacological reasons may have a psychological component because they include motivation, memory, learning, decision-making, attentional, and attitudinal factors connected with poor prescribing practices and insufficient knowledge about drugs like narcotics. There are also important psychosocial as well as medical reasons why pain relieving drugs may not be given sufficiently often or in a large enough dose to maintain the patient in a pain free condition. Key studies reviewed by Macrae (1991) indicate that nurses do not give as much as is prescribed because they are afraid of addictive dependency and respiratory depression. They may also use stereotypes about certain social categories of patient who are assumed not to need analgesia or much of it, for example men are commonly treated as more stoical. Structurally, the organization may not be adequately staffed to meet the needs of seriously ill patients by giving them sufficient analgesia and at the right time. But the main psychological reasons associated with this area are that staff themselves do not notice that the patient is in pain or ask about pain. They may allow routine procedures to take priority over the provision of pain relief or do not care enough to act. In addition to inexperience and fears about addiction, abuse, or overuse, staff may have expectations—realistic or unrealistic—about how much suffering should be expected from a person with a particular illness or trauma and this may influence the way they respond to patients. Furthermore, a study by Choinere *et al.* (1990) has shown that nurses tended to overestimate the success of analgesia in 46% of cases and no analgesia at all was given in a startling 25% of cases, where pain was present.

Staff have varied attitudes towards patients in pain (Winn 1991). Some believe that pain is not important because it is not life threatening. Another common attitude is that 'doctor (or nurse) knows best', which makes patients feel anxious or wimpish if they ask for more relief. A third set of attitudes arise when staff ignore individual differences between patients in their need for analgesic and assume that 'one dose suits all'. Lastly, there is the mistaken assumption that a patient who is quiet cannot be in pain, which ignores copious findings showing that withdrawal and helplessness is a common reaction to severe pain.

These common beliefs and actions among staff are explained in part by Donovan *et al.* (1987) who found that patients often did not report their pain immediately when asked or articulate their need for pain relief. They found that staff often devalued the pain by relegating it to distress and in using this explanation, it then acted as a deterrent to providing more analgesic. Donovan *et al.* also showed that contrary to popular belief among staff that patients would be avid consumers of analgesic if only allowed to do so, patients in fact take smaller doses of analgesic than expected. The basis for staff concern about addiction is negligible. Mistaken beliefs that patients who sleep cannot be in a lot of pain and that pain is well controlled in hospitals also mitigate against proper provision (Donovan *et al.* 1987). So staff who are working with cancer patients would do well to develop self-awareness individually and in groups about their own attitudes, motives, and behaviour in providing or withholding analgesics from those who are in pain. These findings present a strong case in favour of continuing to examine how staff treat patients in pain as well as looking at the patients themselves as a patient's behaviour is best understood within this context.

Support in families

Families can be substantially affected by the presence of a loved one who is in chronic pain but not all families are in this situation. Turk *et al.* (1987) found that some families cope 'surprisingly well'. Consequently, health professionals must be sensitive to this diversity as it would be mistaken psychologically as well as from a resource point of view, to provide care for families who do not need it. However, in families where well-being is affected there are commonly reports of fatigue, nervousness, tiredness, tension, and poor physical health. Rowat and Knafl (1985) found that 60% of the partners of pain patients expressed uncertainty, 83% reported some kind of health disturbance, 69% said they were sad, fearful, depressed, nervous, or irritable, and 40% expressed helplessness about relieving their partners pain. Such results suggest that families need help too if they are to be successful sustaining their own mental and physical well-being as well as assisting the person in pain. Particularly at the time they are giving help and support to a dying family member, caregivers may be struggling to maintain their own psychological health, and the presence of pain is known to be an important factor here. Miaskowski *et al.* (1997) investigated 86 family caregivers of cancer patients in pain and compared their mood with 42 where the person was pain-free. Results from this profile of mood states showed that in cases where a family member was in pain, the family had significantly higher levels of tension, depression, and mood disturbance than in pain-free families, thus demonstrating the powerful effect of the presence of pain on the mood of the caregivers.

Given that there is a move to care for cancer patients in their homes, especially during the final stages of palliative care, there is a need to know how well family members are able to assess the pain and discomfort of their loved one during this period. This is particularly important if communications with the patient deteriorate or cease, for example due to unconsciousness. Pain is a subjective phenomenon and its experience and report are highly influenced by personal meanings and interpretations that are very difficult to discern, even for those who are closely related. Rowat and Knafl (1985) found that 38% of spouses were unable to describe their partner's pain and where they could do this, they tended to describe it in sensory terms, so ignoring the important emotional qualities of chronic pain. Despite this gloomy success rate, some studies show that as a rule, women are more sensitive to their partner's pain than men (Romano *et al.* 1989). As women are more likely to be informal caregivers of those with painful cancers then the success rate of these judgements is more likely to be higher under difficult proxy conditions. Pain is a private and personal experience that is only partially communicable to other people. In studies that have compared the pain assessments of health professionals and patients, it is commonly found that the association between the two sets of judgements is relatively poor—the correlation coefficient typically reaches about 0.3, on a scale from 0 to 1.

Where communication between patient and carer is not a problem, Elliott *et al.* (1996) showed that family members consistently assessed the pain and disability of their family member as much higher than the patients did themselves probably because they had different information available to them. In this study, the amount and type of information available to family carers was investigated; those who had more factual information about pain and its treatment and had fewer misconceptions about it, perceived that their patients had less pain. In particular, those who were most accurate expressed a cluster of distinctive beliefs. They knew that there was no ceiling for the amount of opioid needed for effective pain relief and that the management of cancer pain was possible. They were not concerned about addiction and thought that non-medical interventions could significantly help to relieve the pain. Elliot *et al.* point out that misunderstandings by other members of the family may continue to prevent patients from receiving appropriate pain management. In this way the whole family may be implicated in the pain outcomes of a particular patient. Such findings make a powerful case for new interventions to target the whole family and not just the primary caregiver at home.

There is no suitable substitute for asking the patient how much pain they feel and accepting that report at face value, and the best measures of pain are those that have been designed for self-administration. The success of using good measures depends on the ability of health professionals to suspend their own beliefs, assumptions, stereotypes, and suspicions about those in their care, in order to administer appropriate and sufficient analgesic, delivered at the right time to relieve that pain. Only with good instruments is it possible to monitor the success or failure of care, treatments, and interventions. This approach has been most successful in the field of pain where assessment, the design of interventions and clinical practice often go hand in hand.

Support for patients

Emotional support is central to the needs of those with chronic illness generally and those with a malignancy in particular; however people cope with their illness in different ways. Not everyone wants to join a social support group; in a US study Taylor *et al.* (1984) found that only 10% of breast cancer patients wanted to join. Furthermore they reported that those who joined many types of social support group tended to be white, female, and from higher socioeconomic groups. Consequently the establishment of social support groups means that we are only providing a service to a small self-selected section of the community. Four types of social support have been identified. Perhaps most important is support arising from liking, sympathy, or love which is often represented by good listening skills and genuine concern. Support may also take the form of providing instrumental aid, goods, or services, such as money or labour. There is informational support where advice is on offer and lastly, there are appraisals and feedback which can assist the person with self-evaluation (Thompson and Pitts 1992).

However not all support is helpful even though it may be well intended. Dunkel-Schetter *et al.* (1992) found that messages that convey negative meanings, such as those that imply blame, failure, or incompetence, are unlikely to be helpful. Messages that minimize or trivialize the cancer can also be harmful because they suppress further discussion and dampen the communication flow. Less self-evident perhaps, is the finding that where informal caregivers are very closely involved with the sufferer, this can also be an impediment. This is because excessive attention may be seen as intrusive, over solicitous, or representing undue concern. At best, a sensitive balance of helpful support is required.

In a study of support for cancer patients, Taylor *et al.* (1986) found that some cancer patients were indeed given high levels of support from their own social groups after receiving a diagnosis. But some felt very isolated often because of rejection, while others, who appeared to be receiving support from their family, friends, or health professionals, were in fact not receiving the sort of support that they most needed. Health professionals should be aware of this diversity of situations, especially the latter case where support appears to be given, but because it is not the right sort, may cause even more distress than no support at all. Taylor *et al.* (1986) also discovered that those who attended social support groups had a special set of characteristics. They were more likely: to have consulted a mental health professional about their cancer, suggesting that they had a greater interest in their psychological health than most; read books about cancer and its treatment, with a view to trying to solve their own problems; and to have been previously involved in other types of support groups. Those who attended social support groups were also found to be no more distressed than those who did not attend. On the contrary, they were just more interested in and concerned about their cancer (Taylor *et al.* 1986) and wanted to share it with other people who were in a similar position (Medvene 1992).

Technological facilities supplied by the internet are currently being tested with the view to using it as a vehicle to bring support to people with cancer pain, especially in situations where there are large geographical distances between people and the health care that they need. One-hour teleconferencing workshops were established for men with painful advanced prostate cancer, in a study by Glajchen and Moul (1996). They targeted men in ethnic minority groups where the disease is prevalent and the predisposition to seek treatment low. Although 88% of those who answered the post-test questionnaire said that the session had been useful and most of these showed high levels of knowledge and information, they only represented half of the total sample. Furthermore, no pre-test baseline of prior information was obtained. Nevertheless, this serves as an interesting model for how health care might be delivered better under difficult circumstances and for this reason deserves replication using a more rigorous design.

Conclusion

In this chapter we have considered a variety of ways in which psychological factors, assessment, and treatment can influence the pain of people with a malignancy. However psychological influences pervade many aspects of the management and treatment of this group of patients. Some are psychosocial features connected with the administration of physical and pharmacological treatments. Others are about applying existing psychological interventions known to manage disability associated with pain to those with cancer. These require high quality controlled large scale studies to investigate their efficacy and provide reliable answers. New psychological techniques are now needed to relieve the different types of pain arising from the malignancy, the treatment, and any phantom sensations, if those techniques already in existence cannot be satisfactorily tailored to relieve this suffering. Much greater use of psychological expertise could be made in palliative care where the biopsychosocial approach to dealing with patients and their families has already been admirably developed by the health-care team but where psychological care is largely carried out by non-psychologists. Good treatment follows from accurate assessment, and the development of excellent measures must continue to be a high clinical priority. Their first class psychometric properties must be used to direct selection over and above other priorities if their pragmatic qualities are to be fully appreciated.

References

Bookbinder, M., Coyle, N., Kiss, M., Layman Goldstein, M., Holritz, K., Thaler, H., et al. (1996). Implementing national standards for cancer pain management: program model and evaluation. *Journal of Pain and Symptom Management*, **12**, 334–47.

Bowers, K. (1968). Pain, anxiety and perceived control. *Journal of Consulting and Clinical Psychology*, **32**, 596–602.

Buller, M.K., and Buller, D.B. (1987). Physician communication style and patient satisfaction. *Journal of Health and Social Behaviour*, **28**, 375–88.

Cassel, E.J. (1982). The nature of suffering and the goals of medicine. *New England Journal of Medicine*, **306**, 639–45.

Choinière, M., Melzack, R., Girard, N., Rondeau, J., and Paquin, M.J. (1990). Comparisons between patients and nurses assessment of pain and medication efficacy in severe burn injuries. *Pain*, **40**, 143–52.

Classen, C., Abramson, S., Angell, K., Desch, C., Vinciguerra, V.P., Rosenbluth, R.J., et al. (1997). Effectiveness of a training program for enhancing therapists' understanding of the supportive-expressive treatment model for breast cancer groups. *Journal of Psychotherapy Practice and Research*, **6**, 211–18.

Cleeland, C.S., Serlin, R., Nakamura, Y., and Mendoza, T. (1996). Effects of culture and language on ratings of cancer pain and patterns of functional interference. *Proceedings of the 8th World Congress on Pain* (ed. T.S. Jensen, J.A. Turner and Z. Wiesenfeld-Hallin), pp. 35–52. IASP Press, Seattle.

Crisson, J.E., and Keefe, F.J. (1988). The relationship of locus of control to pain coping strategies and psychological distress in chronic pain patients. *Pain*, **35**, 147–54.

Dalton, J.A., and Feuerstein, M. (1988). Biobehavioural factors in cancer pain. *Pain*, **33**, 137–47.

Donovan, K. (1993). Breaking Bad News. In Communicating Bad News. *Behavioural Science Learning Module*, Division of Mental Health, World Health Organization, Geneva.

Donovan, M., Dillon, P., and McGuire, L. (1987). Incidence and characteristics of pain in a sample of medical-surgical inpatients. *Pain*, **30**, 69–78.

Doyle, D., Hanks, G.W.C., and McDonald, N. (1993). What is palliative medicine? In *Oxford textbook of palliative medicine* (ed. D. Doyle, G.W.C. Hanks, and N. McDonald), pp. 3–8. Oxford Medical Publications.

Dunkel-Schetter, C., Blasband, D.E., Feinstein, L.G., and Herbert, T.B. (1992). Elements of supportive interactions: when are attempts to help effective? In *Helping and being helped: naturalistic studies* (ed. S. Spacapan and S. Oskamp) pp. 83. Sage.

Elliott, B., Elliott, T.E., Murray, D.M., Braun, B.L., and Johnson, K.M. (1996). Patients and family members: the role of knowledge and attitudes in cancer pain. *Journal of Pain and Symptom Management*, **12**, 209–20.

Fernandez, E., and Turk, D.C. (1989). The utility of cognitive coping strategies for altering pain perception: a meta-analysis. *Pain*, **38**, 123–36.

Fordyce, W.E. (1976). *Behavioural methods for chronic pain and illness*. Mosby, St. Louis.

Glajchen, M., and Moul, J.W. (1996). Teleconferencing as a method of educating men about managing advanced prostate cancer and pain. *Journal of Psychosocial Oncology*, **14**, 73–87.

Huskisson, E.C. (1983). Visual analogue scales. In *Pain measurement and assessment*, (ed. R. Melzack) pp. 33–7. Raven, New York.

Ickes, W.J., and Kidd, R.F. (1976). An attributional analysis of helping behaviour. In *New directions in attribution research*, Vol. 1 (eds. J.H. Harvey, W.J. Ickes and R.F. Kidd) Laurence Erlbaum, Hillsdale, New Jersey, pp. 311–34.

Jensen, M.P., Karoly, P., and Braver, S. (1986). The measurement of clinical pain intensity: a comparison of six methods. *Pain*, **27**, 117–26.

Kleinman, A.R. (1988). *The illness narratives: suffering, healing and the human condition*. Basic Books, New York.

Lawson, K., Reesor, K.A., Keefe, F.J., and Turner, J.A. (1990). Dimensions of pain-related cognitive coping: cross-validation of the factor structure of the Coping Strategy Questionnaire. *Pain*, **43**, 195–204.

Liebskind, J.C. (1991). Pain can kill. *Pain*, **44**, 3–4.

Linton, S.J. (1986). Behavioural remediation of chronic pain: a status report. *Pain*, **24**, 125–141.

Macrae, W.A. (1991). *Why is pain treated so badly?* Paper to the Edinburgh International Science Festival, Royal College of Surgeons, Edinburgh.

Medvene, L. (1992). Self-help groups, peer helping and social comparison. In *Helping and being helped: naturalistic studies* (ed. S. Spacapan and S. Oskamp), pp. 49. Sage.

Melzack, R. (1975). The McGill pain questionnaire: major properties and scoring method. *Pain*, **1**, 277–99.

Melzack, R. (1987). The short-form McGill pain questionnaire. *Pain*, **36**, 191–7.

Melzack, R., and Wall, P.D. (1965). Pain mechanisms—a new theory. *Science*, **150**, 971–9.

Melzack, R., and Wall, P.D. (1982). *The challenge of pain* (1st edn). Penguin Harmondsworth.

Miaskowski, C., Kragness, L., Dibble, S., and Wallhagen, M. (1997). Differences in mood states, health status and caregiver strain between family caregivers of oncology outpatients with and without cancer-related pain. *Journal of Pain and Symptom Management*, **13**, 138–47.

Moorey, S., and Greer, S. (1989). *Psychological therapy for patients with cancer: a new approach*. Heinemann Medical Books, London.

Pither, C.E. (1989). Treatment of persistent pain. *British Medical Journal*, **229**, 12.

Ray, C., Fisher, J., and Lindop, J. (1984). The surgeon–patient relationship in the context of breast cancer. *International Review of Applied Psychology*, **33**, 531–43.

Reader, G.G., Pratt, L., and Mudd, M.C. (1957). What patients expect from their doctors. *The Modern Hospital*, **89**, 88.

Rodin, J., and Salovey, P. (1989). Health psychology. *Annual Review of Psychology*, **40**, 533–79.

Romano, J.M., Turner, J.A., and Clancy, S.L. (1989). Sex differences in the relationship of pain patient dysfunction to spouse adjustment. *Pain*, **39**, 289–95.

Rose, M., and Adams, D. (1989). In *Evidence for pain and suffering in other animals. Animal experimentation: the consensus change* (ed. G. Langley) Macmillan, New York, Chapter 3.

Rosensteil, A.K., and Keefe, F.J. (1983). The use of coping strategies in chronic low back pain patients. *Pain*, **17**, 33–44.

Rowat, K.M., and Knafl, K.A. (1985). Living with chronic pain: the spouses perspective. *Pain*, **23**, 259–71.

Skevington, S.M. (1990). A standardised scale to measure beliefs about controlling pain (BPCQ). *Psychology and Health*, **4**, 221–32.

Skevington, S.M. (1995). *Psychology of pain*. John Wiley, Chichester.

Sloan, P.A., Donnelly, M.B., Scwartz, R.W., and Sloan, D. (1996). Cancer pain assessment and management by housestaff. *Pain*, **67**, 475–81.

Spiegel, D., and Bloom, J.R. (1983). Group therapy and hypnosis reduce metastatic breast carcinoma pain. *Psychosomatic Medicine*, **45**, 333–9.

Stephenson, J. (1996). Researchers hope techno-teaching will improve cancer pain treatment. *Journal of the American Medical Association*, **276**, 22, 1783–6.

Sternbach, R.A. (1983). Ethical considerations in pain research in man. In *Pain measurement and assessment*, pp. 259 (ed. R. Melzack) Raven Press, New York.

Syrjala, K.L., and Chapko, M.E. (1995). Evidence for a biopsychosocial model of cancer treatment and related pain. *Pain*, **61**, 69–79.

Syrjala, K., Donaldson, G.W., Davies, M.W., Kippes, M.E., and Carr, J.E. (1995). Relaxation and imagery and cognitive-behavioural training reduce pain during cancer treatment: a controlled clinical trial. *Pain*, **63**, 189–98.

Taylor, S.E., Lichtman, R.R., and Wood, J.V. (1984). Attributions, beliefs about control and adjustment to breast cancer. *Journal of Personality and Social Psychology*, **46**, 489–502.

Taylor, S.E., Falke, R.L., Shoptaw, S.J., and Lichtman, R.R. (1986). Social support, support groups and the cancer patient. *Journal of Consulting and Clinical Psychology*, **54**, 608–15.

Telles, J.L., and Pollack, M.H. (1981). Feeling sick—the experience and legitimation of illness. *Social Science and Medicine*, **15A**, 243–51.

Thompson, S.C., (1981). Will it hurt less if I can control it? A complex answer to a simple question. *Psychological Bulletin*, **90**, 1, 89–101.

Thompson, S.C., and Pitts, J.S. (1992). In sickness and in health: chronic illness, marriage and spousal caregiving. In *Helping and being helped: naturalistic studies* (ed. S. Spacapan and S. Oscamp) pp. 115. Sage.

Turk, D.C., and Feldman, C.S. (1992). Non-invasive approaches to pain control in terminal illness. *Hospice Journal*, **8**, 1–23.

Turk, D.C., Flor, H., and Rudy, T.E. (1987). Pain and families I: etiology, maintenance and psychosocial impact. *Pain*, **30**, 3–27.

Twycross, R., Harcourt, J., and Bergl, S. (1996). A survey of pain in patients with advanced cancer. *Journal of Pain and Symptom Management*, **12**, 273–82.

Wallace, K.G. (1997). Analysis of recent literature concerning relaxation and imagery interventions for cancer pain. *Cancer Nursing*, **20**, 79–87.

Wallston, K.A. (1989). *Control in chronic illness*. Paper to the International Conference on Health Psychology, Cardiff.

Weinman, J., and Higgins, P. (1975). How doctors try their patients. *Psychology Today*, **3**, 49–54.

WHO (1990). *Cancer pain relief and palliative care*: report of a WHO expert committee. Technical report series 804, World Health Organization, Geneva.

Williams, D.A., and Thorn, B.E. (1989). An empirical assessment of pain beliefs. *Pain*, **36**, 351–8.

Wilson, J.J., and Gil, K.M. (1996). The efficacy of psychological and pharmacological interventions for the treatment of chronic disease-related and non-disease-related pain. *Clinical Psychology Review*, **16**, 573–97.

Winn, D. (1991). Pain. Interview with A. Spence and C. Pither. *Nursing Times*. **24** February.

Wortman, C.B., and Silver, R.C. (1989). The myths of coping with loss. *Journal of Consulting and Clinical Psychology*, **57**, 349–57.

Dedication

This chapter is dedicated to the memory of my mother, Margaret Skevington (1911–1998).

Acknowledgement

I would like to thank Dr James Brennan for thoughtful and generous comments on the chapter.

FOUR

Spiritual help

DAVID STOTER

Introduction

The nature of spiritual care

Spiritual care as a concept has attracted growing attention in recent years, but still generates uncertainty for many carers and a range of often confusing definitions from writers. One thing is paramount, that whatever the approach, the nature of spiritual help required has to start from a consideration of the spiritual need of the person concerned whether that person is a patient, relative, or professional carer. It involves accepting each person together with all their attitudes, hopes, and fears and with all related feelings and emotions.

In the context of cancer pain it involves whole areas of devastation for the person concerned and there is a distinguishing factor to do with the commonly held view that cancer is the 'big ogre'. There is often a perception of hopelessness once the diagnosis is given which is associated with changing expectations of life and future plans with possible stigma and also with the fear of pain and discomfort related to the known forms of treatment.

Good spiritual help and care means acceptance of the individual whoever and wherever they are, together with all related feelings, and offers a 'place of safety' where the situation can be explored and where all emotions and feelings can be expressed as powerfully as necessary. It means offering a place for 'letting go' which for many patients is not to be found with friends and relatives for fear of 'losing face' or adding to their distress. This 'safe place' allows for inner tensions that have built up to be released safely. This in itself is helpful in facilitating the relationships between patients, family, and friends where misunderstandings can develop if tension builds over time and then explodes in volcanic-like eruptions after a long period of fear and repression.

Spirituality and spiritual need

The starting point is to be found in an understanding of what is meant by spirituality and spiritual need, which is essential for anyone offering spiritual care. Many current definitions appear obscure to a practitioner in search of guidance, but it is widely recognized that the spiritual dimension is universal and thus everyone has spiritual needs. The spiritual dimension of man is distinct from the religious dimension which relates to religious beliefs and practices and is not necessarily universal as a person may not have a particular religious belief of faith. Smith (1996) describes the spiritual dimension as complementing the physical and psychological dimensions which give meaning to life.

The spiritual dimension is that part of the personality linking the other parts, integrating and transcending the physical, social, and emotional aspects where they all meet (Stoter 1995). It is the dimension through which a search for meaning in life is facilitated and is a basis for beliefs and values and a sense of purpose in life. The nature of the spiritual dimension is influenced by a person's background; by life experiences, ethnic, cultural factors, and education making each person unique. It is the part of the personality through which relationships between individuals are made, and therefore is important in relation to the partnership between patient and carer (Socken and Carson 1987). It follows that the spiritual needs of each individual will vary and the nature of spiritual care given will differ, indicating a need for individual assessment for each person. The mix of ethnic groups in today's society can give rise to complex and diverse elements in spiritual needs, particularly with the complexity of inter- and intra-cultural aspects to be considered.

Spiritual care

The quality of care depends first of all on a good assessment of a person's individual need. Although some needs are common to all, the recognition of an individual's particular needs is essential for effective care. Spiritual care is not to be seen as something to be given only by religious leaders, and no individual carer should be seen to carry the sole responsibility for giving spiritual care, which should be an integral part of assessment of need and management of each care programme. All members of the team and family are involved in working together with the patient in this holistic approach to care. Communication skills are important together with inter-personal and interpretive skills which enhance the quality of the all important relationship with the patient who may feel most at ease in relating to one or more particular members of the team, a situation which needs to be accepted with trust by others. The nature and provision of spiritual care will be explored in detail later in this chapter.

Spiritual pain

Recognition of spiritual pain and understanding its nature is one of the most demanding aspects of spiritual care, which requires a high level of maturity and skill. There is a deep inter-relationship between physical and spiritual pain; they affect each other so closely that it is almost impossible to define the boundaries. Spiritual care is about care for the whole person and not just a matter of treating the disease but rather one of treating the '*dis-ease*' which arises as a result of the illness and manifests itself through pain, internal suffering, and distress. To consider the disease only, has the effect of depersonalizing an individual. Pain and suffering are synonymous—they go together as Herman Hesse (1984) points out 'suffering is suffering—there is no argument about it—it hurts, it is painful'.

Spiritual pain is a particularly debilitating and disabling pain. A study by Warden *et al.* (1998) shows that nurses in particular show 'neutral' attitudes to 'suffering' and their pain management was ineffective. They concluded 'a value neutral culture of health care is not conductive to recognition and subsequent relief of suffering'. It is more than a question of something hurting the body or mind, it is a deep 'hurt of the person' bringing a feeling of 'destruction' of the person. It can be exacerbated by anxiety, fear, and the effects of previous experiences and often manifests itself in physical pain. It saps energy, and destroys belief and confidence both personally for the patient, and in others and may soon destroy perceptions of values. A major influence in the consideration of spiritual pain is that of cultural/familial or societal pressures. The way people respond to or express pain is often governed by customs and the expectations of their culture and family. In some cultures it is desirable to express pain and grief loudly while in other groups it is more acceptable to present a stoical front and keep silent.

Cancer pain

Pain related to cancer care

All these responses may be exacerbated in the context of pain related to cancer. Apart from any physical pain related to the specific form of the disease there are aspects which are potentially associated with cancer. Cancer is seen by many as a disease which brings destruction of the person and their hopes and expectations, as a destroyer of relationships and quality of life. There are some who fear cancer (even the name) who put off seeking help thus reducing the effectiveness of treatment. The associated fear and spiritual pain can effect the perception of physical pain and may lead to feelings of isolation and loss of self worth. One patient was heard to comment 'I am just a slab of meat on a table being bombarded by radiation'.

The nature of a patient's spiritual pain is heavily influenced by the person's view of themselves and the view held of success or failure in life, personal relationships, work and by wider society. So often self evaluation is seen in the level of achievement, which at the best of times is fragile, focusing on failure rather than the positive aspects of success achieved. This is an important aspect of pain management in the care programme.

Loss of body image is another important component of spiritual pain, one that is often overlooked or undervalued by professionals for one or other of two reasons; either by comparing what the person's situation would have been without treatment with the disfigurement, or by assuming that what cannot be seen, or what can be disguised by prostheses, is no longer a problem. A patient who had had a mastectomy three years previously said to someone who said 'you'd never know', 'every time I get out of the bath I see myself and am revolted!'. As human beings, people see their own imperfections in stark detail, as in the reaction to developing a spot on the face.

The element of hopelessness so often associated with cancer creates a constant fear that the physical pain can only get worse. This happens particularly where patients are not given any indication of the kind of effective treatment available. The unspoken fear is 'if they cannot control my pain now, what is it going to be like later on?'. This is why it is so important to have a clear diagnosis of the source of fear, as there are associated levels of spiritual pain which no analgesics can reach and which no treatment can cure.

The importance of maintaining hope for the patient is well recognized. Elsdon (1995) sees caring as a way to do this and suggests that one cure for spiritual pain is to be 'found in the experience of pain itself'. She sees spiritual pain not so much as a problem to be solved, but a 'question to be lived'.

The effects of pain

Physical pain that is not well managed has an isolating effect which is cumulative and can spiral into an invasive and dominating problem; this increases in severity as the person becomes less hopeful of relief and more tense. The experience of such dominating pain can have a negative effect on family and personal relationships and also leads to growing resentment towards professionals expected to be able to relieve pain. The loss of ability to function as in the past again compounds the feelings of hopelessness leading to general feelings of despair. It is here that pain undermines feelings of self worth and may lead ultimately to self destructive modes of thinking when no adequate interventions are taken.

So the spiritual and physical aspects of pain are deeply interdependent and each cannot be treated in isolation. An integrated approach to pain management is essential and co-operation between all members of the caring team is vital leading to a cohesive and integrated care programme.

Spiritual help and interventions in pain management

General principles of intervention

Pain, whenever and however it occurs and whatever the cause, is like a raw open wound which by its very nature if constantly rubbed or frequently touched feels raw and sore. Spiritual care as a form of intervention means first of all identification of the carer(s) with the person suffering. It involves the carer in a relationship of sharing in anothers' pain, often with a realization that there are no clear solutions to areas of pain which are inaccessible to analgesic control. In some cases the pain may never be completely resolved, any resolution only being possible as the person concerned is able to discover a way through. Acceptance is an important part of the approach, acceptance of what is happening together with realistic aims, hopes and plans for the future and good communication with significant family and friends and others in their lives. Carer's are involved in establishing agreed patterns of management treatment and care which are acceptable to the patient and family.

Defining the territory

This real partnership in care gives the patient the dignity of not only having a voice but also having control and setting the goals. The carer enables him to discuss and use his personal resources and strengths to the full, 'so the patient not the caregiver defines the territory' (Saunders 1969).

The caregiver's role in this as in the whole management of spiritual care is firstly one of identification and assessment of need. Any interventions, unlike those associated with physical pain, are 'inactive' because the most important mode of intervention demands a capacity to lay aside any authoritative professional mode of control, coming alongside the patient with 'empty hands' and just 'being there'. Any subsequent course of action will be fully accepted by the patient as it arises from and responds to the personal expression of need and desire to be helped, and is followed by acceptance of the help offered. Secondly it is important to hear what the patient is saying, to listen to the person in all aspects of their expression, not only verbal but including body language, unspoken words, eye contact, reflective listening, etc. This requires a high quality of communicative and interpretive skills together with self awareness, confidence, and self control on the part of the carer.

Once the basic rapport is established 'other interventions' become possible where they are acceptable to the patient. One example is the use of touch which can further increase a feeling of safety and deepen the level of interaction and may in time release deeper feelings and previously hidden fears. This may enable a process of exploration of those deep feelings in a safe environment which may lead to greater self awareness and help to bring a sense of regaining control of life. Flowing from this the way may open up for other forms of intervention such as helpful alternative therapies, aromatherapy, acupuncture, imagery, visualisation, and reflexology—in fact, any provision of benefit to the individual which may involve personal cultural or religious expression; all interventions which give a sense of value to the patient.

As severe pain can undermine self value and worth, it can lead to self destructive modes of thinking which in the extreme can exclude all other considerations including: the ability to relate to others; the pain is often more than physical; there is an element of perceived loss of dignity, status and expectations in many ways, loss of the free relationship with close friends, or even acquaintances; there may be embarrassment of coming face to face with limitations at awkward moments; and the reality of facing one's mortality of what life has or has not been. Even high achievers may experience a sense of failure in the light of what they could have been or what others expected of them.

Listening

All modes of intervention begin with listening which is essential for forging the trusting relationship as the base line for spiritual care. The skills of reflective and interpretive listening are essential, avoiding unnecessary and inappropriate interventions. The ability to remain silent and share the moment and what is being communicated is often healing and deepens the rapport and trust so easily destroyed by many professional carers' seeming compulsion to have to give answers!

Interpretive and listening skills in particular involve 'being with' not just physically but in empathy with the patient. For some touch is important which, if accepted, may further deepen the care felt by the patient. As the patient may communicate the nature and depth of the pain experienced through a variety of different forms of expression, the skilled listener will recognize and acknowledge them appropriately and avoid platitudes and glib answers.

Handling spiritual pain

An important aspect of handling spiritual pain and selecting appropriate interventions lies first in making an accurate assessment of the origins of pain and the patients' need. There may have been a history of uncertainty, fear, and unease, or just chronic debilitating ill health with symptoms which may have caused much distress. Part of the assessment process is the identification of what is caused by the disease process and what is caused by the dis-ease which is spiritual suffering and pain.

This early assessment and diagnosis of spiritual pain demands considerable skill from the carer and time for each patient to talk about what is happening to them together with what they are doing for themselves. This cannot be done by direct question and answer approach, but through the formation of the spiritual bond between the patient and carer in which the patient knows there is full acceptance. Within this comfortable relationship, problems and worries surface and may often 'gush' out in utter relief; it doesn't mean others have *not* listened but rather that the patient has not *felt* heard.

An assessment of spiritual need

This basic assessment of spiritual need thus requires a range of observations which may not all be possible in one single meeting but will be a picture built up and emerging as a result of careful observation and use of interpretive skills. The kinds of observations to record will include:

- The patient's own perception of self image.
- Understanding of what the situation is, what is happening.
- The nature of support available from family, friends, and others.
- The nature of their family relationships, hopes, fears, and expectations of life ahead.
- Their own views and beliefs.
- Their life experiences.
- Religious affiliation—if any.
- Their cultural and ethnic background.
- Their willingness to receive help.
- An assessment of their coping mechanisms and personal strengths.
- Assessment of general emotional well-being.

Assessment of this kind will build up a picture of the person's individual need and capacity for relationships and will assist the carer in making an accurate and helpful diagnosis of approach needed and the place reached on life's journey. It will suggest the kinds of intervention likely to be most successful in relieving pain whatever its nature and origin (Elsdon 1995; Stoll 1979; Stoter 1995).

The roots of pain may then become apparent, opening the way to plan spiritual care to suit the personal needs. The importance of this spiritual assessment in diagnosis is often overlooked, as it is not thought to need specific diagnosis. Sometimes the professional response is that it needs an orthodox or religious approach or a non-religious but equally platitudinous response and a decision may be made to move too quickly and for wrong reasons down an anti-depressant route of treatment when spiritual care might make this intervention unnecessary.

To feel heard at the heart of spiritual pain is deeply therapeutic because it brings a sense of hope and relief from feelings of abandonment as the beginning of a partnership is established with a companion to share the journey into an unknown and crucial point in life.

There may be cultural and ethnic complexities in making this kind of diagnosis, especially where cultural or religious perspectives and background colour the patient's real needs and misinterpretations are possible. Words have different meanings in different cultures and lead to quick responses or snap judgements threatening the relationship, exacerbating the pain and can be misinterpreted as racial/cultural prejudice. For example, in some cultures or religions, pain is seen as judgement for past misdeeds or as something inevitable to be accepted and suffered in silence.

Ethical aspects

Skills involved with intervention

High levels of communication skills are essential to the whole process of caregiving, particularly where communicating information about a diagnosis is concerned. The expression 'breaking bad news' gives the impression that this is a one off event, something unpleasant for both patient and carer, to be done as quickly as possible, whereas it is a process, needing time and regular follow up as a natural part of the caregiving process. A horticultural analogy might be appropriate here as seen in planting a seed to grow into a healthy plant. The process begins with choosing the best situation followed by soil preparation, digging and fertilizing the ground before planting. This has to be continued with watering, protecting the tender shoots from frost, supporting the plant until it is well established. One difficulty for the person who realizes theirs is the responsibility to give unwelcome information is that they may slip into a 'bad news mode'. They feel uncomfortable, apprehensive of the likely response to the nature of the communication and in their anxiety to 'get it across' they may become authoritative and not establish the kind of rapport needed. The process will be affected by what has gone before, for example in the way the situation and information given has been handled (or not given) by the GP, experience in outpatients departments or on the ward. All this has a profound effect on the expectations and receptivity of the patient. It is coloured by the levels of fear and apprehension. Fear is a powerful inhibitor in receiving the reality of a situation as well as having a powerful effect on the perception and severity of pain.

The timing and place for giving information is important in setting the scene and also signals how 'available' the communicator is, whether there is time to stay with the patient allowing the patient to be 'in control' and take in the information at a manageable speed with an opportunity to consider and ask questions which arise, or whether this is just given as a 'piece of information'. Time is needed to allow the process to develop, rather than giving an unwelcome statement and leaving the person alone to take it in. The need to see this as a process and not an event can be gauged by the number of those who have 'been told' but who still complain of 'not being told anything!'

Once all the initial information has been given there will be a need to follow up, to revisit the situation to allow for the process of coming to terms with its significance, to take it in and to ask questions about the possible outcomes and treatment. This is a critical aspect of pain management in which pain can be needlessly exacerbated, alternatively critical aspects of rapport and partnership and trust can be established. The way in which the process is handled can have a profound impact on spiritual pain and thus the response necessary in handling pain related to dis-ease. All of this process is mirrored in communications with family and relatives and can affect their attitudes towards openness in their relationships with the patient, with staff and thus their part in relieving or exacerbating spiritual pain.

The ethical aspects of communication are important in ensuring information is given early, truthfully, and honestly, and if it is to be effective in a way that can be understood. The control of the flow of communication needs to be in the hands of the patient. To enable the person to say what they know or expect is helpful as this knowledge can be built upon. It is essential that truth is adhered to if trust is to be maintained and important that there is team approval and knowledge of what information has been given, together with how the patient responded. In the end the patient has the right to control, to accept, or reject the information.

Openness about the truth is essential for all concerned. Once distrust or dishonesty is suspected, effective communication is lost, often arousing feelings of anger, resentment, and even abandonment, with loss of confidence and increased fear leading to more pain. This may compound producing a powerful sense of isolation leading to despair as the patient feels devalued and not trusted to face reality about what is happening. When important information is given badly there is a most damaging effect on opportunity for the future relationship and for the process of coming to terms with reality. When it is given well, openness and honesty pave the way for further trust, interdependence and mutual sharing of the situation which is creative.

Skills involved with other interventions

Once the rapport has been established between the persons concerned, the way is open to consider other forms of possible intervention. These may be found and met within the team or it may be necessary to consider bringing in professionals with other specialist skills, to effect a reduction in stress levels which in turn may lead to pain reduction (Stoter 1995).

The use of complementary therapies such as aromatherapy, massage, and reflexology may have a part to play in reducing stress levels and enhancing a sense of wellbeing. There is real value in the fact that someone is giving personal time, skill, and attention which enhances a sense of well-being. The use of aromatic oils or burning perfumed candles can be valuable particularly where there is a sensitivity about unpleasant odours. These therapies all bring a sense of well-being and relaxation and help to restore a sense of self worth. All such therapies creatively used have a value in pain reduction (Stoter 1995). Many of the relaxing therapies can be carried out also by family and friends if they are willing to be involved. This may be useful in creating a shared relaxing atmosphere in the home.

For some individuals help and relief comes through religious groups or leaders, praying or laying on hands where it is requested. Within all faiths there are elements designed to bring comfort and relief to those in pain. Relief from guilt through confession or absolution may reduce stress and pain and help to restore relationships through forgiveness and acceptance. Some find the practice of meditation or imagery has a value in pain relief and when appropriately introduced can be practised by an individual whenever the need arises (Elsdon 1995).

A caring environment can provide a sense of restfulness and personal memorabilia or favourite foods brought into a hospital surrounding may be appreciated as a sharing of love and care. The use of flowers, or a single flower, a background providing favourite music are all demonstrations of thoughtfulness beyond words showing that the person is valued. These are actions often lost or overlooked in institutional life or even in the sick room at home; they can be given by any person who is observant and sensitive to need and not only by professional carers. However because it is difficult to be specific about detail and because they are so personal, they make a clear statement that the carer has something to share with a person who matters and the sense of well-being can help to relieve the concentration on pain (Twycross 1991).

There is one other skill which can sometimes be used appropriately by a very skilled person. This is in the form of a confrontational intervention to break through barriers of isolation and self-negation or damaging denial of reality, for example when essential decisions need to be taken. This approach should only be used after careful thought, when there is sufficient time for the process and by someone skilled in this process. The skill of all forms of care lies in recognizing the most appropriate and acceptable mode of approach, and the right of the individual to respond or not and to remain in control of the situation.

Staff support in giving spiritual care

To share the pain of another person can be a very costly experience for the carer, as Cassidy demonstrates so clearly (1991). She speaks of the 'terrible agony in watching someone "hollowed out"'. She also describes those who listen to others so exposing themselves to anothers' pain, as being part of the healing process (Cassidy 1991). The effects of cancer pain can be threatening to both professional and lay carers. Providing good spiritual care is very demanding and requires total concentration from the carers.

This quality of care demands of the carer an ability to understand and respect the beliefs, values hopes and fears of the patient and members of the family. In turn this demands a maturity from the carer, of self knowledge and awareness of one's own spirituality and vulnerability together with understanding the whole process of coming alongside, unconditionally and without judgement, with a willingness to respond to needs. It demands a willingness to facilitate interventions which may at times be in conflict with the carer's own beliefs (Stoter 1997).

Coping skills are important for carers when faced with a threatening situation such as impending death. For some, total denial can be a short term defence (Cox 1985) but in the longer term this strategy may be pathological. If the carers are inadequately supported when placed in threatening situations they can thus develop coping strategies inappropriate to this kind of care (Weisman 1981).

This calls for change in professional training and development to give time for learning to understand the process of spiritual pain and care. Carers need to acquire an understanding and awareness of their own spirituality and needs as an integral part of education, training, and development. Alongside this special training in self-development there needs to be a supportive attitude in the professional team promoting a recognition of and sensitivity to each other's needs and pressures and how this in turn affects relationships with patients and families. This awareness of the quality of relationships may disclose knowledge of the fact that patients are receiving adequate help from a particular member of staff or from someone outside the team and that situation needs respect, acceptance, and maturity from colleagues (Stoll 1979; Stoter 1997).

It is essential for team members to use every opportunity to share what is happening including all aspects of spiritual care in case reviews. These opportunities can be used to support each other when situations become perplexing or distressing; support of this kind coming as informal groups meet, during team meetings, or case conferences. It requires sensitivity and discerning leadership within the team. Support is found through:

- One to one support.
- Good communication channels.
- Management and organizational recognition.
- Encouraging staff to participate in and feed into decision making processes.
- A stated staff support policy.
- Team discussions.
- Support groups.
- Provision of relaxation/time out facilities.
- A safe and healthy working environment.
- The general ethos of caring where staff are valued.
- Services through counselling, occupational health, chaplains etc.
- In-service training including self-awareness and development.

It is important to know what junior staff are experiencing and hearing as they are often on the receiving end in hearing the deepest cries of pain from patients, particularly at night when feelings often surface and whoever is around has to listen and respond.

Spiritual care is a component of all care given whatever the professional discipline or level of seniority. It is also an integral part of staff care and family care and central to the cultural ethos.

To ignore or minimize spiritual care means the focus is on the disease and the

dis-ease is not being recognized or adequately responded to. In recognizing the importance of spiritual care the dis-ease is seen and responded to often making the management of the disease easier, particularly pain control. Thus spiritual care is not an
optional extra but an integral part of good care.

References

Cassidy, S. (1991). *Good friday people*, Dart, Longman and Todd, London.

Cox, T. (1985). *Stress*. McMillan Publishers Ltd, Hants.

Elsdon, R. (1995). Spiritual pain in dying people: the nurse's role. *Professional Nurse*,
10, (10), 641–3.

Hermann, H. (1984). *Narziss and Goldmund*. Penguin Books Ltd.

Saunders, C. (1969). The moment of truth, care for the dying patient. In *Death and
dying, current issues in treatment of the dying person* (ed. Pearson, L.) Press of Cape
Western University, Cleveland.

Smith, A.B. (1996). *The God shift*. New Millennium, London.

Socken, K.L., and Carson, V.J. (1987). Responding to the spiritual need of chronically
ill. *Nursing Clinics of North America*. University of Baltimore (Maryland) **22**, 3,
pp. 603–11.

Stoll, R. (1979). Guidelines for spiritual assessment. *American Journal of Nursing*, **79**,
1574–77.

Stoter, D. (1995). *Spiritual aspects of health care*. Mosby International, London.

Stoter, D. (1997). *Staff support in health care*. Blackwell Science, Oxford.

Twycross, R. (1981). In *Mud and stars*. Report of a working party. Sobell Publications,
Oxford.

Warden, S., Carpenter, J., and Brockopp, D. (1998). Nurses' beliefs about suffering
and their management of pain. *International Journal of Palliative Nursing*, **4**,
No. 1, pp. 21–25.

Weisman, A. (1981). Understanding the cancer patient, the syndrome of caregivers
plight. *Psychiatry*, **44**, 161–8.

Further reading

Edwards, B. (1995). Management of spiritual distress. *Emergency Nurse*, **3**, (2).

Farmer, E. (1996). *Exploring the spiritual dimension of care*. Mark Allen Publishing
Ltd, Wiltshire.

Gill, J. (1995). Spiritual care of the terminally ill. *Community Nurse Journal. Palliative
Care Section*, pp. 23–24.

Harrington, A. (1995). Spiritual care: what does it mean to RN's? *Australian Journal of
Advanced Nursing*, **12**, (4), pp. 5–14.

Narayanasamy, A. (1996). Spiritual care of chronically ill patients. *British Journal of
Nursing*, **5**, (7).

Oldnall, A. (1996). A critical analysis of nursing: meeting the spiritual needs of patients. *Journal of Advanced Nursing*, **23**, 138–44.

Penson, J., and Fisher, R. (1991). *Palliative care for patients with cancer*. Edward Arnold.

Reed, P.G. (1987). Spirituality and well-being in terminally ill hospitalised adults. *Research in Nursing and Health*, **10**, 335–44.

FIVE

Nursing issues

LORNA FOYLE

Come blessed peace, we once again implore,
and let our pains be less, our power more

Alexander Brome '*The Riddle*' (1646)

The holistic nature of nursing provides nurses with an unparalleled opportunity to make a significant contribution in the management of cancer pain.

Nursing beliefs and models of care are based on the concept of the holistic nature of illness, where the assessment of the individual is centred on understanding and responding to the needs of the whole person as a unique individual (Penson and Holloway 1989). Cancer pain management is a fundamental component of nursing practice which precisely reflects this philosophy. In a similar vein, the concept of total pain (Saunders 1967) was based on observations that an individual's experience of pain is a combination of emotional, spiritual, and social pain as well as physical pain.

These ideas were expanded into a multidimensional conceptualization of cancer related pain (Ahles and Blanchard 1988; McGuire 1987). This multidimensional framework suggests six separate dimensions that contribute to the patient's experience of pain and consists of the following components:

- Physiological (organic causes of pain).
- Sensory (intensity, location, quality).
- Affective (depression, anxiety).
- Cognitive (manner in which pain influences a person's thought process. How the individual interprets the meaning of pain).
- Behavioural (pain-related behaviour).
- Socio-cultural components (demographic, social, and cultural factors that are related to the experience of pain).

This multidimensional view of cancer pain requires a broad approach to assessment and management and involves a team approach from a range of health-care providers. Medical specialities such as; oncology, radiotherapy, anaesthetics, orthopaedics, neurosurgery, and psychiatry have a role in the assessment and management of pain (Richardson 1997). Other professions such as physiotherapists, social workers, occupational therapists, and pharmacists have responsibilities in managing cancer pain, but generally nurses have the most opportunity to develop close and fulfilling professional relationships. Nursing has a repertoire of interventions to offer as part of pain management, one of which is good communication skills. Good communication is equally important not only with the patient and family but with other health-care team members.

Communication

Cancer pain and its significance for the person experiencing it has the potential to isolate, but effective communication can dissipate some of those feelings of isolation. As patients search for meaning after receiving a diagnosis of cancer, their perception of pain may increase. Therefore, assisting patients in expressing and exploring the causes of their pain empowers patients to assume an active role in pain assessment and management which can diminish pain. This helps to distinguish the feelings or meaning attributed to pain from those beliefs about death (Ferrell and Dean 1995). This group of vulnerable patients may be incapable of expressing their pain because of their fears about what it may mean prognostically.

Effective communication is central to any interaction with the patient suffering from cancer pain. The nurse–patient relationship relies on the skills of the nurse to communicate with the patient and carers. These skills include; listening, observing, interpreting, questioning, and informing.

Uncertainty that is synonymous with a cancer diagnosis incurs feelings of loss of control over ones life and loss of initiative and sense of identity can transform a responsible, independent person into a passive and dependant patient (Abrams 1990). The ability to communicate is potentially powerful and it is the patient's right to be fully active in any decision making process.

Nurses may experience difficulties when communicating with cancer patients, especially those who are dying: these difficulties can lead nurses to impose blocking mechanisms. Nurses may be able to identify distressing symptoms yet make little attempt to elicit the intensity of each symptom or the degree to which it affects the patient (Wilkinson 1991); this can impact on pain management. Other communication difficulties encountered relate to patients' reluctance to discuss their pain and lack of continuity in nurse–patient relationship activity (Hawthorn and Redmond 1998) which may be attributable to shift patterns in the hospital setting. Similarly, the pain experience can destroy language making it impossible for patients to convey the reality of their experience (Scarry 1985). A patient's inability to speak English as a first language or because of cognitive or physical impairment can create other communication barriers and appropriate measures need to be taken to overcome this. In cancer pain management the nurses' role is integral in informing and supporting patients and their relatives.

Communication between nurse and patient is fundamentally important but communicating the patient's pain and experience and results of interventions to other health-care professionals is one of the most important, if not the most important responsibility of the nurse.

Nurses' role

Cancer pain management is the responsibility of a multi-disciplinary team, each discipline bringing its own expertise. However, it is the nurse who plays a pivotal role in the success or failure of any key pain management strategy for, especially in the acute setting, it is the nurse who more than any other member of the team, spends a consistent time period with the person in pain.

As nurses are key workers in this process, clarification of their scope of practice is essential. Most trained nurses should be able to achieve certain basic core competencies but it is inherent on senior nurses to devise guidelines for clinical practice so that each nurse understands their role in the pain management strategy. For example; in a non-specialist cancer ward, nurses need a cancer knowledge base that enables appropriate assessment, development, implementation, and evaluation of a pain management strategy. Swift consultation with other professionals when appropriate is essential nursing practice.

A clinical nurse specialist should have more advanced theoretical knowledge and clinical expertise in cancer pain management to enable assessment, diagnosis, analysis of complex problems and be able to use relevant research and theories where appropriate. It is imperative that nurses are able to identify their own boundaries of expertise in order to refer to a more experienced practitioner when necessary.

The training of pre-post registration nurses often creates dilemmas as they need to gain the necessary training and expertise to become skilled practitioners. These training needs may compete with the goal of protecting patients from unnecessary intrusion and pain from inexperienced practitioners (Fordham and Dunn 1994). To clarify some of these concerns the United Kingdom Central Council's Code of Professional Conduct (UKCC 1992) states that the nurse should; 'ensure that no action or omission on his/her part or within his/her sphere of influence is detrimental to the condition or safety of patients and clients'.

However, in the absence of any agreed criteria or guidelines regarding levels of competency, the responsibility lies with the individual nurse. The UKCC (1992) recommend that nurses should; 'acknowledge any limitations of practice and refuse in such cases to accept delegated functions without first having received instructions in regard to those functions and having been assessed as competent'.

Responsibilities around procedures

Despite differing levels of expertise and competence, every nurse has fundamental roles and responsibilities that must be utilized in cancer pain management. These responsibilities parallel those for any patient in pain. Nurse duties and responsibilities in cancer pain management need to allude briefly to those involving oral medication.

For those patients unable to self-medicate if they are prescribed regular analgesia, it is imperative that the patient in pain receives these exactly on time. This is the responsibility of all qualified nurses. Controlled drugs need to be prescribed in writing, kept in safe custody and recorded in registers. Examples of schedule two control drugs are morphine, diamorphine, and pethidine (Sofaer 1998). Demands on nurses in the hospital setting are increasing and it is tempting to defer the administration of controlled drugs until a less hectic time. The timing of the administration of drugs should not be compromised by the practitioner: medication requires precise timing to ensure the patient gains maximum benefit.

The majority of cancer patients obtain relief from a combination of pharmacological and non-pharmacological strategies. Unfortunately approximately 5%–10% continue to suffer (Foley 1985) despite these measures. Alternative methods are needed to treat this population of patients. Referral of the patient to pain consultants or anaesthetists may result in the decision to initiate special procedures. There is a range of these procedures (King and Jacob 1993):

- Cryoanalgesia
- Radiofrequency lesioning
- Facet block
- Epidural analgesia
- Caudal block
- Spinal blockade
- Coeliac plexus block
- Stellate ganglion block
- Splanchnic nerve block
- Lumber sympathetic blockade
- Regional intravenous sympathetic block
- Intercostal nerve blockade
- Upper limb blocks (brachial plexus and supra-capsular block)
- Lower limb blocks (femoral, sciatic, obturator, lateral, and peripheral nerve blocks)
- Trigger point injections
- Others.

Prior to all these procedures the patient should be informed of the nature of treatment, including the common adverse effects and complications that can arise (King and Jacob 1993). This provides an opportunity to alleviate some of the patient's anxieties and ensure that informed consent has been given for the particular procedure.

During the procedure the nurse's prime responsibility is for the comfort and reassurance of the patient. This can be achieved by providing a calm relaxed atmosphere in which nurses use listening skills and are there to provide reassurance. A secondary role is to assist the doctor to perform the procedure under aseptic conditions. Monitoring patient's vital signs may be required and the nurse should record these.

After the procedure is completed, the procedure should be recorded in a book. The details documented should include: the patient's name, doctor and nurse present, drugs used, and any complications (King and Jacob 1993). The recording of vital signs will be maintained until the patient's condition appears to be stable and there are no adverse reactions.

A specialist nurse may be required to carry out skills not acquired in basic training, for example spinal top-up procedure, when the doctor may not be available and there is a need to ensure continuing comfort for the patient. Nurses may want to extend their role but should remember that this procedure should only be carried out with a high level of theoretical knowledge and practical skill.

Since each nurse is individually responsible and accountable for their actions, nurses who take on these duties will need to update their knowledge and competence. Therefore it is advisable that nursing and medical staff have an agreed policy, encompassing a formal assessment of the nurse wishing to undertake spinal administration.

Further information on nursing and duties and responsibilities relating to special procedures can be found in Carroll and Bowsher (1993).

Assessing the patient's pain

An accurate assessment of the patient's pain is an essential nursing responsibility and is crucial to implementing the appropriate pain management strategy. If the causes of pain have not been identified clearly then it may take longer to control the patient's pain. It must be remembered that there are multiple dimensions of cancer pain which contribute to the total pain experience and will require a multi-professional approach.

Assessment is the vital first step towards the control of cancer pain (WHO 1986). When cancer patient's present with pain many factors must be taken into account on the first assessment (Donovan 1987). These factors include:

- Location
- Intensity
- Duration
- Factors influencing the occurrence of pain
- Effects of pain
- Psychosocial effects
- Aggravating factors
- Alleviating factors
- Effects of therapy
- Associated symptoms (e.g. nausea etc).

Pain assessment and measurement levels are useful in providing information. Few pain assessment tools currently available fulfil all these informational factors but some tools offer a greater contribution to the management of cancer pain than others. By the very nature of its presentation, cancer pain has meaning or significance to the person suffering. For example, it may signify that cancer is progressing.

Patients may only be able to tolerate assessment and measurement of their cancer pain for short periods. In the following section a number of valid and reliable tools available to measure pain are presented. Nurses must understand that each of these tools has advantages and disadvantages and for the patient the tool must be user friendly.

Visual analogue scale

A visual analogue scale consists of a 10 cm line that is anchored at either end with extremes of pain using words such as 'no pain' and 'worst pain imaginable' (Fig. 5.1). The scale may also have specific points along the line which may be numbered and is known as a numeric graphic rating scale, but this is likely to introduce significant bias into the result. A verbal graphic rating scale (Fig. 5.1) uses the line principle but substitutes words for numbers. The patient identifies the point along the line which signifies his or her perceived experience of pain. This is less reliable than a verbal rating scale without linear form.

Pain Rating Scales

No pain |-------------------------------------| Worst pain imaginable

Numeric Graphic Rating Scale

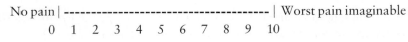

No pain | ------------------------------------- | Worst pain imaginable
        0   1   2   3   4   5   6   7   8   9   10

Verbal Rating Scale

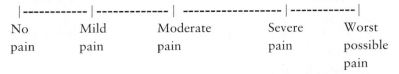

No	Mild	Moderate	Severe	Worst
pain	pain	pain	pain	possible
				pain

Fig. 5.1 Visual analogue scale

Although easy to administer the visual analogue scale is time consuming to score and thus provides opportunity for error (Schofield 1995). A careful explanation of the scale can reduce failure rate (Scott and Huskisson 1976) but it requires time to explain its use in monitoring pain. A visual analogue scale places few demands on sick patients and is sensitive to changes in pain intensity (Choinere *et al.* 1990; Melzack and Katz 1994). It is reported to be more accurate in reflecting those changes (Ohnhaus and Adler 1975) than the verbal rating scale. When using a verbal rating scale one problem that may be encountered is that the patient may be illiterate or English is not their first language.

Body diagrams

Body diagrams enable the patient to identify the location and distribution of pain which is particularly relevant to the cancer patient as the patient may be experiencing pain at a number of different sites (Hawthorne and Redmond 1998). Clinicians or patients can complete the body diagrams but additional information, for example, the area which hurts the most, should be included. Body diagrams are easy to use and visually demonstrate the extent and sites of pain. However the limitation on body diagrams is that they only record a small part of the pain experience.

Pain questionnaires

Pain questionnaires combine a number of approaches such as open and closed questions, rating scales, and body diagrams to measure the pain experience. A range of pain questionnaires (listed below) are in use but not all are used in the assessment of cancer pain.

- McGill Pain Questionnaire (Melzack 1975)
- Wisconsin Brief Pain Questionnaire (Daut *et al*. 1983)
- The London Hospital Pain Investigation Chart (Raiman 1986)
- Edmonton Symptom Assessment System (Bruera *et al*. 1991)
- Initial Pain Assessment tool (McCaffrey and Beebe 1994).

The McGill Pain Questionnaire (MPQ) (Melzack 1975) is a popular pain assessment tool, used mainly in specialist pain clinics, to measure the sensory, affective, and evaluative dimensions of the pain experience (Melzack and Katz 1994). Additional information gleaned from the MPQ may include the location of pain, the intensity and periodicity of pain, the accompanying symptoms, the effects on sleep, activity and eating, and the pattern of analgesic use (Richardson 1997).

A short-form McGill Pain Questionnaire (SF-PQ) has been developed where time to collect information is limited (Melzack 1987). Both formats of the questionnaire can discriminate between different types of pain and the effect of treatment on that pain (Hawthorne and Redmond 1998). One of its disadvantages is that it requires a degree of concentration which renders it unsuitable for sick people. Some of the words used in the questionnaire are complex and may not be understood by all patients (Chapman *et al*. 1985; Deschamps *et al*. 1988) which restricts its use in some cancer pain patients.

Another pain questionnaire used with cancer patients is the London Hospital Pain Observation Chart (Raiman 1986). This incorporates a body chart and pain rating scale which has a facility to record nursing and pharmacological interventions.

The Brief Pain Questionnaire was developed mainly for clinical use with patients who were too ill to be subjected to longer exhausting assessment techniques; it was formerly known as the Wisconsin Brief Pain Questionnaire (Daut *et al*. 1983). Patients identify the location of their pain on a drawing, whilst explaining other issues concerning duration and cause of pain. The questionnaire provides a list of descriptors to assist the patient in describing the nature of the pain.

The tools cited in this section represent some of the wide variety of pain assessment tools available to the nursing profession. Despite growing evidence that pain measurement tools ensure that patients receive higher quality of pain relief (Carroll 1993) they are still not widely used in nursing practice. Perhaps it is the very existence of so many tools that deters nurses from even selecting one. To be useful, an assessment measure should be multidimensional, valid, reliable, sensitive, easy to administer, and not place undue demands on the patient or the nurse (Schofield 1995).

Nurses need to have a knowledge of most pain assessment tools and be prepared to adapt the selected tool to individual patient's needs and environment. Regardless of which tool is used, the nurse must remember that it is the patient's own report of the pain experience that is vital to the assessment process. Cancer patients should always receive an initial assessment modified to their particular condition at that time. These pain assessment activities can be used to provide a firm basis for the planning of nursing interventions as part of the multi-professional, patient-centred pain management plan.

Nursing interventions in pain management

The experience of pain can be modified by non-pharmacological methods, many of which are closely related to nursing's scope of practice. Research-based knowledge is sparse regarding the use and efficacy of these methods (Fordham and Dunn 1994) and in the clinical setting these interventions have not been tested thoroughly (Synder 1985).

The nursing interventions included in this chapter do not affect the underlying pathology or alter the sensation of patients' pain. However, these techniques can furnish individuals with an opportunity to be involved in the management of their pain, sometimes reducing feelings of helplessness. It may also restore an element of control that cancer patients express as having lost and may already be part of the patient's repertoire to deal with the pain.

Nurses have several responsibilities with regard to these techniques. They must have a reliable knowledge base in order to anticipate side-effects and be able to monitor, evaluate, and accurately document the efficacy of the treatment. Communication with the patient and family is crucial. In particular, it is important that the nurse maintains a balance between not raising the expectations of the patient whilst inspiring confidence in the proposed pain management measures.

Some of the measures nurses can instigate in the management of cancer pain are outlined below.

Heat

The application of heat can reduce pain associated with muscle spasms, joint stiffness, inflammation, oedema, ischaemia, and effusion (Lehman and Lateur 1982). The reduction of pain can be potentially attributed to vasodilation increasing blood supply to a local area and enhanced muscle relaxation, thus relieving muscle spasm, for example; in colic (Fordham and Dunn 1994). Applying heat to a local area often involves water, either by immersing the affected part, for instance; hands in water; or the heat may be applied in the form of a hot water bottle or heating pad. These should be wrapped in a protective cover, such as a towel, and applied to the affected area.

Heat should be applied for twenty minutes. The nurse should be mindful that some disease processes may be altered as in those individuals where bleeding or the potential for bleeding may occur, for example; patients with fungating lesions or leukaemia. Heat is often a practical remedy which patients and their carers can use in their own surroundings.

Cold

Cold is another method of pain management that is often ignored, yet it has been demonstrated to be more effective than heat (LaFoy and Geden 1989). Cold produces vasoconstriction which may decrease sensitivity to pain by creating numbness (Michlovitz 1990). The patient's skin should be protected from direct exposure of the cold source by using at least one layer of towelling (Spross and Burke 1993). The cold source can be in the form of ice cubes, ice packs, and packs of frozen vegetables. The patient's comfort should be of prime importance, so if the patient cannot tolerate the application of cold immediately, additional layers of towelling can be laid between the cold source and the skin until the patient adapts to the cold.

Peristalsis of the gastrointestinal tract seems to increase with cold application and decrease with heat application (Lehman and Lateur 1989). Therefore the application of cold is inadvisable for those patients complaining of colic.

Heat and cold can be used alternatively. Its effect should be evaluated after each use and documented. Heat and cold are usually part of a total pain management strategy but prior to use should be discussed with the patient, particularly those who have communication difficulties due to decreased or absent sensations. These techniques should be discontinued if there is no evidence of pain relief after several applications. Both applications are also contra-indicated in areas which have been previously treated with radiotherapy (Hawthorn and Redmond 1998) and cold should not be used on extremities.

Massage

Massage is described as the touching or application of forces to the soft tissues, usually muscles, tendons, or ligaments without causing movement or a change in the position of a joint. The nurse must receive specific training and have time to practise before using massage as a form of treatment for the patient. A number of different treatments are employed in massage, including stroking or effleurage, connective tissue massage, kneading and petrissage, friction, and deep massage (Haldeman 1989).

Stroking and effleurage consist of gentle stroking movements that are applied in the direction of the flow of blood and lymphs through the venous and lymphatic system (Spross and Burke 1993) in a rhythmic manner. Kneading and petrissage requires the nurse to grasp, lift, and knead the tissues being massaged. The skin should move with the hands over the underlying tissues (Pearce 1993).

Concern has been expressed over using massage for people with cancer. This concern is based on the belief that massage may encourage the spread of cancer (McNamara 1994). There is no evidence to support this belief (Hawthorne and Redmond 1998). Nurses experienced in massage techniques report that for patients with advanced cancer, massage is best confined to those areas of the body that are easily accessible, for example; hand and arm, foot and calf, or neck, and shoulders (Pearce 1993).

Massage directly over a palpable tumour should be avoided. Other contra-indications for the use of massage in patients with a diagnosis of cancer are those who also have deep venous thrombosis, thrombophlebitis, and bleeding disorders. Areas of open lesions and tender skin should be avoided (Horrigan 1995).

The benefits of massage for cancer patients in managing pain are often surprising. One study demonstrated that after a thirty minute massage in a population of cancer patients, heart and respiratory rate as well as pain and anxiety rates decreased (Ferrell-Tory and Glick 1993). Nurses using massage view it as a powerful means of opening communication channels which have been previously closed by conveying feelings of calming, compassion, support, and empathy.

In a highly technical, often depersonalized environment massage can often communicate reassurance to patients and decrease the effects of hospitalization and depersonalization associated with illness (Simms 1986). Nurses using massage must exercise caution when initiating it as part of a pain management strategy. Touch is not always acceptable to all patients and discussion with the patient on how comfortable the patient is with physical touch is essential before treatment commences. Any signs of anxiety and discomfort by the patient should discourage the use of massage. On the other hand, the fact that massage is a therapeutic intervention with clearly defined boundaries, may make it acceptable for these patients (McNamara 1994).

Other physical measures

Appropriate positioning of the patient in pain can alleviate the intensity of the pain experience and nurses should endeavour to assist patients to find a favoured comfortable position and not move them unless necessary. Pillows or other supports should be provided to help maintain a favoured position (Wilkie *et al.* 1989). Elevating painful limbs can reduce pain.

Maintaining a balance between activity and rest is viewed as a problem by cancer patients. They are driven by a strong desire to maintain activities in their environment which were part of their role in normal living. Nurses need to encourage them to rest and to discuss their feelings of frustration and loss of control. Rest can be facilitated by careful planning, whichever environment the patient inhabits. Environment is crucial to resting and rest can be facilitated by the provision of appropriate lighting, temperature, and ventilation (Fordham and Dunn 1994).

Lack of privacy may also inhibit a person's expression of pain and act as a barrier to communication (Fager-Haugh and Strauss 1977). Nurses can be instrumental in organizing the environment by organizing quiet times, scheduling investigations and interventions appropriately, and facilitating visiting times to suit the patient's needs.

These strategies generally fall into three categories, physical, cognitive, and behavioural, which can be used individually or simultaneously. The physical category includes the application of heat, cold, massage, and transcutaneous electronic nerve stimulation (TENS), discussed in detail in Chapter 13.

Reducing the perception of pain

Treatment strategies aimed at reducing the perception of pain can be classified as cognitive, behavioural, or cognitive-behaviour. They are particularly relevant for the cancer patient's pain where the psychosocial factors contribute to the pain experience. The nurse can facilitate the patient acquiring a range of behavioural and cognitive skills which provide them with a greater sense of control over the pain (Turk and Meichenbaum 1989). Cognitive behavioural strategies range in complexity from simple distraction to hypnosis. Each nurse must be aware of their level of expertise and practice within those boundaries.

The following are techniques that all trained nurses should aspire to use either in their own practice or involving those with the appropriate expertise. They are distraction, guided imagery, relaxation, music, and humour therapy.

Distraction

Distraction removes pain from the focus of attention, thus increasing the individual's pain tolerance. Most patients in pain have generally already devised distractions from their pain but nurses may need to discuss these. Distraction should only be used if the patient is committed to its use and if they feel physically able as it does require some effort to sustain it. When distraction interventions are completed, patients may experience increased awareness of pain and an increase in fatigue and irritability (McCaffery and Beebe 1994). Other interventions should be offered at this point to prevent the pain worsening.

Relaxation

There are several methods of inducing physiological and psychological relaxation (Richardson 1997). They include awareness of control of breathing and relaxation of muscle groups in sequence (Horrigan 1993). By concentrating the mind on a specific physical function the mind is distracted from the pain. Relaxation can be performed in any position but the activity is enhanced if the patient is lying on a supportive soft surface (Horrigan 1993). Always support painful joints and muscles before beginning the exercise (Cook 1986; Levin *et al*. 1987; McCaffery 1990).

Guided imagery

Guided imagery is a technique which uses one's mind to create an experience, a mental image which distracts away from the pain. Often nurse-led at the outset, patients soon embark to imaginary places that hold special and comfortable memories for them. It is important for them to have identified their own memories as some standard scenarios can evoke poignant and unpleasant experiences which can be upsetting for the patient.

Nurses utilising these techniques need to feel confident in their use and know of their limitations in practice. They should also be aware of other techniques to assist in controlling pain and where to access the practitioners with the expertise. These other strategies include; focusing, reforming, music therapy, biofeedback, and systematic desensitization. More details and clinical examples of these techniques are detailed in the book *Pain* (McCaffery and Beebe 1994).

Conclusion

Pain is a multidimensional phenomenon. The management of cancer pain is a multi-disciplinary challenge requiring close collaboration between health-care professionals and demands an integrated approach combining pharmacological and non-pharmacological techniques (Hawthorn and Redmond 1998). This approach to pain control is recommended by WHO (1990) referring to a team which includes; doctors, nursing and other health professionals.

Nurses are focal in the health-care teams; they are in the most pertinent position to collect and record comprehensive information about the cancer patient's pain experience. Nurses require knowledge of pain assessment, pharmacological and non-pharmacological methods of pain relief, and management techniques. Equally essential is evaluation of these techniques and responses by the patient to them are of paramount importance.

Undoubtedly a nurse's pre and post registration education is crucial to improve nursing knowledge and skills in the management of cancer pain. Despite a burgeoning interest and literature in this field there appears little evidence of standardized nursing input in pain management techniques and therefore success remains haphazard. Research has highlighted nursing knowledge deficits and inconsistent responses in many areas related to pain (Clarke *et al*. 1996).

In contrast, there have been some encouraging findings. Fothergill-BourBonnais and Wilson-Barnett (1992) compared the knowledge of nurses working in intensive therapy and hospice settings. The findings, suggested that although hospice nurses were more knowledgeable in pain management both groups demonstrated a lack of knowledge in specific content areas.

Nurses should be aware of the deficits in their knowledge and seek to fill them in order to ensure continuity of pain management for all cancer patients. Nursing practice needs to advance its knowledge and skills but retain its essence of providing care and support. The impact of incurable disease, such as cancer, inevitably means that nurses attend patients at times of extreme distress and provide intimate physical and emotional care (Copp 1986). This ultimately leads to the nurse having a deeper knowledge of the patient. An opportunity to develop an open and trusting relationship exists which can add significantly to the patient's pain management and quality of life.

The nurse is in the best position to teach, support, and empower the patient with a cancer diagnosis and their families to ease their pain. Only when nurses are part of a patient-focused, holistic, multi-professional approach to pain management can patients receive the quality of care they truly deserve.

References

Abrams, N.A. (1990). A contrary view of the nurse as patient advocate. *Ethics in nursing: an anthology* (ed. Pence, T. *et al.*) National League for Nursing Publications.

Ahles, T.A., and Blanchard, E.B. (1983). The multi-dimensional nature of cancer related pain. *Pain*, **17**, 277–28.

Bruera, E., Kuehn, N., Miller, M.J., Selmser, P., and Macmillan, K. (1991). The Edmonton symptom assessment system (ESAS). A simple method for the assessment of palliative care patients. *Journal of Palliative Care*, **7**, 6–9.

Carroll, D. (1993). Pain. In *Pain management and nursing care* (ed. D. Carroll and D. Bowsher) Butterworth-Heinemann, Oxford, pp. 1–4.

Carroll, D., and Bowsher, D. (1993). *Pain management and nursing care* (ed. D. Carroll and D. Bowsher) Butterworth-Heineman, Oxford.

Chapman, C.R., Casey, K.L., Dubner, R., Foley, K.H., Gracely, R.H., and Reading, A.E. (1985). Pain measurement: an overview. *Pain*, **10**, 221–31.

Choinere, R., Melzack, R., Girard, N., Rondeau, J., and Pacquin, M.J. (1990). Comparisons between patients and nurses assessment of pain and medications efficacy in severe burn injuries. *Pain*, **40**, 143–52.

Clarke, E.B., French, B., Bilodeau, M.I. *et al.* (1996). Pain management knowledge, attitudes and clinical practice. The impact of nurses' characteristics and education. *Journal of Pain and Symptom Management*, **11**, 18–31.

Cook, J.D. (1986). Music as intervention in the oncology setting. *Cancer Nursing*, **9**, 23–8.

Copp, L.A. (1986). The nurse as an advocate for vulnerable persons. *Journal of Advanced Nursing*, **11**, 255–65.

Daut, R., Cleeland, C., and Flanery, R.C. (1983). Development of Wisconsin brief pain questionnaire to assess pain in cancer and other diseases. *Pain*, **17**, 197–203.

Deschamps, M., Banur, R., and Coldman, A.J. (1988). Assessment of adult cancer pain: short-comings of current methods. *Pain*, **32**, 133–9.

Donovan, M. (1987). Clinical assessment of cancer pain. In *Cancer pain management* (2nd edn) (ed.) D.B. McGuire and C.H. Yarboro, pp. 105–31.

Fager-Haugh, S.Y., and Strauss, A. (1977). *Politics of pain management: staff patient interaction*. Addison-Wesley, New York.

Ferrell, B.A., and Dean, G. (1995). The meaning of cancer pain. *Seminars in Oncology Nursing*, **1**, 17–22.

Ferrell-Torry, A., and Glick, O. (1993). The use of therapeutic massage as a nursing intervention to modify anxiety and the perception of cancer pain. *Cancer Nursing*, **16**, 92–101.

Foley, K. (1985). The treatment of cancer pain. *New England Journal of Medicine*, **313**, 84–95.

Fordham, M., and Dunn, V. (1994). *Alongside the person in pain*. Baillière Tindal.

Fothergill-BourBonnais, F., and Wilson-Barnett, F. (1992). A comparative study of intensive care unit and hospice nurse knowledge on pain management. *Journal of Advanced Nursing*, **17**, 362–72.

Haldeman, S. (1989). Manipulation and massage for the relief of back pain. In *Textbook of Pain* (2nd edn) (ed. P. Wall and R. Melzack) pp. 942–51. Churchill Livingstone, Edinburgh.

Hawthorne, J., and Redmond, K. (1998). *Pain cause and management*. Blackwell Scientific Publications, Oxford.

Horrigan, C. (1993). Massage. In *The nurses handbook of therapies* (ed. D. Rankin-Box) pp. 125–32. Churchill Livingstone, Edinburgh.

King, and Jacob, P. (1993). Special procedures. In *Pain management and nursing care* (ed. D. Carroll and D. Bowsher) Butterworth-Heineman, Oxford, 206–49.

Lafoy, J., and Geden, E.A. (1989). Post episiotomy pain: warm versus cold site baths. *Journal of Obstetrics and Neonatal nursing*, **18**, 399–403.

Lehman, J., and Lateur, B. (1982). Therapeutic heat. In *Therapeutic use of heat and cold* (ed. J. Lehman). Williams & Williams, Baltimore.

Lehman, J., and Lateur, B. (1989). Ultrasound, shortwave, microwave, superficial heat and cold in the treatment of pain. In *Textbook of pain* (ed. P.D. Wall and R. Melzack) pp. 932–41. Churchill Livingstone, Edinburgh.

Levin, R., Malloy, G.B., and Hyman, R.B. (1987). Nursing management of postoperative pain: use of relaxation techniques with female cholecycystectomy patients. *Journal of Advanced Nursing*, **12**, 463–72.

McCaffery, M. (1990). Nursing approaches to non-pharmacological pain control. *International Journal of Nursing Studies*, **27**, 1–5.

McCaffery, M., and Beebe, M. (1994). *Pain: clinical manual for nursing practice* (2nd edn). Moseby, London.

McGuire, D.B. (1987). Coping strategies used by cancer patients with pain. *Oncology Nursing Forum*, **14**, 123.

McNamara, P. (1994). *Massage for people with cancer*. Wandsworth Cancer Support Centre, London.

Melzack, R. (1975). The McGill Pain Questionnaire. Properties and scoring methods. *Pain*, **1**, 295–9.

Melzack, R. (1987). The Short-form McGill Pain Questionnaire. *Pain*, **30**, 191–7.

Melzack, R., and Katz, J. (1994). Pain measurement in persons in pain. In *Textbook of Pain* (3rd edn) (eds. P.D. Wall and R. Melzack) pp. 337–56. Churchill Livingstone, Edinburgh.

Michlovitz, S. (1990). The use of cold as a therapeutic agent. In *Thermal agents in rehabilitation* (ed. S.L. Miccholvitz). Davis, Philadelphia.

Ohnhaus, E.E., and Adler, R. (1975). Methodological problems in the measurement of pain: a comparison between the verbal rating scale and the visual analogue scale. *Pain*, **1**, 379–84.

Pearce, C. (1993). Care of the dying. In *Pain management and nursing care* (ed. D. Carroll and D. Bowser) Butterworth & Heineman, Oxford, 68–89.

Penson, J., and Holloway, I. (1989). Fringe benefits: alternative medicine in patient care. *Senior Nurse*, **9**, 9–10.

Raiman, J. (1986). Towards understanding pain and planning for relief. *Nursing*, **11**, 411–23.

Richardson, A. (1997). Cancer pain and its management. In *Pain its nature and management* (ed. V. Thomas). Baillière Tindal.

Saunders, C.M. (1967). *The management of terminal illness*. Hospital Medical Publication.

Scarry, E. (1985). *The body in pain: the making and unmaking of the world*. Oxford University Press, New York.

Schofield, P. (1995). Using assessment tools to help patients in pain. *Professional Nurse*, **10**, 703–6.

Scott, J., and Huskisson, E. (1976). Graphic representation of pain. *Pain*, **2**, 175–84.

Simms, S. (1986). Slow stroke massage for cancer patients. *Nursing Times*, **82**, 47–50.

Sofaer, B. (1998). *Pain, principles, practice and patients* (3rd edn). Stanley Thomas.

Spross, J., and Burke, M. (1993). Non-pharmacological measurement of cancer pain. In *Cancer pain management* (ed. D. McGuire, C. Yarboro and B. Ferrell) Jones & Bartlett Publications.

Synder, M. (1985). *Independent nursing interventions*. John Wiley, New York.

Turk, D., and Meichenbaum, D. (1989). A cognitive behavioural approach to pain management. In *Textbook of pain* (2nd edn) (ed. P.D. Wall and R. Melzack) pp. 1001–9. Churchill-Livingstone, Edinburgh.

United Kingdom Central Council for Nursing, Midwifery & Health Visitors (UKCC). (1992). *Code of professional conduct* (3rd edn). UKCC, London.

Wilkie, D., Lovejoy, N., Dodd, M., and Tessler, M. (1988). Cancer pain control behaviours: description and correlation with Intensity. *Oncology Nursing Forum*, **15**, 723–31.

Wilkinson, S. (1991). Factors which influence how nurses communicate with cancer patients. *Journal of Advanced Nursing*, **16**, 677–88.

World Health Organization. (1986). *Cancer pain relief*. WHO Geneva.

World Health Organization. (1990). *Cancer pain relief and palliative care: a report of WHO expert committee* Technical Report Series, No. 804, WHO Geneva.

SIX

Physiotherapy

BETTY O'GORMAN AND ANN ELFRED

'Chronic pain is experienced by about one third of all cancer patients and by 70–90% of those with advanced disease.' (Portnoy 1992)

'A significant portion of terminally ill patients with pain do not receive adequate pain relief from pharmacological agents alone.' (Ahles and Martin 1992)

Traditionally in palliative care and oncology pharmacology has played the major role in the management of cancer pain (Baines 1989), but this approach may be insufficient to achieve optimal pain relief. Many units have included physiotherapy since their inception; in one modern hospice unit this is longer than 30 years. Expertise has developed from this small base as a speciality of physiotherapy in oncology and palliative care. Physiotherapy practice covers many modalities which may be of use in the alleviation of pain in cancer patients. Many patients have co-existing conditions that may contribute to their overall pain picture. Multiple pathologies of both malignant and non-malignant origin are common.

The chartered physiotherapist has various techniques available e.g. manual, electrotherapeutic, exercise and complementary. Some of these, such as transcutaneous electrical nerve stimulation (TENS) and acupuncture are dealt with in Chapter 13 and will therefore not be explored in depth although they form a regular part of a physiotherapist's treatment regimen.

Pain is frequently accompanied by feelings of anger, helplessness, and loss of control (Bonica *et al*. 1990). Anxiety and frustration are the most important predictors of pain unpleasantness (Vingoe 1994). Such feelings need to be acknowledged and attempts made to address them as part of a treatment regimen. Dame Cicely Saunders describes physical, emotional, psychosocial, and spiritual elements combining to form a picture of 'total pain' (Saunders 1967). Addressing only the physical component will not bring about pain relief and, therefore, the physiotherapist together with other professionals need to take a holistic approach, whilst not neglecting a thorough physical assessment using specific modalities to target each component of the pain experience (Ahles *et al*. 1983).

Approaches which help the patient to regain control can enhance self-esteem and are often the most effective. Patients may have been passive recipients of a series of unpleasant interventions and may welcome the opportunity to take a more active role in their own pain management (de Wit *et al*. 1997). Psychological welfare is enhanced where individuals believe that they have some ability to control their emotions and physical symptoms (Thompson *et al*. 1993). The perception of having control over pain relates highly to satisfaction with pain relief (Pellino and Ward 1998). Most of the techniques described here are within the control of the patient and many of them require the patients active input rather than the passive role they may have had to adopt previously. Active coping strategies have been associated with positive adjustment, whereas passive coping strategies have been linked with maladaptive outcome measures such as increased pain and depression (Snow-Turek *et al.* 1996).

General principles

When assessing patients and planning treatment regimens, certain guidelines should always be observed (O'Gorman 1994).

- Consider the patient totally.
- Commence treatment as soon as possible and continue on a regular basis.
- Be realistic. Try to be as positive as possible, but don't make false promises.
- Safety is paramount. Over-vigorous treatments may exacerbate symptoms or even cause new problems such as pathological fracture.
- Listen to the patient—don't make assumptions.
- Be sensitive to a deteriorating condition. Adapt treatment regimens appropriately, but be prepared to continue.
- Be prepared to involve friends and relatives in planning goals and achieving these.

A number of modalities may be considered and combined as part of a treatment regimen.

Assessment

Before commencing treatment careful assessment of the patient is essential. An accurate history should be taken from the patient and previous treatment records should be read. Details of the patient's pain should include onset, site, severity, quality (e.g. aching, shooting, burning, stabbing), frequency, and duration. It is also necessary to ascertain the effect of the pain upon the patients life, for example their functioning and social interactions. Ongoing assessment is essential, both to monitor the effect of interventions as well as to adapt to a fluctuating or deteriorating condition. The therapist must be prepared to alter their strategies as the situation changes, which may be daily as disease advances.

Positioning and handling

Physiotherapy is essentially a 'hands-on' profession and good physical skills underpin all modalities. The approach must be confident and with explanation if the patient is to trust the therapist. Words can be crucial in the treatment of pain either to positive or negative effect (Staats *et al.* 1998). Limbs need to be held in a gentle yet secure manner with the hands moulded and sensitive to the structures beneath them. Sudden, jerky, or rigid handling is likely to tense the patient and exacerbate pain. Special care must be taken where there is altered sensation, for example allodynia or hyperalgesia. It is essential to ensure that the patient is in a comfortable, well-supported position both 'generally' and 'locally'. The effects of gravity on the body must always be considered. If a patient's trunk is allowed to be positioned in front of the line of gravity then it will be increasingly difficult to support it and make the patient comfortable. Therefore patients should be reclined back from the vertical at the hips which will minimize the effect of gravity on the body. By doing this either in bed or reclining in a wheelchair or armchair, the line of gravity will then pass in front of the head and neck through the thorax.

The patient's overall position and comfort must be considered.

- Is the patient well supported?
- Warm enough or too hot?
- Is the top pillow of a stack soft?
- Are the sheets wrinkled?
- Is the clothing unduly tight or restrictive?

Attention to such details gives the patient confidence, a feeling of their very specific needs being addressed and can greatly enhance the efficiency of treatment because they feel 'cared for'. Specific problems may need particular measures. This may be as simple as a weak limb supported on a pillow or foam wedge or may require custom-made splints or supports.

Exercise

Therapeutic exercise is generally considered as a part of rehabilitation but may also make an important contribution to pain relief. Prolonged illness or pain often leads to lengthy periods of bed rest and fear of movement. This may cause joint stiffness, short-ened soft tissues, and weak muscles, all of which may lead to further pain and reluct-ance to move, establishing a vicious cycle. Exercise may help to break this cycle and re-establish a more normal pattern of movement. For those who are weak, frail or paralysed, exercise will need to be passive, that is performed by the therapist and not under the patient's voluntary control. Also, the part to be moved must be held securely yet gently. Initially, the range of joint movement should be small, with the aim of grad-ually increasing it to as near full as possible. Movements should be slow and rhyth-mical and should not elicit pain. Passive stretching of soft tissues may also be used. Care must be taken not to force or over-extend structures which may be poorly protected because of weakness, paralysis, or general frailty. The combination of these techniques may help to maintain or restore normal range of movement, reduce muscle spasm, and improve soft tissue extensibility. For those who are able, active exercise is the method of choice. Specific exercise schemes should be taught to address the particular needs of the individual. Exercise should be within patient's tolerance and stamina and will usually start simply and progress gently. It is often helpful to write exercises down, both to encourage the patient to practise on their own and to enlist the help of willing friends and relatives. Frequently a combination of active and passive exercise will be required to achieve optimum effect. As well as treating presenting pain, exercise is important in preventing the pains associated with joint stiffness and soft tissue inelasticity which can lead to deformity and loss of function. A simple regimen of exercises, supervised by the therapist and practised regularly, can greatly enhance feelings of control and well-being as well as having positive physical effects.

General mobility

Man was meant to be ambulant and general immobility may cause pain in any area of the body through inactivity or pressure. Maintaining or improving general mobility is therefore important to minimize this effect. The rapid provision of a suitable walking aid and encouragement may facilitate this. Aids should be assessed on an individual basis—needs vary from a stick, through crutches and tripods, to a rollator. Where ambulation is not possible, a wheelchair may be provided. Whilst this will not counteract the physical effects of immobility, it does help to minimize frustration and enhance independence which may be important in maintaining feelings of control.

Massage

Massage may reduce pain via the spinal gating mechanism (Melzack and Wall 1988) and by increasing the production of endogenous opioids (Staats *et al.* 1998). Most people find massage a pleasant experience which helps to induce relaxation and improve their sense of well-being. A regional massage, for example of the back or neck and shoulders, may be very soothing for the patient who is anxious, distressed, or in 'total pain'. Local massage has a part to play in a number of circumstances such as oedema or muscle spasm. Oedema may occur from various causes leading to painful, distended tissues. Massage improves venous and lymphatic return and may help to alleviate this feeling (Wood and Becker 1981). Lymphoedema requires a particular technique based on the principles of manual lymphatic drainage (Mortimer *et al.* 1998). Abdominal massage may be a useful adjuvant treatment in the management of constipation, which can cause considerable pain. It is not suitable in the on-going management of intestinal obstruction. Local massage can also be used to alleviate pain arising from muscle spasm, as in an acute stiff neck. Care should be exercised if underlying pathology is suspected, as with the protective spasm that may surround spinal cord compression. In all cases, care must be taken that techniques are gentle and used with caution, avoiding damage to de-vitalized tissues. Aggressive techniques and manipulations are generally contra-indicated in this patient population.

Relaxation

Relaxation is a state which decreases the activity of the sympathetic and motor nervous systems (Benson *et al*. 1974). It is the opposite of the 'fight-or-flight' response which produces both physiological changes (increased blood pressure, muscle tension, and raised heart and respiratory rates) and psychological effects of stress and irritability, which may combine to increase pain (Melzack and Wall 1988). Thus by inducing relaxation in an individual, pain may be alleviated. Benson and his colleagues describe the 'relaxation response' where muscle tone is reduced, blood pressure and respiratory rate decreased, and pupils constricted. One study in an American centre confirmed that relaxation training reduced pain in patients undergoing bone marrow transplant for cancer (Syrjala *et al*. 1995).

A small study of individual relaxation sessions carried out at the writer's centre (Howell and Kelly 1995) identified a number of benefits, which included

- patients perceived a reduction in distress and anxiety which lead to a positive influence on other symptoms, for example pain and dyspnoea;
- skilled positioning resulted in increased comfort;
- it was useful to be able to offer a pleasant, non-invasive treatment to frail patients, even when close to death;
- being taught how to relax gave a feeling of control.

A number of techniques have been described for inducing relaxation (e.g. contract—relax, progressive relaxation, autogenic training, guided imagery). The method chosen will reflect both the preferences and response of the patient as well as the training of the therapist. It can be very helpful to support individual teaching sessions with the provision of an audiotape for the patient to use on their own or with relatives and carers.

Heat and cold

Both heat and cold have traditionally been used as methods of relieving pain for thousands of years. Melzack & Wall (1988) suggest that they work by producing sensory modulation of pain via a spinal gating mechanism. Both heat and cold have circulatory effects. An increasing number of methods are available for their application but research into the effectiveness of any particular method is scanty. What is offered in any unit will depend on the preferences and experience of the therapist and the equipment available. In many though not all circumstances, heat and cold may be interchangeable and patient preference may also be taken into account. Application of heat produces a rise in tissue temperature which in turn produces a therapeutic effect. Alleviation of pain may result from:

- spinal gating effect (Melzack and Wall 1988);
- circulatory effects—by improving ischaemia which may lead to muscle spasm and removing the chemicals released by inflammation;

- by increasing the extensibility of collagen fibres. This may be especially useful; where joint stiffness or soft tissue shortening are a feature (Palastanga 1994).

A number of methods of application are available and the simple should not be despised: a warm bath can be a very effective way of applying general heat and will also help to induce relaxation, or may be combined with simple exercises. Simple hot packs or electrically heated pads are extremely convenient and can be lent to or purchased by patients for use at home. More sophisticated electrotherapeutic equipment may also be available but is beyond the scope of this text. Application of heat is contra-indicated if skin sensation is reduced or absent because of the risk of burns. Its use should also be avoided where patients are paralysed and therefore unable to move away from the heat source should it become uncomfortable. Care should be used where oedema is a feature as localized heat may exacerbate this; in these circumstances, cold may be more effective.

The application of cold to the skin may also produce pain relief by circulatory effects, initially producing vasoconstriction followed by vasodilation, and via the spinal gating mechanism. Cold also has neural effects, slowing the conduction of peripheral nerves (Ernst and Fialka 1994). This provides a powerful sensory stimulus which may reduce muscle hypertonia and spasm (Palastanga 1994). When using cryotherapy the skin should be protected. Crushed ice wrapped in wet towels is a very effective method though re-usable gel packs may be more convenient. For patients at home, a bag of frozen peas is both effective and convenient. Ice massage can be very beneficial on localized areas.

Electrotherapy

The practice of physiotherapy has traditionally encompassed a number of electrotherapeutic modalities, the scope of which are beyond this text. Many of these are used to heat the tissues, as described in the previous section. Some techniques, such as interferential and ultrasound, cause mechanical and electrical disturbance within the tissues which is said to produce a therapeutic effect (Low 1994). The effects of such currents on neoplastic tissue have not been well evaluated but it has been suggested that they may accelerate growth or cause metastases. Their use is, therefore, contra-indicated directly over tumours. The most commonly used technique in oncology and palliative care, and in the writer's experience the most beneficial, is probably transcutaneous electrical nerve stimulation (TENS) which is dealt with in Chapter 13.

Aids to daily living (ADLs)

Patients who are living with pain or disability may be helped by a variety of equipment, the provision of which may be the remit of a physiotherapist or occupational therapist. This is a huge subject which cannot be dealt with comprehensively here—a vast number of catalogues are available and professional advice should be sought in making suitable choices. A balance must be struck between the early provision of ADLs to maximize function and maintain safety whilst not taking over functions which the patient is still capable of managing. Where their condition is fluctuating or deteriorating, the therapist must continually re-evaluate equipment and be prepared to change it as necessary. Examples of simple equipment which may be helpful are:

- a leg lifter (manual or electrical), to ease the effort of lifting a heavy or painful lower limb;
- a mattress variator (electrically operated backrest) to enable the patient to change their position easily;
- thick-handled cutlery to facilitate grip where it is weak, painful, or stiff.

Collars and splints

Collars and splints may aid pain relief by providing support in a number of circumstances but their value needs to be carefully assessed in order not to inconvenience the patient more than they help (O'Gorman 1994).

- A soft collar may help to alleviate pain where there is spasm or weakness of neck muscles. At times a more rigid collar may be required if there is structural instability or weakness is extreme.
- Foot drop is a commonly encountered problem which can cause pain on the dorsum of the foot, extending proximally when resting, with reciprocal tightness of posterior structures. This can be alleviated by a splint which supports the ankle at 90° when resting. To prevent painful sprains or other injury when ambulant, an ankle-foot orthosis which fits into a shoe may be used.
- Reduced tone or weakness of the rotator cuff can lead to subluxation of the glenohumeral joint which is a very painful condition. The support of a suitable gutter sling or shoulder immobilizer can prevent or alleviate this.
- A cock-up splint for wrist drop may prevent pain in the extensors of the wrist and prevent shortening of the flexors. In some circumstances it may also improve grip.

Physiotherapy and lymphoedema

Secondary lymphoedema is a common problem amongst cancer patients which may result both from the disease itself or from treatment. In one study, the incidence of lymphoedema of the upper limb following surgery for breast cancer with axillary clearance plus radiotherapy was found to be 38.3% (Kissen *et al.* 1986). Lymphoedema of the lower limbs may result from a number of causes, including any pelvic tumour.

Lymphoedema has often been regarded as a painless problem but studies have shown that around 50% of patients presenting with lymphoedema also complain that it is painful (Carroll and Rose 1992). This pain may result from a number of causes

(Vecht 1990): Conservative treatment may significantly improve this pain. In an audit of lymphoedema sufferers at the writer's centre, 77% complained of pain. Physiotherapists are ideally placed to carry out conservative treatment for lymphoedema as the main elements of such regimens include their core skills. Elements of treatment for lymphoedema following full assessment may include:

- massage/manual lymph drainage;
- graduated, multi-layer compression bandaging;
- containment hosiery;
- exercises;
- skin care;
- general advice on risk factors, lifestyle etc.

A number of texts are available giving details of such regimens (Gillham 1994, Mortimer *et al.* 1998).

Rehabilitation

The aim of all the interventions discussed has been to relieve pain and discomfort. Once this is achieved the patients focus will almost certainly change. What then? The therapist may now be faced with an immobile, bored, or frustrated patient. Rehabilitation has been described as making a patient into a person again (Doyle 1998). Applied to oncology and palliative care, this means the maximization of potential at whatever level the patient is functioning. Realistic goals need to be agreed with the patient and the treatment regimen reassessed to achieve them.

Psychological support and the ability to do things for oneself are the two main factors contributing to quality of life (Martlew 1996). Following physiotherapy 100% of patients interviewed felt they had been given psychological support, 80% had improved function, and several felt more in control of their situation.

Multi-disciplinary working

'No one individual can possess the range of skills necessary to provide a comprehensive programme of pain management' (O'Brien 1993).

The ongoing care of cancer patients with pain can be both rewarding yet stressful. To sustain the necessary level of input, professionals need to take support from each other. At different times varying members of the multi-disciplinary team may need to take the lead, according to circumstances. Although doctors and nurses often fulfil this role, at times other professionals such as the physiotherapist, chaplain, or social worker may take the lead and this may change throughout the course of the disease. Optimal pain relief may only be achieved by a combination of two or more therapies (Bonica *et al.* 1990).

In true multi-disciplinary working, professional boundaries may be blurred—there is no room for professional possessiveness.

'We must hang together, or we will surely hang separately.' Benjamin Franklin.

Case study 1

Mr C. aged 67 was diagnosed with multiple myeloma and vertebral metastases affecting T12–L4, with collapse at T12. He had been treated with a single fraction of radiotherapy to this area and was admitted to the hospice for further symptom control.

His main complaints were of generalized aches and pains with a moderate to severe band of pain in the lumbar region which was controlled at rest but troublesome on movement. The cause of this was identified as a combination of bone disease, nerve compression, and muscle spasm with a considerable anxiety overlay. He described his main distress as 'not being able to walk about more freely'. His pain relief was managed with epidural medication and a syringe driver.

When first seen by the physiotherapist, he was on a low air loss bed. He was rather vague and uncertain about recent events but knew that he had not been mobile for several weeks. He had quite good muscle power (lower limbs 4/5 Oxford Scale) but was very fearful of any movement. Initially he was assisted and encouraged to change his position in bed and given assisted active exercises which were performed gently and within pain free range. He was also taught simple active exercises to practise on his own: These exercises were progressed gently and without eliciting pain. After three days he was hoisted out into a wheelchair which enabled him to move around for the first time in several weeks.

After one week, he felt confident enough to try standing with two therapists and started to practice balance and postural exercises. He continued with a daily programme of exercises and commenced walking practice in the parallel bars, progressing to a rollator. Mr C. continued to be very anxious but this gradually decreased as his mobility and confidence improved. He was eventually able to mobilize independently and manage stairs. A home assessment was performed and he was discharged home one month after his admission.

Eighteen months later, Mr C. was re-referred for physiotherapy with chronic low back pain. He was loaned a TENS machine and taught how to use this with good effect. Two and a half years after his original referral, Mr C. remains independently mobile and pain-controlled at home.

Case study 2

Mr A. a 52 year old had a history of cancer of the thyroid gland which had been treated with radical excision, radioiodine therapy, and external beam radiotherapy. He was referred for physiotherapy treatment of lymphoedema of his neck accompanied by feelings of 'hardness' and 'pressure' together with pain on movement. On examination, he had loss of cervical lordosis with a poking chin and 'dowager's hump'. There was marked radiation fibrosis of the whole of the cervical and suprascapular area. All neck movements were extremely limited and painful.

Mr A. was treated with a course of massage to the fibrotic areas using gentle finger kneading. Active exercises and posture correction were taught in front of a mirror together with gentle stretches added at the limits of range of movement. A semi-rigid head support, the headmaster collar, was provided. This gave support under the chin and allowed a small amount of stretch anteriorly whilst not compressing the throat: This was only worn for short periods at first. A soft collar was also used for relief when tired. Mr A. was encouraged not to wear a collar all the time and was weaned off these again towards the end of the course of treatment.

Mr A. was treated twice weekly for two months during which time his range of movement increased, his posture improved and his tissues softened, resulting in an overall diminution of pain and discomfort. He was taught an ongoing programme of active exercise and stretching to continue at home.

Acknowledgements

The authors wish to thank Sue Mason for her enthusiasm, help, and attention to detail in typing this chapter.

References

Ahles, T., Blanchard. G., and Ruckdeschel, J. (1983). The multi-dimensional nature of cancer related pain. *Pain*, **17**, 277–88.

Ahles, T., and Martin, J. (1992). Cancer pain: a multi-dimensional perspective. *The Hospice Journal*, **8**, 25–48.

Baines, M. (1989). Pain relief in active patients with cancer: analgesic drugs are the foundation of management. *British Medical Journal*, **298**, 36–8.

Benson, H., Beary, J., and Carol, M. (1974). The relaxation response. *Psychiatry*, **37**, 37–46.

Bonica, J., Ventafridda V., and Twycross, R. (1990). Cancer pain. In *The management of pain*, **1**, (2nd edn) (ed. J. Bonica, V. Ventrafridda, and R. Twycross), pp. 400–58. Lea & Febiger, Philadelphia & London.

Carroll, D., and Rose, K. (1992). Treatment leads to significant improvement: effect of conservative treatment on pain in lymphoedema. *Professional Nurse*, Oct., 32–6.

De Wit, R. van Dam, F. Zandbelt, L., van Buuren, A., van der Heijden, K. Leenhouts G., and Loonstra, S. (1997). A pain education program for chronic cancer pain patients: follow-up results from a randomised controlled trial. *Pain*, **73**, 55–69.

Doyle D. (1998). Introduction to rehabilitation. In *Oxford textbook of palliative medicine* (2nd edn). (ed. D. Doyle, G.W.C. Hanks and N. MacDonald) pp. 817–18. Oxford University Press.

Ernst, E., and Eialka, V. (1994). Ice freezes pain? A review of the clinical effectiveness of analgesic cold therapy. *Journal of Pain and Sympton Management*, **9**, 56–9.

Gillham, L. (1994). Lymphoedema and physiotherapists: control not cure. *Physiotherapy*, **80**, 835–43.

Howells, W., and Kelly, M. (1995). An exploratory study to consider the benefits of relaxation therapy as carried out by physiotherapists in palliative care. Unpublished.

Kissin, M., Querci della Rovere, G., Easton, D., and Westbury, G. (1986). Risk of ly phoedema following the treatment of breast cancer. *British Journal of Surgery*, **73**, 580–4.

Low, J. (1994). Electrotherapeutic modalities. In *Pain management by physiotherapy* (2nd edn) (ed. P.G. Wells, V. Frampton, and D. Bowsher) pp. 140–76. Butterworth Heinemann.

Martlew, B. (1996). What do you let the patient tell you? *Physiotherapy*, **82**, 558–65.

Melzack, R., and Wall, P. (1988). *The challenge of pain* (2nd edn). Penguin Books.

Mortimer, P.S., Badger, C., and Hall, J. (1998). Lymphoedema. In *Oxford textbook of palliative medicine* (2nd edn) (ed. B. Doyle, G.W.C. Hanks and N. MacDonald) pp. 657–65, Oxford University Press.

O'Brien, T. (1993). Symptom control. In *The management of terminal malignant disease* (ed. C. Saunders and N. Sykes). Hodder and Stoughton, London.

O'Gorman, B. (1994). The management of cancer pain in terminal care. In *Pain management by physiotherapy* (2nd edn) (ed. C.D.J. Wells, V. Frampton and D. Bowsher), Butterworth-Heineman.

Palastanga, N.M. (1994). Heat and cold. In *Pain management by physiotherapy* (2nd edn) (ed. C.D.J. Wells, V. Frampton, and D. Bowsher) pp. 177–86. Butterworth Heinemann.

Pellino, T., and Ward, S. (1998). Perceived control mediates the relationship between pain severity and patient satisfaction. *Journal of Pain and Sympton Management*, **15**, 110–16.

Portnoy, R. (1992). Cancer pain: pathophysiology and syndromes. *Lancet*, **339**, 1026–31.

Saunders, C.M. (1967). *The management of terminal illness*. Hospital Medicine Publications. London.

Staats, P., Hekmat, H., and Staats, A. (1998). Suggestion/placebo effects on pain: negative as well as positive. *Journal of Pain and Sympton Management*, **15**, 235–43.

Syrjala, K., Donaldson, G., Davis, M., Kippes, M., and Carr, J. (1995). Relaxation and imagery and cognitive-behavioural training reduce pain during cancer treatment: a controlled clinical trial. *Pain*, **63**, 189–98.

Snow-Turek, A., Norris, M., and Tan, G. (1996). Active and passive coping strategies in chronic pain patients. *Pain*, **64**, 455–62.

Thompson, S., Sobolew-Shubin, A., Galbraith, M. Schwankovsky, L., and Cruzon, D. (1993). Maintaining perceptions of control: finding perceived control in low-control circumstances. *Journal of Personality and Social Psychology*, **64**, 293–304.

Vecht, G. (1990). Arm pain in the patient with breast cancer. *Journal of Pain and Sympton Management*, **5**, 109–17.

Vingoe, F. (1994). Anxiety and pain: terrible twins or supportive siblings. In (ed. Gibson, H.B.) *Psychology, pain and anaesthesia*, pp. 282–307. Chapman & Hall.

Wood, E., and Becker, P. (1981). *Beards massage* (3rd edn). WB Saunders Company.

SEVEN

Non-pharmacological methods for the treatment of pain in children

C. WOOD, M. VIEYRA, AND P. POULAIN

There is increasing interest in the use of non-pharmacological methods for alleviating pain in children. This interest does not imply that the aetiology of children's pain is psychological in nature. The Cartesian dichotomy between the 'psyche' and the 'soma', and the resulting 'psychosomatic' ideas about the psychological aetiology of physical pain have been largely abandoned, in favour of a more multi-factorial biopsychosocial model. The gate control theory explains the complexity in the modulation of pain which is located at 3 levels: the gating of the oncoming nociceptive input in the dorsal horn of the spinal cord; the modulation at the level of the limbic system through descending pathways to the dorsal horn; and modulation at the level of the cerebral cortex by a range of cognitive (understanding, meaning, expectation, control, and attention) and affective factors (depression, anxiety, and fear) that can affect the pain experience (Tarbell 1999). This model of pain modulation makes it possible to understand the variability of pain response across individuals and to take into account cognitive and emotional factors in the assessment of pain perception. It also makes clear how physical and psychological strategies can be used to modify the perception of pain at the cortical level.

Different methods can be used, either alone or combined (in most cases) with medical methods of pain control. According to McGrath (1990) these non-pharmacological methods can be categorized as physical, behavioural, or cognitive.

Physical methods

Function is of prime importance for a child. A thorough assessment is necessary before focusing on physical methods. One must get to know how the child is managing, getting to school, spending leisure time, dealing with every day chores. Physical methods of pain control can be quite useful for children, because they can alter the sensory aspects of pain. The goals are to be established by the therapist and the patient. They focus on pain reduction, restoration of physical function, management of daily activities, and patient and family education. These methods can be administered by nurses, physiotherapists, occupational therapists or even by the parents (Allen *et al*. 1993).

Exercise: Exercise has not only physical but also psychological benefits in pain patients, especially children. Therapeutic exercise programs are prescribed according to the initial assessment. Active and resistive exercise can help strengthen weak muscles, improve posture, local and systemic circulation, increase bone density and general endurance (Allen *et al.* 1993). Passive or active assisted motion is necessary when the patient is unable to move a limb because of pain or weakness but can also be helpful to mobilize tightened structures. It can also help a frightened child in gaining confidence with movements. Exercise and physiotherapy (walking, swimming) help the child to readapt progressively and are also an excellent way of reducing stress and increasing relaxation. Children with recurrent pain syndromes (headaches, migraines, recurrent abdominal pain) may benefit greatly from exercise particularly if it is performed on a regular basis.

Physiotherapy and massage have been helpful for muscular pain. These strategies also produce relaxation and promote blood circulation. When the child accepts this physical contact it creates a level of therapeutic relationship or rapport which becomes an important component of the therapy.

Heat therapy by heat applications, heating pads, or ultrasound is also helpful for chronic pain and chronic muscular conditions. Unfortunately, the paediatric literature is scant in this area.

Cold therapy by cold compresses or ice massage can be used to reduce pain in acute conditions.

Contrast bathing: combining heat and cold has been administered.

Acupuncture There is little literature on its use in children (Yee *et al.* 1993).

Transcutaneous electrical nerve stimulation (TENS) is a safe method, which should be associated with other treatment methods. Even though children like the use of it (it looks like a walkman apparatus), little research has been done in paediatrics (Eland 1993; Lander and Fowler-Kerry 1993).

Touch, massage, and holding: children are often deprived of affective and therapeutic touch. Blackburn and Barnard (1985) showed that the mean number of loving touches in a neonatal unit was about five touches per 24 hours. Other authors have shown the benefit of touch and holding (Jay 1982; Field 1990). Touch and massage can be seen as a way of communicating empathy, and concern. It may be performed by the parents or by the nurses and can be particularly helpful (Field *et al.* 1997).

Psychological methods

Different psychological methods can be used to alleviate pain in children. The two methods are: behavioural strategies (including relaxation, biofeedback, operant conditioning, modelling and desensitization) and cognitive methods (including distraction/attention, imagery, thought-stopping, hypnosis).

Behavioural methods

One important way of identifying and assessing pain is through observing behaviour. Behaviour can also either exacerbate or reduce pain. Behaviour therapy is generally used to modify those symptoms that interfere with an individual's adaptive functioning. Different emotional, behavioural, familial, and situational factors influence the perception of pain. Therefore pain can be changed by modifying any of these factors. The principle goal of behavioural techniques involves the modification of any behaviours, engaged in by both the child and those in his or her immediate environment (parents, teachers, carers, medical practitioners), that may provoke, maintain, or exacerbate the child's experience of pain.

Operant conditioning

The behaviours of children who experience pain are inevitably shaped by the reaction of those in their environment. Pain behaviours, anxiety, and fear can be inadvertently positively reinforced by sympathy or concern from family members, or friends. Pain complaints (crying, seeking reassurance, grimacing, etc.) that are rewarded by special attention, the escape from undesired responsibilities of school, avoidance of difficult social or familial situations, or lowered expectations for performance will, as a result, be more likely to be maintained and recur. Behaviours leading to positive outcomes have a greater chance of recurring than behaviours leading to a negative outcome. Pain behaviours can also be reinforced when pain medication is taken only when the pain behaviour occurs rather than on a fixed variable schedule.

These conditioned behaviours may lead to exaggerated pain symptomatology as well as increased pain perception. This is particularly true for recurrent and chronic pain, because these children experience frequent episodes of strong, sometimes unexplained pain. Since parents often fluctuate between ignoring these complaints and providing excessive attention to them, children may learn that they need to express stronger complaints in order to convince their parents that they need the same level of support that they occasionally receive (McGrath 1990).

In children with recurrent pain syndromes, the development of conditioned pain triggers—environmental stimuli or situations that may provoke a painful episodes—is quite common. These triggers may have been associated with painful episodes in time or location, and therefore come to trigger anticipatory anxiety in children, which then can lead to pain.

In the use of operant conditioning paradigms to treat paediatric pain, it is necessary to identify verbal and nonverbal pain behaviours and to determine the reinforcing consequences maintaining the behaviour (e.g. parents, family, school, work; Masek *et al*. 1984). The responses of these significant persons must then be modified in order to minimize the occurrence of the maladaptive pain behaviours and to maximize the occurrence of adaptive behaviours (coping strategies). Operant conditioning is usually one component in an integrated multifaceted pain management program.

Relaxation

Relaxation, yoga, and meditation are used to alleviate or reduce anxiety, stress, and pain in adults as well as in children. Relaxation may be defined (McCaffery and

Beebe 1994) as a state of relative freedom from both anxiety and skeletal muscle tension, a quieting or calming of the mind and muscles during which physiological changes occur such as decreased oxygen consumption, respiratory rate, heart rate, muscle tension, and blood pressure, accompanied by increased skin resistance and production of alpha waves (Benson *et al.* 1974). Relaxation has specific benefits, for example it helps a patient go to sleep, reduces skeletal muscle tension, decreases diurnal fatigue, and distracts from pain. It increases effectiveness of other pain relief measures and decreases fear of painful procedures (McCaffery and Beebe 1994). Several techniques have been used for children, including progressive muscle relaxation, autogenic phrases, suggestion–relaxation, and meditation. Most practitioners use a combination of methods, integrating breathing exercises and progressive muscle relaxation. Children learn to relax their bodies when breathing deeply and calmly, and the deeper their breathing becomes the more they feel relaxed. Children are taught to tighten and relax various muscle groups, focusing on increasing relaxation and decreasing muscular tension. Often these directions are accompanied by imagery to help children more effectively perform the exercise. For example, a child might imagine that he is squeezing lemons with both fists and then dropping the lemons and shaking out the juice in order to tense and relax muscles in the hands and arms better. These techniques have been used for acute pain, procedural pain (Powers 1999), cancer pain, sickle cell disease, arthritic pain (Walco *et al.* 1999), burns, headaches (Engel *et al.* 1992; Holden *et al.* 1999), recurrent abdominal pain (Janicke and Finney 1999), and dental pain. They constitute an effective coping strategy for procedural, chronic and on-going pain, and can be performed several times a day (McCaffery and Beebe 1994; Janicke and Finney 1999).

Relaxation should only be taught to a child after the technique has already been explained and prepared. The type of relaxation should be guided by the child's interests and preferences (Hobbie 1986). Specific directions for relaxation and suggestions for pain control need to be adapted to the child's age and cognitive level. In the same manner it is useful to know what sort of relaxation technique is best suited for each child (active, passive, visual imagery, auditory or kinaesthetic). It is therefore important to talk with patients of places and things they enjoy before starting a session. Relaxation can be an unpleasant experience for some children or adolescents who might experience feeling of being out of control. It is fundamental that the health-care team does not misinterpret the success of relaxation as meaning that the pain is of psychological origin.

Biofeedback

Biofeedback can be very useful in children, often as a tool in conjunction with relaxation. It enables children to distinguish through auditory or visual signals the difference between relaxed and tense body states. Normally non-observable physiological activity (heart rate, muscle tension, body temperature of extremities) is monitored electronically, amplified and translated into an observable auditory or visual signal, usually displayed on a computer screen. Children can learn how to modify these physiological responses, and thereby reduce pain levels.

Biofeedback also enables the patient to realize how their body can respond to stressful events. The contemplation or discussion of events that may be unrecognized sources of stress (difficulties in school, with friends or family conflict) may in fact be shown to increase heart rate or muscle tension. These areas can then become targets of intervention. The specific mechanism of action of biofeedback has been the object of debate. Some authors suggest the mechanism of clinical improvement by means of specific visceral or skeletal muscular training. Others suggest that the effect is an indirect one involving relaxation or cognitive change (Tarler-Benlolo 1975; Meichenbaum 1976).

Different authors have demonstrated the importance of this technique for recurrent pain states such as headaches (Bussone *et al*. 1998; Hermann *et al*. 1997; Womack *et al*. 1988), fibromyalgia, reflex sympathetic dystrophy, juvenile rheumatoid arthritis (Lavigne *et al*. 1992), sickle cell disease (Cozzi *et al*. 1987).

Biofeedback is particularly appropriate for children whose pain is caused or exacerbated by physiological changes associated with a stressed or tense state (McGrath 1990).

Modelling

Modelling involves learning by observing another person's behaviour in a particular situation. Learning is accomplished by imitation rather than by direct instruction. This strategy has been shown to be useful in reducing fears and avoidance behaviours, including those related to painful procedures. In watching another child cope successfully with a painful procedure, an observing child can learn to be less fearful and thus to cope more effectively. This observational learning is even more effective when coupled with 'guided practice' in which the child can practice the modelled behaviours in progressively more realistic circumstances (Bandura 1976). The therapist assists and reinforces the child's efforts. Modelling for pain management can be useful for children requiring medical and dental procedures, especially with younger children or those with more limited verbal skills (McGrath 1990). It has been shown that modelling works best if the model is quite similar in age and sex to the the child and if the child observes a model who learns to cope, rather than one who automatically reacts in an 'ideal' manner.

Desensitization

This is a learning procedure in which an individual is gradually exposed to an anxiety provoking object or situation, until their anxiety decreases. Children learn a response that is incompatible with anxiety (relaxation) which is paired with the anxiety producing stimulus. This strategy can be quite effective in reducing conditioned fears and anxiety related to repeated invasive procedures (e.g. needle phobia).

Cognitive approaches

Cognitive methods include distraction, imagery, thought stopping, and hypnosis. The primary objective in most cognitive techniques involves having patients become completely and selectively focused on a thought or an image, so that they are unable to attend to or to perceive pain in their usual manner.

Distraction and attention

Distraction is the most common method for reducing everyday pains and is often performed spontaneously by parents to focus the child's attention on something different and interesting (McCaffery and Beebe 1994). Distraction actively alters the perception of pain. The more the child is absorbed by something the more the pain can be reduced. It is thought that rather than being a simple diversionary tactic in which the child still experiences pain but does not pay attention to it, distraction results in the actual attenuation of neuronal impulses evoked by a noxious stimulus. The child is therefore actually reducing their pain rather than ignoring it (McGrath 1990).

The choice of strategy used is very important, since in order to be effective, it must help the child to concentrate on something else. It must therefore be of interest to the child, adapted to their cognitive age and energy level, and must try to stimulate all the other sensory modalities (hearing, vision, touch, movement) adapted to the child's preferences. Different strategies can be used according to the age of the child, their developmental capacities and favourite activities such as holding a familiar object, singing, describing a favourite place or toy or cartoon, playing video games, watching a cartoon or the TV, blowing bubbles, breathing out, listening to stories or music, hand squeezing (Twycross *et al.* 1998). For infants and young children it is preferable to use concrete external events or interesting objects, toys, or intriguing things. For older children, mental activities or physical activities are more adapted to their developmental capacities (McGrath 1990).

Imagery

Imagery involves the use of imagination to modify the response to pain (Doody *et al.* 1991). The individual concentrates on the image of an experience or a situation and recalls the sensation and perceptions that are associated with that experience. It is a sort of day dreaming process. Therapeutic imagery makes use of pleasant and agreeable situations, places or experiences, and can be either images actually experienced by the patient or ones that they may create using imagination. Imagery results not only in distraction but also in relaxation and in a modification of the physiological state. Imagery can be guided in such a way that children imagine things related to their pain that will help to reduce it (pain floating away, or ice on a burn). Children can also use imagery to imagine their analgesics or other drugs going around their body to the places where the pain is and taking it away (Carter 1994).

The technique must also be adapted to the age of the child: for a young child: animals or heroes; for older children: more sophisticated methods. For instance a child can imagine being a favourite superhero, strong and powerful, not bothered by the tiny pinch of a 'mosquito bite' during a procedure. A child can also be involved in a story which is being told or read to him; e.g. being asked what happens next which new character can come into the story.

Thought stopping

This technique of identifying negative thoughts and substituting coping or positive statements was modified by Ross (1984) to reduce anticipatory anxiety and increase control during painful events. It is used when children who anticipate pain related to medical procedures have negative thoughts. They are taught to substitute positive thoughts and therefore develop independant coping strategies. When the child begins to think of the event, he is asked to stop his activities and repeat all the positive statements he has previously learned. Thought-stopping has been a useful method to reduce anxiety for dental treatment and procedural pain (Ross 1984).

Hypnosis

Children have been found to be more adept than adults in using hypnotherapy for the control of pain (Wakeman and Kaplan 1978). There are a number of studies reporting the successful use of self-hypnosis techniques for painful procedures (Zeltzer and LeBaron 1982) as well as for a variety of chronic illnesses including malignancies, haemophilia, diabetes, sickle cell disease, migraines, and juvenile rheumatoid arthritis (Olness and Kohen 1996; Zeltzer *et al*. 1991). Some authors find hypnosis to be superior to other cognitive techniques (Zeltzer and LeBaron 1982; Zeltzer *et al*. 1991; Kuttner 1993).

The clinical use of hypnosis requires some training and experience. A therapist who does not believe in the efficacy of hypnoanalgesia or who lacks faith in the child's ability to overcome pain is unlikely to succeed in helping the child (Erickson 1991). Confidence, enthusiasm, and rapport generated by the therapist are important factors in achieving clinical states of hypnosis (Scott Smith and Womack 1987).

Induction techniques can be used in combination and should be tailored to the interests and attitudes of the child. They must also be adapted to the developmental or cognitive level. At the preverbal age, rocking, auditory stimulation or visual stimulation are useful. Between the age of 2 and 4, the therapist can speak to the child through a doll or toy; or ask him to be like floppy Raggedy Ann. At preschool and early school age one can start telling a story, speak of a favourite place, or use pop-up books. The middle aged child may want to be on a magic carpet, or be riding a bike, or listening to his favourite music. Classical hypnotic inductions such as eye fixation or arm rigidity can also be used. An adolescent might see himself driving a car, playing his favourite sports activity, or being in a favourite place. Classical inductions can also be employed. It is important that the therapist enquires about the child's interests, his likes and dislikes and that he adapts himself to what the child desires. This implies imagination but also knowledge of the current TV heroes, video games, or popular films. Explanations have to be made so that the child understands what is going to happen and what is expected from him. Once the child accepts the technique, practice is essential and the help of the parents can be very useful.

The advantage of hypnosis over relaxation techniques is the possibility of incorporating therapeutic suggestions. It is therefore a very useful method for analgesia, in acute conditions but also for chronic pain. For pain control different techniques have been used such as direct suggestions for hypnoanalgesia, as a request of numbness or of glove anaesthesia. Distancing suggestions can also be used such as transferring the pain away from self or to another part of the body. Other suggestions concern the feeling of comfort, or relaxation. Time distortion and other distraction techniques can also be used.

Training needs

Many of these non-pharmacological methods can be used by health-care professionals with little training. Others such as hypnosis, behavioural therapy require recognized qualification. A multi-disciplinary team is necessary to promote such skills. There are an increasing number of training programs, whose purpose is to train nurses and other front line health professionals to administer and use a number of these strategies (Solomon and Saylor 1995).

Summary

There are many non-pharmacological methods for the treatment of pain, including methods that can be characterized as physical and those that are best described as psychological. Physical strategies include exercise, massage, physiotherapy, heat and cold therapy, acupuncture, and TENS. Psychological approaches include behavioural strategies such as relaxation, biofeedback, operant strategies, modelling, and desensitization, as well as cognitive approaches such as distraction, imagery, and hypnosis. All of these non-pharmacological methods of pain control should be employed as often as required in conjunction with analgesic drugs. These non-medical methods may alleviate or reduce pain through central cortical processes or by decreasing fear, anxiety, and muscle tension associated with pain. Another proposed mechanism of action involves increasing the perception of control the child has over his pain and his body's reactions, which in turn has an effect on fear, anxiety, and muscular and autonomic responses. Generally these strategies have been applied in combination. Research has progressed somewhat in matching intervention to type of clinical problem. However, there is still much work to do in trying to develop our understanding of which types of interventions work for which children, with which type of pain in which circumstances (McGrath 1999). Finally, while dissemination of these techniques has progressed, more work needs to be done on teaching primary carers (nurses, parents, educators) about these techniques and how they can be applied to children in pain.

References

Allen, J., Jedlinsky, B.P., Wilson, T.L., and McCarthy, C.F. (1993). Physical therapy management of pain in children. In *Pain in infants, children and adolescents* (ed. N.L. Schechter, C.B. Berde, and M. Yaster), pp. 317–29. Williams and Wilkins, Baltimore.

Bandura, A. (1976). Effecting change through participant modelling. In *Counseling methods* (ed. J.D. Krumboltz and C.E. Eiser) pp. 248–65. Holt, Rinehart and Winston, New York.

Benson, H., Biary, J.F., and Carol, M.P. (1974). The relaxation response. *Psychiatry*, 37, 37–44.

Blackburn, S., and Barnard, K.E. (1985). Analysis of care giving events in preterm infants in the special care unit. In *Infant stress under intensive care* (ed. A.W. Gottfreid and I. Gaiter) 84, pp. 31–3. University Park Press, Baltimore.

Bussone, G., Grazzi, L., D'Amico, D., and Andrasik, F. (1998). Biofeedback-assisted relaxation training for adolescents with tension-type headache: a controlled study. *Cephalagia*, **18**, 463–7.

Carter, B. (1994). *Child and infant pain: principles of nursing care and management*. Chapman and Hall, London.

Cozzi, L., Tryon, W., and Sedlacek, K. The effectiveness of biofeedback-assisted relaxation in modifying sickle cell crisis. *Biofeedback and Self Regulation*, **12**, 51–61.

Doody, S.B., Smith, C., and Webb, J. (1991). Non pharmacological interventions for pain management. *Critical Care Nursing Clinics of North America*, **3**, 69–75.

Eland, J. (1993). The use of TENS with children. In *Pain in infants, children and adolescents* (ed. N.L. Schechter, C.B. Berde, and M. Yaster) pp. 331–9. William and Wilkins, Baltimore.

Engel, J.M., Rapoff, M.A., and Pressman, A.R. (1992). Long-term follow-up of relaxation training for paediatric headaches disorders. *Headache*, **32**, 152–6.

Erickson, C.J. (1991). Applications of cyberphysiologic techniques in pain management. *Pediatric Annals*, **20**, 145–56.

Field, T. (1990). Alleviating stress in newborn infants in the intensive care unit. *Clinics in Perinatology*, **17**, 1–9.

Field, T., Hernandez-Rief, M., Seligman, S., Krasnegor, J., and Sunshine, W. (1997). Juvenile rheumatoid arthritis: benefits from massage therapy. *Journal Paediatric Psychology*, **22**, 607–17.

Hermann, C., Blanchard, E.B., and Flor, H. (1997). Biofeedback treatment for paediatric migraine: prediction of treatment outcome. *Journal of Consulting and Clinical Psychology*, **55**, 611–16.

Hobbie, C. (1986). Relaxation techniques for children and young people. *Journal of Paediatric Health Care*, **3**, 83–7.

Holden, E., Deichmann, M., and Levy, J. (1999). Empirically supported treatments in paediatric psychology: recurrent paediatric headache. *Journal of Paediatric Psychology*, **24**, 91–109.

Janicke, D., and Finney, J. (1999). Empirically supported treatments in paediatric psychology: Recurrent abdominal pain. *Journal of Pediatric Psychology*, **24**, 115–28.

Jay, S. (1982). The effects of gentle human touch on mechanically ventilated very-short-gestation infants. *Maternal-Child Nursing Journal*, **11**, 198–256.

Kuttner, L. (1993). Hypnotic interventions for children in pain. In *Pain in infants, children and adolescents* (ed. N.L. Schechter, C.B. Berde, and M. Yaster), pp. 229–36. William and Wilkins, Baltimore.

Lander, J., and Fowler-Kerry, S. (1993). TENS for children's procedural pain. *Pain*, **52**, 209–16.

Lavigne, J., Ross, C., Berry, S., Hayford, J., and Pachman, L. (1992). Evaluation of a psychological treatment package for treating pain in juvenile rheumatoid arthritis. *Arthritis Care and Research*, **5**, 101–10.

McCaffery, M., and Beebe, A. (1994). *Pain: clinical manual for nursing practice*. Ed Mosby.

McCaffery, M., and Wong, D. (1993). Nursing interventions for pain control in children. In *Pain in infants, children and adolescents* (ed. N.L. Schechter, C.B. Berde and M. Yaster), pp. 295–316. William and Wilkins, Baltimore.

McGrath, P.A. (1990). *Pain in children*, pp. 132–72. Guilford Press, New York.

McGrath, P.A. (1999). Commentary: psychological interventions for controlling children's pain: challenges for evidence-based medicine. *Journal of Pediatric Psychology*, **24**, 172–4.

Masek, B.J., Russo, D.C., and Varn, J.W. (1984). Behavioural approaches to the management of chronic pain in children. *Pediatrics Clinics of North America*, **31**, 1113–1131.

Meichenbaum, D. (1976). Cognitive factors in biofeedback therapy. *Biofeedback Self Regulation*, **1**, 201–16.

Olness, K., and Kohen, D.P. (1996). *Hypnosis and hypnotherapy with children*. Guilford Press, New York.

Powers, S. (1999). Empirically supported treatments in paediatric psychology: procedure related pain. *Journal of Pediatric Psychology*, **24**, 131–46.

Ross, D.M. (1984). Thought-stopping: A coping strategy for impending feared events. *Issues in Comprehensive Pediatric Nursing*, **7**, 83–9.

Scott Smith, M., Womack, W.M. (1987). Stress management techniques in childhood and adolescence. *Clinical Pediatrics*, **26**, 581–5.

Solomon, R., and Saylor, C. (1995). *National Cancer Institute's pediatric pain management: a professional course*. Michigan State University.

Tarbell, S. (1999). *Complementary methods of chronic pain control in children pain*, pp. 237–44. An updated review. IASP Press.

Tarler-Benlolo, L. (1975). The role of relaxation in biofeedback training: a critical review of the literature. *Psychology Bulletin*, **85**, 727–55.

Twycross, A., Moriarty, A., and Betts, T. (1998). *Paediatric Pain Management: a multidisciplinary approach*, pp. 95–104. Radcliffe Medical Press Ltd.

Wakeman, R.J., and Kaplan, J.Z. (1978). An experimental study of hypnosis in painful burns. *American Journal of Clinical Hypnosis*, **21**, 3–12.

Walco, G., Sterling, C., Conte, P., and Engel R. (1999). Empirically supported treatments in paediatric psychology: disease related pain. *Journal of Pediatric Psychology*, **24**, 155–67.

Womack, W.M., Smith, M.S., and Chen, A.C.N. (1988). Behavioural management of paediatric headache: a pilot study and case report. *Pain*, **32**, 279–83.

Yee, J.D., Lin, Y.C., and Aubuchon, P.A. (1993). Acupuncture. In *Pain in infants, children and adolescents* (ed. N.L. Schechter, C.B. Berde and M. Yaster), pp. 341–8. Williams and Wilkins Baltimore.

Zeltzer, L., and Le Baron, S. (1982). Hypnosis and nonhypnotic techniques for reduction of pain and anxiety during painful procedures in children and adolescents with cancer. *Journal Pediatrics*, **101**, 1032–5.

Zeltzer, L.K., Dolgin, M.J., LeBaron, S., and LeBaron, C. (1991). A randomized controlled study of behavioural intervention for chemotherapy distress in children with cancer. *Pediatrics*, **88**, 34–42.

EIGHT

Nerve blocks—simple injections, epidurals, spinals, and more complex blocks

HARALD BREIVIK

The skilful practice of diagnostic and 'prognostic' local anaesthetic nerve blocks, followed by selective neurolytic blocks with ethanol or phenol, was the basis for the pioneering anaesthesiologists' involvement in relief of 'intractable' pain (Bonica 1953; Swerdlow 1983). During the last three decades knowledge of the pharmacology and toxicology of opioid analgesics has improved. At the same time development and availability of more effective forms of administration of opioid analgesic drugs has also contributed to improved medical management of severe cancer pain (Twycross 1994).

The modern palliative care movement was ushered in by Dame Cicely Saunders when she founded St Christopher's Hospice in 1967. Subsequent efforts from WHO (1986), organizations such as the International Association for the Study of Pain with its many national chapters (Loeser 1997), professional associations (Ferrante *et al.* 1996), and governments (Jacox *et al.* 1994) at educating health personnel, patients, and health politicians, have greatly improved the general level of knowledge of pain relief. Slowly the availability of drugs for pain relief and resources for palliative care have increased, but only in some affluent western countries (Twycross 1997).

All of this has resulted in a growing awareness of pharmacologic treatment of pain, systematically adminstered according to the WHO-analgesic ladder (WHO 1986). More realistic appraisal of the dangers of opioid drugs and reduction of a widespread 'opioidophobia' have changed attitudes to more liberal use of the effective opioid analgesic drugs. Presently, in many western countries, 70–90% of patients with cancer pain will have satisfactory pain relief from pharmacological methods alone (Zech *et al.* 1995). There is therefore less need for neurodestructive methods such as neurolytic nerve blocks with their many disadvantages (Diamond and Coniam 1991; Twycross 1994).

Nerve blocks when the WHO-analgesic ladder is too short

However, there are still many indications for nerve blocks for cancer pain (Ferrante *et al.* 1996). The following brief review of some of the useful nerve blocks will illustrate that the WHO-analgesic ladder approach should be supplemented with nerve blocks in a comprehensive palliative care approach. The classic WHO-analgesic ladder may turn out to be too short because unacceptable side effects prevent dose escalation, or movement may cause severe breakthrough pain. An overall evaluation of costs and risks in relation to the patient's situation, may indicate that a successful nerve block, such as an alcohol coeliac plexus block or an intercostal nerve block serve the patient best.

Nerve impulse blockade with reversible local anaesthetic drugs

Infiltration of a painful primary or metastatic tumour, interruption of impulse conduction along peripheral nerves from a painful cancerous growth, or interruption of pain impulse conduction pathways in the spinal cord with local anaesthetic drugs result in local or regional anaesthesia and pain relief lasting from 1–12 hours. Not infrequently pain relief may outlast the local anaesthetic effect by days or even weeks (Boys *et al.* 1993). Local anaesthetic infiltrations and simple blocks may therefore have therapeutic effects and should be used liberally (Twycross 1994). The opportunity to completely rest from pain, even if for only a few hours, will be appreciated. It can be prolonged with catheter-techniques.

Diagnostic blocks, but not prognostic blocks

Local anaesthetic blocks will aid in diagnosis and localization of the cause of pain, but systemic effects from absorbed local anaesthetic drug on central and peripheral neuropathic components of pain may confound the prognostic value of blocks done before neurolytic blocks. Local anaesthetic nerve blocks should therefore not be used to predict the effect of neurolytic blocks or other neurodestructive treatment such as thermocoagulation or surgical denervation (Hogan and Abrams 1997).

Infiltration with a local anaesthetic solution

Local anaesthetic into a painful focus will give immediate relief. When this pain focus is a trigger of muscle spasm, reflex, and referred pain, a prolonged effect far beyond the duration of the pharmacological effect of the local anaesthetic occurs. This is more likely to happen if a long acting local anaesthetic like bupivacaine is coadministered with a small dose of a depot corticosteroid (*v.i.*). Many 'simple' painful conditions that are also common in cancer patients, can be relieved in this way:

- trigger point injection in myofascial pain;
- humero-scapular joint or tendon pain;
- sacro-iliac pain;
- postherpetic neuralgia.

Sympathetically maintained pain

Although 'cancer pain' most often is considered acute, nociceptive pain, cancer patients certainly also can develop complex regional pain syndromes in which sympathetically maintained pain often is an important component (Janig and Stanton-Hicks 1995).

Cancer patients with pain must be subjected to a systematic pain analysis, and when appropriate, diagnostic and therapeutic sympathetic blocks must be offered.

Acute relief for severe breakthrough pain and pain emergencies

An acute overwhelmingly intense breakthrough pain, pain from a pathological fracture, or an acutely ischaemic limb, can best be relieved with a regional anaesthetic block. A plexus block, epidural or spinal anaesthetic will give immediate relief and allow time for alternative treatment to be instituted.

Specific spinal cord analgesia

Specific and very potent analgesic effects can be obtained at the spinal cord level by simultaneous application of

- a low concentration of a local anaesthetic drug (which inhibits excitation of nervous tissues and synapses);
- an opioid drug;
- an adrenergic drug; (both of which increase inhibition of synaptic transmission of pain nerve impulses).

When coadministered intrathecally or epidurally at an appropriate spinal level, so that the three drugs reach the spinal cord dorsal horn with its pain regulating interneurons, supraadditive analgesic effects result from doses of each component that otherwise would be subanalgesic. For a review and references see Breivik *et al.* (1995).

Adrenaline, which does have α_2-agonist effects, has an added advantage when coadministered with bupivacaine or fentanyl epidurally; the vasoconstrictive effect on epidural blood vessels decreases epidural blood flow and systemic absorption of bupivacaine and fentanyl, decreasing systemic side-effects, while increasing the amount of analgesic drugs that can diffuse across the dura and into the spinal cord (Baron *et al.* 1996; Niemi and Breivik 1998). In addition adrenaline seems to impede or prevent the development of acute tolerance to opioid analgesics in the spinal cord (Yaksh and Ready 1981).

Continuous epidural catheter infusion of such analgesic mixtures for prolonged pain relief after major surgery is now widespread and popular with patients and nurses alike because of its effectiveness and wide margin of safety (Breivik 1995). This technique can be applied equally effectively for severe pain related to cancer.

Prolonged segmental epidural catheter analgesia

This technique requires that the anaesthesiologist is able to insert an epidural catheter at the appropriate segmental level, from the upper cervical to the upper lumbar level. Also, that there is a system for handling and caring for catheters and infusion devices for prolonged periods at home, in a hospice or palliative care institution, or in a hospital. This again requires investment in equipment, a reliably produced, stable and sterile drug supply together with adequate staff training.

Although serious complications are extremely rare when a system for safe practice of epidural analgesia has been implemented (Breivik 1995), spinal infection and bleeding can occur, with potentially disastrous consequences for the spinal cord. Training of nurses (and patients) to monitor for early signs of these complications, such as back pain and increasing leg weakness, and a system for rapid action should such symptoms occur, is mandatory for treatment of postoperative pain with these methods. For treatment of advanced cancer pain, these risks may be more acceptable.

Technical details of epidural catheter placement and maintenance are well described in anaesthesiological literature and are outside of the scope of this review.

Prolonged spinal catheter analgesia

When epidural analgesia becomes ineffective, insertion of a catheter into the subarachnoid space and slow infusion of a more concentrated local anaesthetic solution containing morphine may give satisfactory analgesia when most other methods have failed (Sjöberg *et al.* 1991). Prolonged treatment is possible, even with the patient at home; but the efforts needed to keep the complication rate low and maintain effect are considerable (Sjöberg *et al.* 1994).

Inflammatory pain treated with injections of local anaesthetic and corticosteroid drugs

Corticosteroids have analgesic effects when administered epidurally, perineurally, or intralesionally. These are in part systemic central nervous system effects, in part local effects on nociceptive nerve endings and inflammatory as well as neurogenic pain mechanisms (Devor *et al.* 1985; Pieretti *et al.* 1992; Twycross 1994).

Segmental epidural application of local anaesthetic drugs give pain relief for several weeks to months in one third of patients; when combined with methylprednisolone in two thirds of patients with radicular nerve root irritation pain (Breivik *et al.* 1976; Breivik and Hesla 1978; Watts and Silagy 1995). This prolonged analgesia may be due to the corticosteroid effect on the proinflammatory contents of intervertebral disc (Olmarker *et al.* 1995) and tissues when a secondary tumour-growth impinges on spinal nerve roots (Twycross 1994).

Perineural injections of a mixture of a local anaesthetic and a corticosteroid cause immediate and prolonged pain relief in nerves made hyperexcitable from local trauma, infiltration of tumour, or inflammatory reactions (Devor *et al.* 1985; Twycross 1994).

Intralesional injection of local anaesthetics and depot corticosteroids similarly may cause immediate and, in some patients, markedly prolonged pain relief, e.g. in multiple myeloma lesions in ribs and rib metastases from breast cancer (Rowell 1988; Twycross 1994).

Neurolytic nerve blocks with ethanol or phenol

The improvements in cancer pain relief with analgesic drugs and neuraxial administration of local anaesthetic and opioid drugs have reduced the need for neurolytic blockade. But there is still a place for some of these techniques. They should not be used in isolation, but as a part of a comprehensive palliative care approach with pharmacological symptom management, antitumour therapy, nursing and psychosocial care.

Advantages of neurolytic blocks

When a single successful intervention can replace chronic administration of multiple drugs, significant savings in costs, side effects, and labour will be realized. Home care and rewarding family life may become possible for a few weeks. A more lucid sensorium and better cognitive abilities will contribute to improved quality of life, the main end point of symptom control in cancer patients. This scenario is more likely to be true after coeliac plexus block than after other neurolytic blocks.

Disadvantages of neurolytic blocks

Possible serious complications from a misplaced injection or injection of an inappropriate dose may cause severe neurolgical deficits.
Duration of analgesia after a neurolytic block is limited, at the most 3–6 months: some blocks can be repeated with success.
Denervation dysaesthetic pain may appear subsequent to a peripheral somatic nerve block with ethanol or phenol. This iatrogenic pain will become a burden to the doctor as much as to the patient.

When should a neurolytic block be performed?

Because of the possibility of severe post-denervation neuropathic pain, most neurolytic blocks of peripheral nerves should be reserved for patients with life expectancy of one year or less. Sympathetic blocks, and possibly subarachnoid neurolysis, are less frequently implicated as causes of lasting deafferentation pain, and may therefore be considered more liberally in patients with longer life expectancy.

Indications for neurolytic blocks

* Upper abdominal visceral pain
    * Coeliac plexus block
    * Splanchnic nerve block
* Pelvic visceral pain
    * Superior hypogastric plexus block
    * Bilateral lumbar sympathetic block
* Perineal pain (in patient with urinary diversion and colostomy)
    * Phenol in glycerol subarachnoid (saddle) block

- Localized chest wall pain
  - Intercostal nerve block
  - Thoracic subarachnoid phenol or ethanol
- Unilateral leg pain (in bed-bound patient)
  - Lumbar subarachnoid phenol or ethanol
- Other localized, severe pain
  - Appropriate peripheral nerve block.

Coeliac plexus block

This undoubtedly is the most effective neurolytic block for cancer pain in selected patients. It has survived criticism of insufficient evidence for effect by those who do not practise coeliac plexus block. This is a case where the request of proof of effect from double blind, placebo controlled, and randomized studies surely will require an unethical withholding of effective treatment from suffering patients (Sharfman and Walsh 1990). In visceral pain from cancer in the upper part of the abdomen, frequently accompanied by nausea and anorexia, opioid therapy is often ineffective and usually complicated by nausea and vomiting.

However, there is one double-blind, randomized, placebo-controlled study of intra-operative coeliac plexus neurolysis which demonstrated that treated patients experienced not only improved pain control, reduction in opioid analgesic consumption and improved function, but also a statistically significant improvement in duration of survival (Lillemo *et al*. 1993). And there is a broad consensus among experienced practioners of regional analgesia that this painful condition can be dramatically relieved by a skilfully executed coeliac plexus block (Swarm and Cousins 1993).

It should not be reserved as the last ditch method: Once step 1 and 2 agents on the WHO analgesic ladder fail to relieve pain, coeliac plexus block should be considered. The quality of pain relief is convincing and side-effects usually tolerable or short lived. Pneumothorax and shoulder pain from ethanol irritation of the diaphragmatic peritoneum may occur. The sympatholysis that results may cause orthostatic hypotension and loose bowels for a few days.

However, possibilities for severe complications exist, paraplegia and intestinal infarction will result if the neurolytic solution is injected into arteries. Epidural, paravertebral, and even subarachnoid injection has occurred with dramatic consequences (Davies 1993; De Conno *et al*. 1993).

The block can be repeated with success if pain recurs after weeks to months. Tumour invasion causing somatic pain will require additional measures for the nonvisceral pain-component.

Indications for coeliac plexus block

Cancer of the pancreas is the classic indication. However, cancer of the stomach, duodenum, liver, gallbladder and choledocal ductus, or any tumour in the upper abdominal cavity causing visceral type pain in the upper abdomen are all indications as well.

Whenever there is abdominal wall involvement or tumour spread to muscles and tissues posterior to the abdominal cavity, pain impulses will also travel through somatic afferent nociceptor fibres of the intercostal nerves. Interrupting the visceral afferent nociceptor fibres passing through the coeliac plexus will in these cases only partly relieve the pain.

Anatomy of the coeliac plexus

The coeliac plexus is the prevertebral sympathetic plexus of ganglia and visceral afferent and efferent nerve fibres that supply the upper abdominal viscera with sympathetic autonomic inervation. It is located in the loose retroperitoneal tissue space anterior to the body of the first lumbar and twelfth thoracic vertebrae. The aorta lies behind, the inferior vena cava and right renal vessels lie in front of the coeliac plexus (Fig. 8.1). The greater, the lesser, and the least splanchnic nerves connect the coeliac plexus via the spinal nerve roots to the thoracic spinal cord.

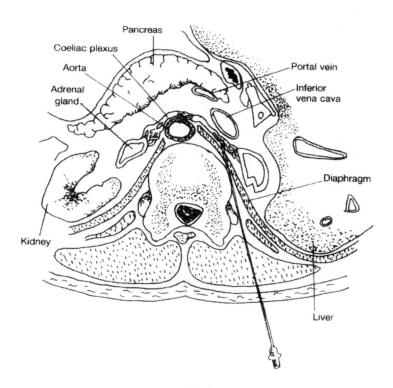

Fig. 8.1 Transverse section at the level of the upper part of the body of the first lumbar vertebra to show the anatomical relationships of the needle position for coeliac plexus block (Reproduced with permission from Diamond and Coniam 1991).

Techniques of coeliac plexus blockade

The coeliac plexus can be injected intraoperatively when the surgeon has determined that the tumour is unresectable (Lillemo *et al.* 1993). However, the block is most often performed percutaneously from the posterior approach, or with computerized tomography scanning (CT)-guidance, with an anterior approach (Patt 1993). Some perform this block with the patient under general anaesthesia and radiographical control of the needle-position (Diamond and Coniam 1991).

I prefer a modification of the technique described by Bonica (1953). With the patient prone, given a small dose of alfentanil intravenously if needed for comfort, but not for complete pain relief, a needle is placed on each side under the midpoint of the 12th rib. With local anaesthetic infiltration the needle is advanced towards the antero-lateral corner of the body of the first lumbar vertebra. When this bone is contacted, the depth marker is moved 1.5–2 cm (depending on the size and build of the patient) from the skin level towards the hub of the needle. The needle is now withdrawn to the subcutaneous tissue, redirected, and advanced 1.5–2 cm beyond the antero-lateral corner of the vertebral body. If the aorta is punctured on the left side, or the vena cava on the right side, the needle is withdrawn till blood stops coming on aspiration.

At this point 5 ml of lignocaine 20 mg/ml is injected in each needle. The patient is now, within a few minutes, able to tell whether his typical pain disappears. He will also be able to inform the anaesthesiologist of any signs of intraspinal or intravascular injection. This is sufficient information to go ahead with injection of 50 ml of 50% ethanol (96% ethanol diluted with bupivacaine 2.5 mg/ml) in each of the two needles.

It should be noted that radiographic imaging of the needle position is no guarantee that the injected neurolytic agent will not cause somatic neurological deficit. Two reported cases of paraplegia following coeliac plexus block in spite of radiographic needle control underscore this important point (Cherry and Lamberty 1984; Woodham and Hanna 1989). Those who perform these blocks with the patient under general anaesthesia or very heavy sedation, obviously will be unable to exploit the indications of correct (or incorrect) needle positioning obtained from a test dose of a small but concentrated dose of local anaesthetic, as described above.

In my experience with about 160 patients, this volume (50 ml × 2) and concentration (50%) of ethanol ensures sufficient spread and effect of the ethanol to denervate the entire coeliac plexus. Some of the reports of poor or shortlasting pain relief from coeliac plexus block (Sharfman and Walsh 1990; Eisenberg *et al*. 1995) may be due to an insufficient injected volume of ethanol.

Side effects of coeliac plexus block with ethanol

The immediate side effect is a drop in blood pressure, which is treated with ephedrine and intravenous colloid-containing fluids. Note that the indirect acting ephedrine is ineffective in patients on long-term treatment with tricyclic antidepressants. These patients are sensitive to the effects of direct-acting vasopressors, so that adrenaline must be used in tiny, titrated doses, for blood pressure support. When orthostatic hypotension persists, blood volume expanding therapy will usually correct this.

Because of the sympathetic denervation of the major part of the gastro-intestinal tract, loose stools may result, often a desirable effect in patients who have been on oral opioids for some time.

The patient should be warned that transient shoulder pain may be a result of the ethanol reaching the diaphragm. Also the full effect may not come on until after one to two days. Too rapid discontinuation of morphine may cause withdrawal symptoms or breakthrough pain. Sometimes the patients may need a reduced dose of oral morphine for residual pain or for pain stemming from tumour invasion of the abdominal wall.

Pain relief from coeliac plexus block with ethanol for pain caused by pancreatic cancer and other upper abdominal malignancies

Percentage good pain relief:

- 73% of 41 patients (Bridenbaugh *et al.* 1964)
- 70% of 57 patients (Black and Dwyer 1973)
- 85% of 136 patients (Brown *et al.* 1981)
- 70% of 160 patients (Breivik 1997—unpublished).

Splanchnic nerve blockade

An easier and safer technique than coeliac plexus block is splanchnic nerve block. In this, the splanchnic nerves are invested with solution above the diaphragm by a technique somewhat similar to that of a lumber sympathectomy. Under X-ray control, one needle from either side is inserted at 10 cm from the mid line where the 12th rib crosses the lateral border of the paravertebral muscles. They are advanced until they strike the T12 vertebral body in the centre. After a small volume (2–4 ml) of contrast material is introduced to show linear spread, the neurolytic (7% aqueous phenol 5 ml) is injected through each needle. As the sympathetic chain is not affected, postural hypotension does not occur and chemical neuritis is a rare occurrence due to the small volume of agent used.

Unusual complications are pneumothorax, chylothorax, or vascular puncture. (Cousins and Bridenbaugh 1988).

Superior hypogastric plexus block and bilateral lumbar sympathetic block

Phenol blocks of the superior hypogastric plexus (Plancarte *et al.* 1990) or bilateral lumbar sympathetic block (Fig. 8.2) (Baxter 1984) may relieve patients with visceral pain from pelvic organs and sigmoid colon. Local extension of common pelvic malignancies such as cervical carcinoma and prostatic carcinoma, will cause somatic nociceptive pain and may limit the effectiveness of chemical lumbar sympathectomies. Perianal and perineal pain, which is mainly of somatic origin and travels via sacral and pudendal nerves, will obviously not be relieved by lumbar sympathetic block.

Subarachnoid (spinal) neurolytic block

Segmental, one sided denervation is obtained by spinal puncture close to the affected nerve roots, followed by subarachnoid injection of 0.3–0.6 ml hypobaric ethanol (96%) with the patient's painful side up; or hyperbaric phenol (5% in glycerol) with the

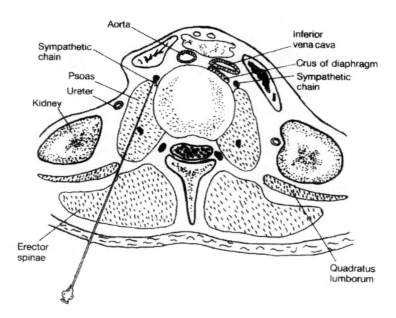

Fig. 8.2 Transverse section at the level of the second lumbar vertebra to show site of injection for lumbar sympathetic block (Reproduced with permission from Diamond and Coniam 1991).

painful side down. This technique is used much less now than up to about 20 years ago, because of dissatisfaction with degree and duration of relief, because of frequent, and sometimes severe side-effects (Twycross 1994), but also because pharmacologic methods now give better pain relief than 20 years ago, and with less risk of severe complications.

Indications for neurolytic spinal block

- Bilateral saddle pain in patients with colostomy and permanent bladder catheter.
- Localized somatic pain of the trunk.
- Unilateral leg pain in a bed-bound patient.

Percentage good pain relief (lasting more than one month)
After subarachnoid block with ethanol:

- 58% in 322 patients (Kuzucu *et al*. 1966)
- 60% in 1908 patients (Drechsel 1984).

Even in experienced hands up to 14% had complications and 15–30% had no pain relief, causing temptation to repeat the block with a larger dose, thereby increasing the risk of neurological complications. A paraplegic patient with urinary and faecal incontinence, but with the same severe perineal and leg pain as before the phenol subarachnoid block, is discouraging indeed.

However, under circumstances with very limited resources, where pharmacological pain relief may be unavailable, the technically simple methods of subarachnoid ethanol or phenol block, which can be performed at the bedside with a needle and a syringe (Stovner and Endresen 1972), may still have a place. It is certainly superior to no pain relief at all in a terminally ill cancer patient.

Subdural and epidural neurolytic blockade

These techniques have been used for cancer pain in the cervical and upper thoracic region where subarachnoid block is less appropriate because of the rapid dilution of injected neurolytic agent (Ischia 1982; Farcot 1983; Korevaar 1988). Experience with these techniques is limited.

Neurolytic blocks of selected peripheral and paravertebral nerves

Neurolytic trigeminal nerve block

This is indicated for head and neck cancer with trigeminal nerve involvement. Less than 1.0 ml ethanol 96% is needed to anaesthetize an appropriate branch or via foramen ovale to the Gasserian ganglion. This usually results in excellent pain relief, also numbness but no motor deficit (Swerdlow 1983).

Neurolytic glossopharyngeal nerve block

This may give good pain relief when pharmacological therapy fails in painful conditions of the mouth and throat. Ethanol is injected at the jugular foramen and may easily also block the vagus, accessory, and hypoglossal nerves, causing dysphagia if bilateral block is performed (Montgomery and Cousins 1972).

Neurolytic intercostal nerve block

Using 1.0 ml of ethanol 96% or phenol 5–6% this block often gives excellent pain relief, lasting, up to a few weeks, if the lesion is localized.

Neurolytic paravertebral spinal nerve blocks

For segmentally well localized somatic pain, this is performed with needle insertion 2–3 cm lateral to the spinous process (of the same vertebra in the lumbar region (Fig. 8.3), but of the vertebra above the segmental nerve to be blocked in the thoracic region). After contact with the transverse process, the needle is redirected below this process and 3–5 ml of the solution is injected. Pain relief may be good, but duration unpredictable.

The block is a simple procedure to perform and should be considered in debilitated and bedridden patients with severe pain not responding well to pharmacological treatment. Consider that an unintended subarachnoid injection, or injection into or close by a radicular artery going to the spinal cord, may cause severe neurological complications.

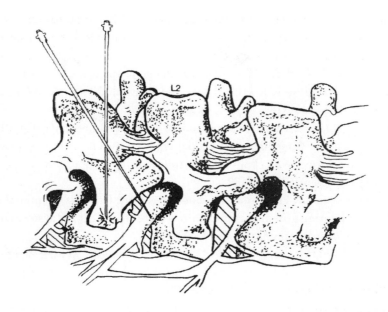

Fig. 8.3 Idealized drawing to illustrate lumbar paravertebral block. The needle on the transverse process is moved caudally to pass a few millimetres below and deeper to where spinal nerve passes (Reproduced with permission from Diamond and Coniam 1991).

Neurolytic transsacral nerve block

This may be indicated when pelvic metastasis cause nerve compression pain which is not well controlled by pharmacological means. The second sacral foramen lies 1 cm below and medial to the posterior superior iliac spine. The fifth sacral foramen lies 1 cm inferior and lateral to the sacral cornua. The 3rd and 4th foramen lie on the line between the 1st and the 5th. The needle is advanced 0.5–1.5 cm beyond the opening of the foramina and about 3 ml of the solution is injected at each site. Note that S2-blockade, even unilateral, may cause urinary incontinence.

References

Baron, C.M., Kowalski, S.E., Greengrass, R. *et al.* (1996). Epinephrine decreases post-operative requirements for continuous thoracic epidural fentanyl infusions. *Anesthesia and Analgesia*, **82**, 760–5.

Baxter, R. (1984). Specialized techniques for the relief of pain. In *The management of terminal malignant disease* (ed. C. Saunders (2nd edn), pp. 91–9. Edward Arnold, London.

Black, A., and Dwyer, B. (1973). Coeliac plexus block. *Anaesthesia and Intensive Care*, **1**, 315.

Bonica, J.J. (1953). *The Management of Pain*. Lea and Febiger, Philadelphia.

Boys, L., Peat, S.J., Hanna, M.H., and Burn, K. (1993). Audit of neural blockade for palliative care patients in an acute unit. *Palliative Medicine*, **7**, 205–11.

Breivik, H. (1995). Safe perioperative spinal and epidural analgesia: Importance of drug combinations, segmental site of injection, training and monitoring. *Acta Anaesthesiologica Scandinavica*, **39**, 869–71.

Breivik, H., and Hesla, P.E. (1978). Epidural analgesia and epidural steroid injections for treatment of chronic low back pain and sciatica. *Tidsskr Nor Lœgeforening* (Norwegian) **99**, 936–9.

Breivik, H., Hesla, P.E., Molnar, I., and Lind, B. (1976). Treatment of chronic low back pain and sciatica: Comparison of caudal epidural injections of bupivacaine and methylprednisolone with bupivacaine followed by saline. *Advances in Pain Research and Therapy*, **1**, 927–32.

Breivik, H., Niemi, G., Haugtomt, H., and Högström, H. (1995). Optimal epidural analgesia: importance of drug combinations and correct segmental site of injection. *Bailliere's Clinical Anaesthesiology*, **9**, 493–512.

Bridenbaugh, L.D., Moore, D.C., and Campell, D.D. (1964). Management of upper abdominal cancer pain. Treatment with celiac plexus block with alcohol. *Journal of the American Medical Association*, **190**, 877.

Brown, D.L., Bulley, C.K., and Quiel, E.L. (1981). Neurolytic celiac plexus block for pancreatic cancer pain. *Anesthesia and Analgesia*, **66**, 869–73.

Cherry, D.A., and Lamberty, J. (1984). Paraplegia following coeliac plexus block. *Anaesthesia and Intensive Care*, **56**, 137–41.

Cousins, M.J., and Bridenbaugh, P.O. (1988). *Neural blockade* (2nd edn), pp. 1171. J.B. Lippincott 6, Philadelphia.

Davis, D.D. (1993). Incidence of major complications of neurolytic coeliac plexus block. *Journal of the Royal Society of Medicine*, **86**, 264–6.

De Conno, F., Caraceni, A., Aldrigetthi, L. *et al.* (1993). Paraplegia following coeliac plexus block. *Pain*, **55**, 383–5.

Devor, M., Govrin-Lippmann, R., and Raber, P. (1985). Corticosteroids reduce neuroma hyperexcitability. In *Advances in pain research and therapy* (ed. H.L. Fields, R. Dubner, and F. Cervero). Vol 9, pp. 451–5. Raven Press, New York.

Diamond, A.W., and Coniam, S.W. (1991). *The management of chronic pain*. Oxford University Press, Oxford.

Drechsel, U. (1984). Treatment of cancer pain with neurolytic agents. *Recent results of cancer research*, **89**, 137–47.

Eisenberg, E., Carr, D.B., and Chalmers, T.C. (1995). Neurolytic celiac plexus block for treatment of cancer pain: a meta-analysis. *Anesthesia and Analgesia*, **80**, 290–5.

Farcot, J.M. (1983). Subdural epi-arachnoid neurolytic block in cervical pain. *Pain*, **17**, 316–7.

Ferrante, F.M., Bedder, M., Caplan, R.A. *et al.* (1996). Practice guidelines for cancer pain management. A report by the American Society of Anesthesiolgists Task Force on pain management, cancer pain section. *Anesthesiology*, **94**, 1243–57.

Hogan, Q.H., and Abrams, S.E. (1997). Neural blockade for diagnosis and prognosis: A review. *Anesthesiology*, **86**, 216–41.

Ischia, S. (1982). Subdural extra-arachnoid neurolytic block in cervical pain. *Pain*, **14**, 347–54.

Jacox, A., Carr, D.B., Payne, R., *et al.* (1994). *Management of cancer pain: clinical practice guideline number 9.* AHCPR publication no. 94–0592. U.S. Department of Health and Human Services, Agency for Health Care Policy and Research, Rockville.

Jänig, W., and Stanton-Hicks, M. (ed.) (1996). Reflex sympathetic dystrophy: a reappraisal. *Progress in Pain Research and Management* (IASP Press, Seattle), **6**, 1–200.

Korevaar, W.C. (1988). Transcatheter thoracic epidural neurolysis using ethyl alcohol. *Anesthesiology*, **69**, 989–93.

Kuzucu, E.Y., Derrick, W.S., and Wilber, S.A. (1966). Control of intractable pain with subarachnoid alcohol block. *Journal of the American Medical Association*, **195**, 541–4.

Lillemo, K.D., Cameron, J.L., Kaufman, H.S. *et al.* (1993). Chemical splanchnicectomy in patients with unresectable pancreatic cancer. *Annals of Surgery*, **217**, 447–57.

Loeser, J.D. (1997). President's address to the 8th world congress on pain. *Progress in Pain Research and Management*, **8**, 3–11.

Montgomery, W., and Cousins, M.J. (1972). Aspects of management of chronic pain illustrated by ninth nerve block. *British Journal of Anaesthesia*, **44**, 383–5.

Niemi, G., and Breivik, H. (1998). Adrenaline greatly enhances sensory blockade and pain relief of a subanalgesic epidural infusion of fentanyl and bupivacaine after major surgery. *Acta Anaesthesiolgica Scandinavica*, 42, (in press).

Olmarker, K., Blomquist, J., Strömberg, J., *et al.* (1995). Inflammatogenic properties of nucleus pulposus. *Spine*, **20**, 665–9.

Patt, R.B. (ed.) (1993). *Cancer Pain.* J.B. Lippincott, Philadelphia.

Pieretti, S., DiGiannuario, A., Loisso, A. *et al.* (1992). Dexamethasone prevents epileptiform activity induced by morphine in vivo and in vitro experiments. *Journal of Pharmacology and Experimental Therapeutics*, **263**, 830–9.

Plancarte, R., Amescua, C., Patt, R.B., and Aldrete, J.A. (1990). Superior hypogastric plexus block for pelvic cancer pain. *Anesthesiology*, **73**, 236–9.

Rowell, N.P. (1988). Intralesional methylprednisolone for rib metastases: an alternative to radiotherapy? *Palliative Medicine*, **2**, 153–5.

Sharfman, W.H., and Walsh, T.D. (1990). Has the efficacy of celicac plexus block been demonstrated in pancreatic cancer pain? *Pain*, **41**, 267–71.

Sjöberg, M., Appelgren, L., Einarsson, S. *et al.* (1991). Long-term intrathecal morphine and bupivacaine in refractory cancer pain: I. Results from the first series of 52 patients. *Acta Anaesthesiologica Scandinavica*, **35**, 30–43.

Sjöberg, M., Nitescue, P., Appelgren, L., and Curelaru, I. (1994). Long-term intrathecal morphine and bupivacaine in refractory cancer pain: I. Results from a morphine and bupivacaine regimen of 0.5:4.75 mg/ml. *Anesthesiology*, **80**, 284–9.

Stovner, J., and Endresen, R. (1972). Intrathecal phenol for cancer pain. *Acta Anaesthesiologica Scandinavica*, **16**, 17– .

Swarm, R.A., and Cousins, M.J. (1993). Anaesthetic techniques for pain control. In *Oxford textbook of palliative medicine* (ed. D. Doyle, G.W.C. Hanks, and N. Macdonald), pp. 204–21. Oxford University Press, Oxford.

Swerdlow, M. (ed.) (1983). *Relief of intractable pain* (3rd edn). Excerpta Medica, Amsterdam.

Twycross, R. (1994). *Pain relief in advanced cancer*. Churchill Livingstone, Edinburgh.

Twycross, R. (1997). The joy of death. *Lancet*, 350 (suppl III), 20.

Watts, E.W., and Silagy, C.A. (1995). A meta-analysis of the efficacy of epidural corticosteroids in the treatment of sciatica. *Anaesthesia and Intensive Care*.

Woodham, M.J., and Hanna, M.H. (1989). Paraplegia after coeliac plexus block. *Anaesthesia*, **44**, 487–9.

World Health Organization (1986). *Cancer pain relief*. World Health Organization, Geneva.

Yaksh, T.L., and Ready, S.V.R. (1981). Studies in the primate on the analgetic effects associated with intrathecal actions of opiates, alpha-adrnergic agonists and baclofen. *Anesthesiology*, **54**, 451–67.

Zech, D.F.J., Grond, S., Lynch, J. *et al.* (1995). Validation of world health organization guidelines for cancer pain relief: a 10-year prospective study. *Pain*, **63**, 65–76.

NINE

Complex interventional therapies

ELLIOT S. KRAMES AND SUNIL K. ROHIRA

In 1986, according to statistics from the American Cancer Society, there were 956 000 new cases of cancer reported; The prevalence of the disease was approximately 1 991 000 patients; and 478 000 patients died of their disease (Bonica 1990). According to Foley, approximately 50% of cancer patients with early disease will complain of pain, however, during the terminal phase of the disease, upwards of 75–80% of these patients will experience pain (Foley 1985). Because cancer pain is so prevalent, especially in the terminal phase of illness, leading to untold suffering of these individuals, it is imperative to address this problem and utilize all of the tools and therapies that are available to caregivers of patients with cancer. It is the intent of this chapter to present complex interventions, including intraspinal analgesic therapy for patients who do not respond to the pharmacological guidelines set out by the World Health Organization Committee on Cancer Pain Management (1986).

Interventional pain management

It has been suggested that 80–90% of cancer related pain syndromes can be well controlled using guidelines established by the World Health Organization; using 1986 statistics that means 280 000–560 000 patients with cancer, do not respond. These patients may be helped by the more complex interventional strategies that are discussed in this chapter.

Why do some patients fail to respond to the WHO guidelines? The reasons for opioid therapeutic failure in the cancer pain population may vary widely. They include the development of opioid non-responsive pain syndromes such as neuropathic pain or the development of pain intensity variability such as the development of incident pain syndromes. They may also include clinician and patient related factors. Clinician factors may include uncertainty about the role of opioid therapy for patients with early disease, indolent metastatic disease, or treatment related disease, and undertreatment of the patient's pain caused by deficiencies of knowledge of opioid therapy, failure of assessment, overestimation of risks of addiction, pharmacologic outcomes, or fears of sanctions by regulatory agencies. Patient related factors leading to opioid therapeutic failure may include ineffectual pain reporting, erroneous fears of addiction to the opioids or beliefs that these drugs are inherently harmful, or inadequate understanding of dosing guidelines (Portnoy 1993).

When implementation of the WHO guidelines fails to provide pain relief for the patient suffering from cancer related pain syndromes, caregivers must not give up seeking alternative pain control techniques for analgesic control. Available therapies for these patients include epidural and intrathecal opioid infusion systems, spinal cord stimulation, local anaesthetic somatic and/or sympathetic nerve blocks, intraspinal conduction blockade with local anaesthetics, intrapleural analgesia, peripheral neurolysis, paravertebral gangliolysis or rhizolysis, lumbar sympathetic neurolysis, superior hypogastric plexus neurolysis, epidural neurolysis, and subarachnoid neurolysis.

Neuromodulatory and some neurodestructive surgical procedures may also assist the patient suffering from intractable cancer related pain. Neuromodulatory procedures include implantation of intraspinal infusion analgesic systems or implantation of spinal cord or peripheral nerve stimulating devices. Some examples of appropriate neurodestructive surgical procedures include cordotomy, pituitary alcohol ablation, rhizotomy, coeliac plexus surgical ablation, superior hypogastric plexus ablation, and myelotomy. This chapter will outline some of the interventional techniques used for cancer pain management.

Nerve blocks

Nerve blocks with local anaesthetic or neurolytic agents are very helpful in the management of intractable cancer pain. Although there is lack of uniformity in the indications for neural blockade, it is generally agreed that 50–80% of patients who receive nerve blocks for cancer pain may benefit (Cousins and Bridenbaugh 1987). They may be useful in the following ways:

- Diagnostic blocks help determine the pain generator and the associated pain pathways.
- Prognostic blocks are indicated in the prediction of the outcome of destructive procedures.
- Pre-emptive analgesic blocks prevent the painful sequels of procedures that may result in conditions such as complex regional pain syndrome.
- Anaesthetic blocks help in the intraoperative management of procedure related pain in cancer patients.
- Therapeutic blocks help in management of painful conditions such as pancreatic cancer that can respond to coeliac plexus block.

Local anaesthetics

Local anaesthetics prevent the opening of the sodium channels or may simply block these channels. The physical and chemical properties of some local anaesthetics are summarized in Fig. 9.1. The two main types of local anaesthetics are esters and amides. Ester local anaesthetics are usually metabolized to yield an alcohol and a para-amino

Agent	Physicochemical Properties			Biologic Properties			Recommended Maximum Single Dose (mg)	Comments	pH of Plain Solutions
	pKa [25°C]	Partition Coefficient	Percent Protein Binding	Equieffective Anaesthetic Concentration	Approximate Anaesthetic Duration (min)	Onset			
Procaine	9.05	0.02	5.8	2	50	Fast	1000	Used mainly for infiltration and differential block	5–6.5
Chloro-procaine	8.97	0.14	?	2	45	Fast	800 (1000 with adrenaline)	Intrathecal injection may be associated with sensory/motor deficits	2.7–4
Tetracine	8.46	4.1	75.6	0.25	175 20	Fast	20	Use is primarily limited to spinal and topical anaesthesia	4.5–6.5
Lignocaine	7.91	2.9	643	1	100	Fast	500 with adrenaline	Most versatile agent	6.5
Mepivacaine	7.76	0.8	77.5	1	100	Fast	50 with adrenaline	Duration of plain solutions longer than lignocaine without adrenaline	4.5
Bupivacaine	8.16	27.5	95.6	0.25	175	Fast	175 (225 with adrenaline)	Lower concentrations provide differential sensory/motor block Ventricular arrhythmias and sudden cardiovascular collapse reported following rapid intravenous injection	4.5–6
Etidocaine	7.7	141	94	0.25	200	Fast	400 with adrenaline	Profound motor block useful for surgical anaesthesia but not for obstetrical analgesia	4.5

Fig. 9.1 Physicochemical properties of local anaesthetics. (From Faust, R.J. (1994). *Anesthesiology review* (2nd edn), p. 316. Churchill Livingstone, Philadelphia.)

butyric acid (PABA) derivative. Some examples of ester local anaesthetics include procaine, chloroprocaine, and tetracaine. Amides are metabolized by aromatic hydroxylation, N-dealkylation and amide hydrolysis. A few examples of amide local anaesthetics include mepivacaine, lignocaine, bupivacaine, and etidocaine. The toxicity of local anaesthetics may be related to one of the following:

• Central nerve system toxicity may result from excessive doses of lignocaine (Reynolds 1987; Reiz and Nath 1986). Symptoms might include numbness of the tongue, light headedness, audio visual disturbances, muscular twitching, unconsciousness, convulsions, and coma. Neurotoxicity with chloroprocaine, in the presence of large amounts of sodium bisulphite and low pH, has been recorded (Ravidrin *et al.* 1980; Moore *et al.* 1982; Gissen *et al.* 1984; Wang *et al.* 1984; Reiz and Nash 1986).

• Cardiovascular toxicity of local anaesthetics results in myocardial depression. Bupivacaine at toxic doses has been associated with refractory ventricular arrhythmia (Reynolds 1987; Reiz and Nath 1986).

• Allergic reactions are more common with ester local anaesthetics than amides. In addition, methylparaben, a preservative may also cause allergic reactions when metabolized to PABA.

Head and neck blocks

Head and neck cancers constitute approximately 4% of all cancers in the United States (Boring *et al.* 1994). Head and neck cancers are often seen in elderly patients who smoke cigarettes or consume alcohol (Davidson *et al.* 1991). Approximately 42 000 new cases of head and neck cancer and additional 25 500 larynx and thyroid cancers were estimated for the year 1994 (Boring *et al.* 1994). Worldwide, approximately half a million new cases of head and neck cancer are projected annually (Boring *et al.* 1994). More recently, younger patients have developed head and neck cancers. There also seems to be a gradual increase in incidence of women developing head and neck cancers (Vokes *et al.* 1993; Boring *et al.* 1994).

Anatomy of trigeminal nervous system and cervical plexus

The trigeminal nerve is a complex cranial nerve that innervates the skin of the face, the anterior two thirds of the tongue, and the oronasal mucosa. In addition, the trigeminal nerve carries motor fibres to the muscles of mastication and tensor tympany and proprioceptive impulses from the temporomandibular joint. The Gasserian ganglion is formed by the fusion of the three major branches of the trigeminal nerve, namely the ophthalmic (**V1**), maxillary (**V2**), and mandibular divisions (**V3**).

The cervical plexus is formed by the anterior primary divisions of the upper four cervical nerves. These anterior primary rami form branches that ascend and descend as well as interdigitate to form a superficial and a deep cervical plexus. The superficial cervical plexus pierces the deep cervical fascia and emerges around the posterior border of the sternocleidomastoid and supplies the anterior cervical region. The deep cervical plexus innervates the deeper structures of the cervical region supplying muscular branches to the sternocleidomastoid, middle scalene, trapezius, and levator scapulae muscles and also supplies branches to the cervical sympathetic chain, phrenic, vagus, and hypoglossal nerves.

Appropriate block determined by dermatomal distribution of pain

Pain caused by cancers of the head and neck can be controlled by blocking the appropriate division of the trigeminal nerve (Fig. 9. 2).

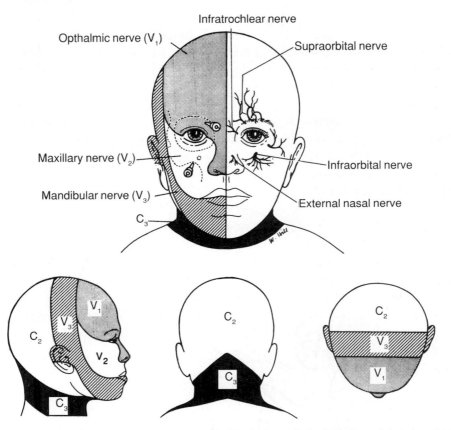

Fig. 9.2 'Dermatome man' showing commonly blocked cutaneous branches of the trigeminal nerve. (From Waldman, S.D. *et al.* (1996). *Interventional pain management* (ed. S.D. Waldman and A.P. Winnie) p. 183. W.D. Saunders, Co., Philadelphia.)

Trigeminal (gasserian) ganglion block

The trigeminal ganglion is formed by fusion of the ophthalmic, maxillary, and mandibular nerves that innervate the head, and course their way to the pons. These nerves may be affected by the tumour itself, radiotherapy, surgery, or local pressure. The trigeminal ganglion is partially contained within Meckels cave, a bony cave within the floor of the cranium. Meckel's cave is formed by a reflection of dura mater within which the trigeminal ganglion is partially contained.

Indications: The principal indication for Gasserian ganglion block is diagnostic prior to neurolysis in patients with facial neuropathic pain.

Procedure: The block may be carried out with 2–4 ml of any local anaesthetic under fluoroscopic guidance. To perform this block, the patient is placed in a supine position with their gaze focused straight ahead. The patient is asked to clench his or her teeth. A skin wheal is raised immediately medial to the masseter muscle and lateral to the lateral fissure of the lips on the side to be blocked. Through this site, a 22 gauge 3 inch spinal needle is advanced cranial, dorsally, and medially toward the foramen ovale. The general direction of the needle should be toward the pupil of the eye in the cranio-caudal plane. The location of the needle tip should be confirmed by fluoroscopy and appropriate paraesthesia to the trigeminal area to be blocked. Subsequently, after negative aspiration of blood or cerebrospinal fluid, 1–2 ml of local anaesthetic may be injected prior to performing neurolysis to confirm appropriate placement of the needle tip. (Fig. 9.3.)

Complications: Inadvertent dural puncture leading to neurotoxicity and death has been reported. Neuritis resulting from alcohol neurolysis can manifest as exacerbation or worsening of the neuropathic pain. Chronic corneal anaesthesia may also follow ganglion neurolysis and may go undetected.

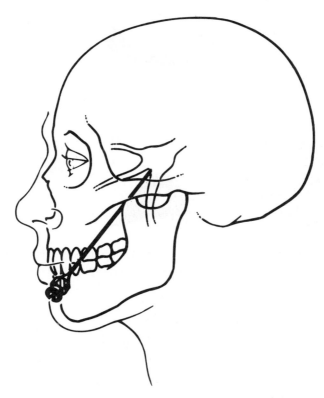

Fig. 9.3 Needle trajectory for gasserian ganglion block. (From Waldman, S.D. *et al*. (1996). *Interventional pain management* (ed. S.D. Waldman and A.P. Winnie) p. 183. W.B. Saunders, Co., Philadelphia.)

Maxillary nerve block

The maxillary nerve forms the second division of the trigeminal nervous system and innervates the dermatomal distribution over the skin of the anterolateral cheek, including the tempero-zygomatic region, inferior portion of the nose, upper lip, upper gums, upper molars, mucosa of the maxillary sinus, lower eyelid, and dura mater of the medial cranial fossa. The nerve divides to form the following end branches: meningeal, zygomatic, infraorbital, nasal, pterygopalatine, and superior labial branches.

Procedure: The maxillary nerve can be blocked through the coronoid notch of the mandible. This is performed with a patient in the supine position and the head turned away from the side to be blocked. The physician palpates the mandibular notch while the patient gently opens and closes his or her mouth. A 22 gauge, 3 inch spinal needle is advanced through the mandibular notch, perpendicular to the notch until the pterygoid plate is reached. The needle is then either redirected in a cephalomedial direction towards the pterygo-palatine fossa, about 1/8 inch past the pterygoid plate for a maxillary nerve block. After careful and negative aspiration for blood, 5 ml of local anaesthetic may then be injected (see Fig. 9.4).

Complications: Local anaesthetic injected into the periorbital region carries the risk of haematoma and/or a block of the cranial nerves to the extraocular muscles.

Mandibular nerve block

The mandibular nerve forms the third division of the trigeminal nervous system. The nerve divides peripherally to form a small anterior and a larger posterior trunk.

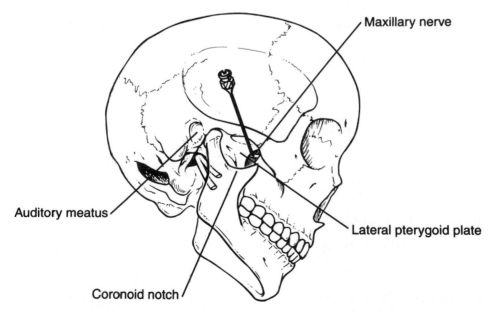

Fig. 9.4 Selective maxillary nerve block. (From Waldman, S.D. *et al.* (1996). *Interventional pain management* (ed. S.D. Waldman and A.P. Winnie) p. 183. W. B. Saunders, Co., Philadelphia.)

The branches from the anterior trunk are the buccinator, masseteric, deep temporal, and external pterygoid nerves. The posterior trunk divides into the auriculo temporal nerve and the inferior alveolar nerve which terminates as the mental nerve. The mandibular division innervates the oral muscles supplied by these nerves, the tympanic membrane, the anterior two-thirds of the tongue, sensation to the lower lip, lower teeth, and mandible as well as the parotid gland. Therefore, pain secondary to cancers of these regions may be alleviated by blocking or destroying the mandibular nerve.

Procedure: The mandibular nerve is blocked in a similar fashion to the maxillary nerve. The patient is placed supine with the head turned away from the side to be blocked. The physician palpates the mandibular notch while the patient gently opens and closes their mouth. A 22 gauge 3 inch spinal needle is advanced through and perpendicular to the mandibular notch to impinge on the lateral pterygoid plate. The needle is then withdrawn slightly and walked off its posterior border. The needle should not be advanced more than half an inch beyond the pterygoid plate. When the needle is in position, 5 ml of local anaesthetic is administered.

Complications: The risks of such an injection include subarachnoid injection, with associated seizure, bleeding and haematoma, and infection.

Supraorbital nerve block

The supraorbital nerve is a branch of the first (ophthalmic) division of the trigeminal nervous system.

Indications: Pain in the dermatome supplied by the supraorbital nerve, namely the skin over the frontal region of the skull including the upper nose, can be blocked by blocking the supraorbital nerve. Pain confined to the unilateral forehead area can be blocked by blocking the supraorbital nerve.

Procedure: This nerve is accessed by entering the supraorbital fossa and eliciting a paraesthesia to the frontal part of the forehead. It is then blocked with either local anaesthetic or a neurolytic agent such as phenol.

Complications: One is cautioned to have the patient close his or her eyes tightly to avoid damage to the patient's eyes.

Infraorbital nerve block

The infraorbital nerve is a peripheral division of the maxillary nerve. It supplies the skin over the anterior upper lip and adjacent cheek.

Indication: Pain in the area inferior to the eye and on the side of the nose can be blocked by infraorbital nerve block. This nerve is blocked as it emerges from the infraorbital foramen.

Superficial and deep cervical plexus block

The superficial and deep cervical plexus is formed by the upper four cervical nerves. The cervical plexus peripherally forms the lesser occipital nerve, the great auricular nerve, the accessory nerve, the anterior cervical nerve, and the suprascapular nerve (Figs 9.5 and 9.6). The superficial cervical plexus is bundled on the posterior border of the sternocleidomastoid muscle. Adequate infiltration of this area with a local anaesthetic can produce an adequate block of this plexus. Neurolytic block may help alleviate chronic pain relating to the distribution of the superficial cervical plexus. Since these nerves are peripheral nerves, alcohol and or phenol neuritis can occur after injection with these neurolytic agents (Burkel and McPhee 1970; Arter and Racz 1990).

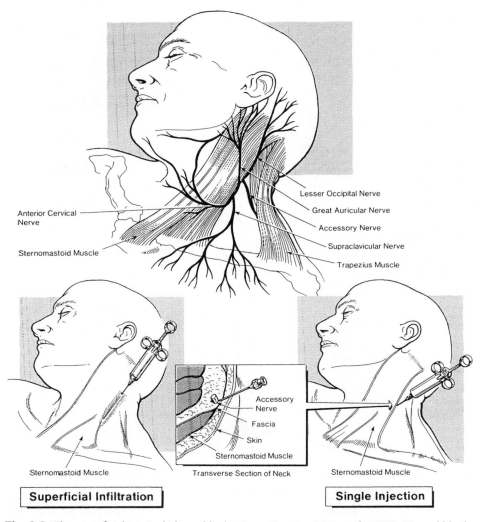

Fig. 9.5 The superficial cervical plexus block. (From Cousins, M.J. *et al.* (1988). *Neural block-ade in clinical anesthesia and management of pain* (2nd edn) (ed. M.J. Cousins and P.O. Bridenbaugh), p. 550. J.B. Lippincott, Philadelphia.)

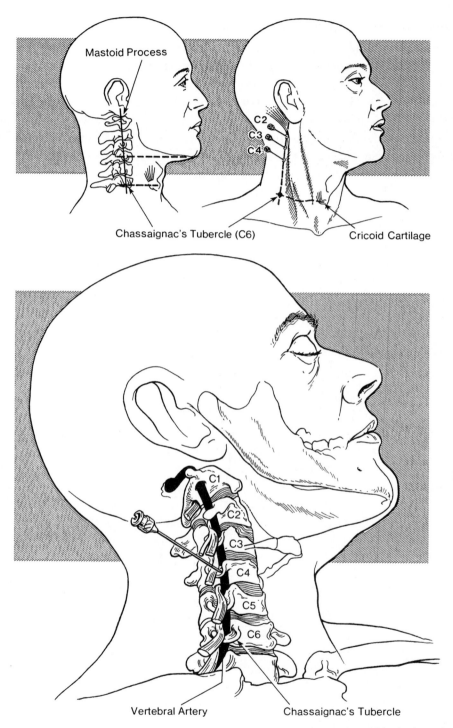

Fig. 9.6 Deep cervical plexis block. (From Cousins, M.J. *et al.* (1988). *Neural blockade in clinical anesthesia and management of pain* (2nd edn) (ed. M.J. Cousins, and P.O. Bridenbaugh), p. 553. J.B. Lippincott, Philadelphia.)

Sympathetic blocks

Sympathetic nervous system anatomy

The sympathetic chain consists of a chain from several sympathetic nervous system plexuses that run along the paravertebral region of the body. These axial sympathetic chains include the cervical, thoracic, and lumbar sympathetic ganglia. The most prominent ganglia are the cervicothoracic (stellate) ganglion, thoracic sympathetic ganglia, splanchnic ganglia, ganglia of the coeliac plexus, and lumbar sympathetic ganglia.

The sympathetic nervous system and pain

The sympathetic system receives afferents nociceptive impulses from the visceral fibres of the head and neck and upper extremities (stellate ganglion): from the cardiothoracic viscera (thoracic sympathetic ganglia): from the abdominal viscera (coeliac plexus): from the uro-genital system and lower extremities (lumbar sympathetic ganglia) and from the pelvic viscera (superior hypogastric ganglia and ganglion of impar).

Pain relating to these cancer pain generators can therefore be controlled by either blocking these ganglia using local anaesthetic or by neurolysis of these ganglia using chemical, radiofrequency thermal lesioning, or cryoneurolysis.

Stellate ganglion block

The stellate ganglion is formed by fusion of the inferior cervical and first thoracic sympathetic ganglia. The ganglion lies over the neck of the first rib. The dome of the pleura is located on its anterior inferior aspect and the vertebral artery on its posterior aspect. For best results of a stellate ganglion block, local anaesthetic solution must fill the space in front of the prevertebral fascia down to at least T2. The stellate ganglion controls sympathetic outflow to the head, neck, and upper extremity.

Indication: The primary indication for this block is the treatment of sympathetically mediated pain of the upper extremities, head, and neck. This block can be used to increase perfusion of the upper extremities, or decrease excessive perspiration of the head, neck, or upper extremities, as in hyperhydrosis.

Procedure: Although this block may be performed utilizing anatomic landmarks, it is safer to use fluoroscopy. The patient is placed in the supine position with the neck slightly extended. After locally prepping and anaesthetizing the area overlying the body of C7, a 1.5 inch, 22 gauge needle is advanced posteriorly and slightly medially while retracting the carotid artery sheath laterally toward the transverse process or antero-lateral border of the vertebral body of C7. When the transverse process or anterolateral border of C7 is reached, the needle is slightly withdrawn approximately 1 mm. After careful and negative aspiration for blood, a few 5 ml of non-ionic radiographic dye added to approximately 10–20 ml of 0.25% bupivacaine is injected. The added radiographic dye enables the surgeon to view the extent of injection anatomically. A post injection Horner's sign only suggests adequate block of the sympathetic nervous system to the head and only post injection increased warmth to the upper extremity suggests adequate sympathetic block to the upper extremity. Pain relief, in the presence of normally maintained sensation, and increased warmth to the upper extremity suggests that the patient indeed has sympathetically maintained pain.

Complications: Serious complications associated with the stellate ganglion block include pneumothorax, local anaesthetic induced seizures from inadvertent injection into the vertebral artery and/or intradural or subarachnoid injections resulting in high spinal anaesthesia, respiratory depression, and even death. Therefore, aspiration prior to injection is an absolute must. Commonly, side-effects of this block might include a feeling of lump in the throat, hoarseness of voice, haematoma, infection, or local muscle tenderness. Rarely pneumothorax or, phrenic nerve palsy may occur.

Coeliac plexus block

Anatomy: Pre-ganglionic neurons from the interomediolateral horn of T5–T12 leave the spinal cord to join the white rami communicans. Instead of synapsing in the sympathetic chain and pre-vertebral sympathetic ganglia, they pass through the chain to synapse at the coeliac plexus. The coeliac plexus lies anterior to the aorta at the level of the L1 vertebral body and anterior to the crura of the diaphragm. The coeliac plexus is the largest of the four great sympathetic plexuses of the thoraco-abdominal region including the thoracic sympathetic plexus, the superior mesenteric plexus, and the superior hypogastric plexus. The coeliac plexus consists of nerves originating from the splanchnic, vagus, and sympathetic post-ganglionic nerves. The coeliac plexus receives afferent nociceptive impulses from all abdominal viscera except the transverse colon, the descending colon, the sigmoid colon and the rectum. Intractable abdominal malignant pain originating from the structures innervated by the coeliac plexus can be blocked by local anaesthetic injection or by neurolysis of the coeliac plexus with alcohol or phenol. The coeliac plexus controls sympathetic flow to the pancreas, liver, gallbladder, omentum, mesentery, and the upper gastrointestinal tract from the stomach to the proximal transverse colon.

Indications: The main indications of this block in cancer relate to malignancy of the pancreas and stomach (Brown 1989; Miller 1985). This block may be performed to reduce the required oral opioid intake of the patient or may be used adjunctively to systemic opioid administration.

Procedure: This block may be performed under fluoroscopic or CT guidance (Hegedus 1979; Miller 1985, Ischia *et al.* 1992; Figs 9.7 and 9.8). To perform this block under fluoroscopy, using a posterior approach, the patient is placed on a fluoroscopic table with a pillow beneath the abdomen. Utilizing fluoroscopy in the oblique, antero-posterior, and lateral projections, 22 gauge needles are advanced bilaterally to the anterolateral

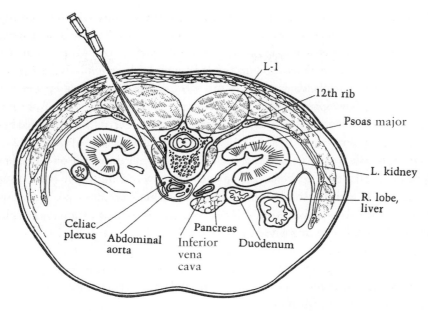

Fig. 9.7 Coeliac plexus block. (From Mulroy, M.F. *et al.* (1996). *Regional anesthesia*, 2nd edn), p. 153, J.B. Lippincott, Philadelphia.)

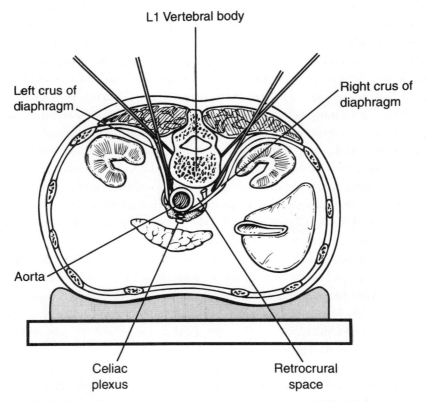

Fig. 9.8 Needle placement for Coeliac plexus block. (From Waldman, S.D. *et al.* (1996). *Interventional pain management* (ed. S.D. Waldman and A.P. Winnie), p. 183. W.B. Saunders, Co., Philadelphia, P.A.)

bodies of L1. The needle on the left side is advanced anteriorly into the aorta aspirating for blood as the needle is advanced. Negative aspiration for blood suggests that the tip of the needle is just posterior to the coeliac plexus. Confirmation of appropriate place-ment of the needles is made by injecting non-ionic radiographic dye through the needles. Appropriate placement of the trans-aortic needle is confirmed by observing a crescent shape of dye spread as the dye spreads around the anterior aorta. Appropriate placement of the retrocrural needle at the anterolateral border of L1 is suggested by dye tracking in the anterolateral border of the vertebral body cephalad to T12. The transaortic needle is place to block the coeliac plexus, while the needle on the right side is appropriately placed to block the splanchnic nerve on the right. Subsequently, through each 22 gauge needle, about 15 ml of 0.25% bupivacaine is injected followed by a neurolytic agent such as 50–100% alcohol. Alcohol is used to destroy the plexus and splanchnic nerve 'permanently'.

Complications: Intractable diarrhoea, profound hypotension, haemorrhage, possible visceral damage, renal trauma with haematuria and intravascular injection. Cord dam-age is also a possibility, albeit rare.

Lumbar sympathetic block

Indications: The indications for lumbar sympathetic blockade in cancer patients include sympathetically mediated pain relating to radiation lumbosacral plexitis, metastasis of the tumour or chemotherapy, phantom limb pain, herpes zoster, neuro-pathic pain of the lower extremity or vascular insufficiency secondary to malignancy. The sympathetic ganglia are located anterolateral to and along side the L2 and L4 ver-tebral bodies bilaterally between the vertebral bodies themselves and anterior and medial to the psoas major muscle. We recommend fluoroscopic guidance to block these ganglia. We use a 20 gauge, 3 inch spinal needle introducer and advance it under fluoro-scopic guidance toward the anterolateral border of L2 to L5 depending on the level that is intended to be blocked. A 25 gauge, 5.5 inch, coaxial, slightly curved spinal nee-dle is advanced through the 20 gauge introducer and through the psoas major muscle to the anterolateral border of the vertebral body. In the anterior-posterior projection of the fluoroscopic beam, the needle tip should lie within the 'eye of the pedicle' or at the same level of the pedicles along an imaginary line drawn in the cranio-caudal direction aligning all of the pedicles. Fluoroscopic dye confirms the location of the needle tip. In the lateral projection of the beam, the needle tip should lie at the anterolateral border. Subsequently, 20–30 ml of 0.25% bupivacaine is injected for diagnostic block. Neuro-lysis can be performed chemically with alcohol or phenol or performed with radiofrequency lesions (Fig. 9.9).

Complications: Lumbar sympathetic blocks carry with them the risk of bleeding, infec-tion, profound hypotension, inadvertent epidural or intrathecal injection, intraneural injection, and inadvertent intravascular injection. Chemical neurolysis with alcohol may be associated with rare damage to the genitofemoral nerve resulting in groin and

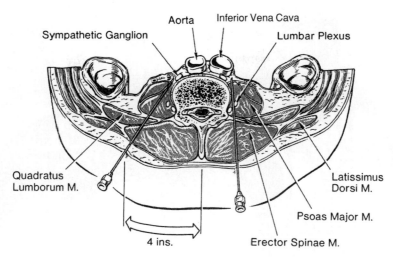

Aorta   Inferior Vena Cava

Sympathetic Ganglion   Lumbar Plexus

Quadratus
Lumborum M.

Latissimus
Dorsi M.

4 ins.   Erector Spinae M.

Psoas Major M.

Fig. 9.9 Lumbar sympathetic block. (From Cousins, M.J. *et al.* (1988). *Neural blockade in clinical anesthesia and management of pain* (2nd edn) (ed. M.J. Cousins, and P.O. Bridenbaugh), p. 483. J.B. Lippincott, Philadelphia, PA.)

flank pain (Haymaker and Woodhall 1945) or damage to the artery of Adamkiewicz resulting in flaccid paraplegia and spinal sensory dissociation (Galizea and Lahiri 1974; Lo and Buckley 1982; Wong and Brown 1995).

Superior hypogastric plexus block

Anatomy: This plexus is located bilaterally at the lower third of the 5th lumbar vertebral body and upper third of S1 vertebral body in proximity to the bifurcation of the common iliac vessels. The pelvic splanchnic nerves arise from the second, third, and fourth sacral nerves. Sympathetic afferents from the distal end of the transverse colon, left colic flexure, the descending colon, the sigmoid colon, and finally the rectum, and parasympathetic afferents from the sacrum ascend to the superior hypogastric plexus via the hypogastric nerves.

Indication: Pelvic visceral cancer pain can be alleviated by blocking the superior hypogastric plexus (Plancarte *et al.* 1990; de Leon-Casasola *et al.* 1993).

Procedure: The patient is placed in a prone position with a pillow beneath the pelvis. The lumbosacral area is prepped in a sterile manner. 22 gauge, 6 inch spinal needles are advanced under fluoroscopic guidance 30° caudad and 45° mesiad from approximately 2 inches from either side of the midline at the L4/5 interspace to lie on the anterolateral aspect of the L5 vertebral body anteriorly. Injection of fluoroscopic dye is used to confirm the location of the needle tip in the retroperitoneal space. At this point after negative aspiration for blood, a total of 20–30 ml of 0.25% bupivacaine with or without a neurolytic agent is injected (Fig. 9.10).

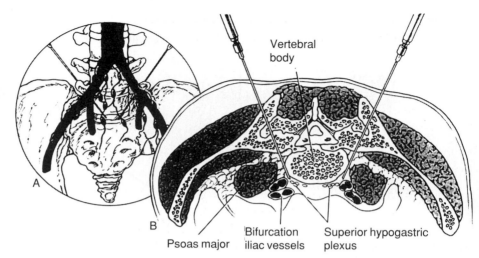

Vertebral body

A

B

Psoas major | Bifurcation iliac vessels | Superior hypogastric plexus

Fig. 9.10 Cross sectional schematic view illustrating bilateral superior hypogastric plexus block and regional anatomy. (From Waldman, S.D. *et al.* (1996). *Interventional pain management* (ed. S.D. Waldman and A.P. Winnie) p. 183. W.B. Saunders, Co., Philadelphia, PA.)

Complications: The complications are similar to those of lumbar sympathetic blocks. Because this block is performed at a lower vertebral level than that for lumbar sympathetic nerve block, the risk of damage to the artery of Adamkiewicz is minimal. Spread of the solution laterally from the anterolateral border of the bodies could result in damage to the genitofemoral nerve.

Interpleural block

Indications: Interpleural analgesia is indicated for pain relief in cancer relating to pancreas, kidney, breast, lung, mesothelioma, and lymphomas. Lung metastases or vertebral body metastases from these tumours might all give rise to pain within the chest cavity (Humphrey *et al.* 1995). Tunneled intrapleural catheters are helpful in the palliation of chronic cancer pain relating to pleuritis, pulmonary fibrosis or pneumonitis (Myers *et al.* 1993; O'Leary and Myers 1997).

Procedure: The patient is placed in a lateral position with the affected side up. An intrapleural catheter is inserted under sterile technique with local anaesthesia and intravenous sedation. The area of insertion is most commonly the T7–8 intercostal space about 3–4 inches from the posterior midline by a technique that allows walking off the top of the rib below. Walking off the top of the rib avoids the intercostal neurovascular bundle and damage to the intercostal nerve. A 17 or 18 gauge Tuohy epidural needle is walked off of the top of the rib and advanced through the intercostal musculature using a loss of resistance technique. Traversing the intercostal membrane, and on entry into the parietal pleura, a loss of resistance is noted. At this point the catheter is introduced through the Tuohy needle about 3–4 inches into the pleural space and the needle is withdrawn over the catheter. A test dose may be used after negative aspiration of blood to prevent an intravascular injection. Subsequently, a local anaesthetic such as 0.25% bupivacaine may be infused in a continuous manner at a rate of 8–10 ml per hour after a bolus dose of 25–50 ml.

Complications: The risk of insertion of such a catheter include pneumothorax, laceration of the intercostal neurovascular bundle, empyema, and formation of a bronchopleural fistula. In addition, local anaesthetic toxicity from an overdose or rapid uptake of local anaesthetic by pulmonary vasculature may occur.

Spinal opioid therapy for malignant pain

The discovery of opioid receptors and opioid compounds in the spinal cord (Pert and Snyder 1973; Hughes *et al.* 1975) provided a rationale for early attempts to deliver opioid drugs intraspinally, first in experimental animals (Yaksh 1978; Yaksh and Rudy 1977) and then in patients with chronic pain (Behar *et al.* 1979; Wang *et al.* 1979). This experience with 'selective spinal analgesia' (Cousins *et al.* 1979) appeared to offer specific benefits to some patients and was followed by trials of continuous spinal opioid infusions using implanted pumps with factory pre-set flow rates (Coombs *et al.* 1981; Onofrio *et al.* 1981). Recent published reports and abstracts in American literature have repeatedly documented the safety and efficacy of implanted non-programmable and programmable pumps for the long-term subarachnoid delivery of opioid drugs in the management of cancer pain (Brazenor 1987; Coombs *et al.* 1983; Krames *et al.* 1985; Shetter *et al.* 1986; Dennis and DeWitty 1987) and nonmalignant pain (Goodman 1981; Varga 1989; Auld *et al.* 1984; Penn and Paice 1987; Barolat *et al.* 1988; Jacobson 1989; Zimmerman and Burchiel 1991; Hassenbusch *et al.* 1991; Krames and Lanning 1993). This documented efficacy, however, may be subject to specific opioid responsive or opioid resistant pain syndromes (Vecht 1989; Arner and Meyerson 1988; Arner and Arner 1989).

Intraspinal opioids: selection criteria for pain of the terminally ill

The selection criteria for the use of intraspinal opioid therapy in patients with cancer related pain is relatively straightforward. Patients with proven opioid responsive pain, who develop intolerable and intractable side-effects after sequential drug trials of strong orally administered opioids are candidates for a trial of infusional spinally administered opioids. Because the cumulative costs of externally administered intrathecal drug infusions (outpatient drug costs, pump costs, nursing costs, etc.) are greater than an implanted system after 3 months (Bedder *et al.* 1989; Lanning and Hrushesky 1990) we recommend that expensive implantable infusion systems be reserved for patients with opioid responsive pain who are going to survive for at least three months. We do not implant intrathecal drug delivery systems in patients who do not have opioid responsive pain such as those with brachial plexopathies or lumbosacral plexus disease or in patients who might have entrapment neuropathies. We recommend that these patients receive epidural analgesia or neuroablative techniques.

If intraspinal analgesic techniques are chosen for these patients, opioids alone may not control the pain. Admixtures of opioids with local anaesthetics and/or clonidine might be effective in patients who do not have opioid responsive pain syndromes.

Trial of spinally administered opioids

There are several approaches to trials for intraspinal opioids. Some practitioners only use the epidural approach, some only the intrathecal approach. Some use daily sequential bolus dosing, increasing the dose daily until the appropriate dose is attained, while others use continuous infusions. Some practitioners believe that the trial should include a single blinded placebo control either given as a bolus or as a continuous infusion. Whatever the method for trial is chosen, it must be adequate for the practitioner to make a rational decision regarding the efficacy of the impending implantation. Questions that must be answered unequivocally include:

- Does the patient's pain respond to opioid therapy?
- Does the patient tolerate the planned intraspinal drug?

A trial should also be designed to mitigate against non specific effects (placebo responses) to the intended therapy. In our practice setting we trial patients by the continuous intrathecal method, as this most accurately mimics the desired end treatment of implanted intrathecal infusion. Because we feel that there is no logic in n-of-one placebo trials, we try, if logistically possible, to extend our continuous intrathecal trial as long as possible to mitigate against the powerful placebo effect of the intrathecal opioid trial. If possible we might trial our patients at least one to two weeks or longer in some patients. During the trial we might, if necessary, do sequential drug trialling of different drugs if our originally intended drug was not efficacious or if there were too many side-effects.

Morphine remains the 'gold standard' of spinally administered opioid therapy because of its long duration of action and relative ease of use. Morphine, the only analgesic approved for intraspinal use, also has history. More is known regarding the use of intraspinal morphine than any other opioid available.

Other opioids such as hydromorphone (Mahler and Forrest 1975; Coombs *et al.* 1986; Shulman *et al.* 1987) meperidine (Maurette *et al.* 1989; Patel *et al.* 1990; Trivedi *et al.* 1990; Thi *et al.* 1992) fentanyl, and sufentanil (Hansdottir *et al.* 1991; Honet *et al.* 1992; Hays and Palmer 1994) have all been used intraspinally, but less is known about these drugs. Although physicians can use these drugs intraspinally, they are not labelled for this use. Time to onset of action, duration of action, uptake and distribution, availability to supraspinal centres and central nervous system side-effects are all governed by the opioids lipid solubility and receptor affinity (Cousins *et al.* 1988a).

Opioids such as morphine with low lipid solubility, enhanced hydrophilicity, and high receptor affinity, cross the dura and enter the substance of the spinal cord slowly but remain bound for prolonged periods of time. Hence, the onset of analgesic action for hydrophilic opioids is slow but the analgesia is generally prolonged. Because of its low lipid solubility and high hydrophilicity, more drug remains in the cerebrospinal fluid and therefore is available to ascend to supraspinal centres through bulk flow of cerebrospinal fluid. Therefore placement of an intrathecal catheter for infusion of a drug anywhere in the thecal sac ensures analgesia anywhere in the body. Risks of cerebrospinal fluid side-effects such as sedation, nausea, and vomiting and respiratory depression are greater when using drugs in this hydrophilic group than in those with higher lipid solubility and higher receptor affinity such as fentanyl and sufentanil.

As expected from its physico-chemical properties, lipophilic drugs such as sufentanil have a rapid onset of action and a prolonged duration of action. Once receptors are saturated with sufentanil, drug becomes available for redistribution through spinal vessel uptake and cerebrospinal fluid bulk flow. Over-sedation may then become a problem. Because lipophilic agents enter the substance of the lipid-containing spinal cord rapidly, and are quickly eliminated from the cerebrospinal fluid, catheter tip placement is essential for optimal analgesia. If lipophilic agents are to be used the intraspinal catheter tip should be placed close to the spinal cord processing and modulating the patients pain as close as possible. Placing the catheter tip over the spinal cord, however, is not without risk of disastrous neurological consequences; in certain rare instances, a granulomatous mass, growing around and including the catheter tip, might develop (North *et al*. 1991; Aldrete *et al*. 1994).

The appropriate dose of an opioid for epidural or intrathecal use depends on the patient's age, pain syndrome, and the systemic dose of the drug, needed for analgesia before the decision to move to intraspinal delivery. As a general rule, patients with neuropathic pain may require higher doses than those with nociceptive pain, and the elderly require fewer doses than younger patients. However, the dosing in all patients should be individualized. Patients with neuropathic pain may require admixtures of opioid and local anaesthetic and/or clonidine for effective relief.

It may be necessary to use other opioid agents besides morphine, even though these agents are not labelled for intraspinal use. Some patients do not tolerate morphine, but may tolerate other hydrophilic agents such as hydromorphone. Sometimes, we may want to use more lipophilic agents such as sufentanil to decrease super-spinal effects such as severe nausea. Because patients on higher systemic opioid doses usually require higher doses of spinally administered opioids than those on lower doses of oral opioids, some clinicians withdraw their patients from all narcotic treatment one to two weeks prior to a trial. This is not our practice. We feel that these 'drug holidays' are unnecessary; they are invariably painful to the patients if alternative pain relief such as epidural anaesthetic blockade is not offered. It is expensive and proof of success of drug holidays in reducing medication requirement for prolonged intervals of time is lacking in both the literature and our experience.

During the trial, the patient's timed oral opioid medications are reduced and the patient is allowed as required medication for breakthrough pain. At the start of the trial we give our patients 50% of their oral opioid requirement as intrathecal infusion and 50% as oral administration. Each successive day of the trial, the oral administration is reduced by 20% and the intrathecal administration is increased by 20%. Complete conversion from high dose oral or systemic opioids to spinally administered opioid will sometimes result in withdrawal symptoms (Tung *et al*. 1980; Messahel and Tomlin 1981).

Because of the length of the trial we most often perform these trials as outpatients after observing our patients for a period of 24 hours in the hospital. We use fluoroscopically-guided 24 gauge paediatric, catheters for our trial, placing our patients on pre and post procedure antibiotic coverage. Because these trials are performed outside of the hospital setting, home infusion for pump rental, nursing, and drug preparation are essential.

Intraspinal admixtures

If patients do not respond to sequential intraspinal opioid trials with different opioids, admixtures combining an opioid with a local anaesthetic and/or alpha adrenergic agent may be considered especially in patients with neuropathic pain. Admixtures of morphine hydrochloride with bupivacaine hydrochloride or clonidine hydrochloride have been shown to be stable in reservoir bags for up to 90 days (Wulf *et al*. 1994).

The addition of bupivacaine to opioids for continuous infusion is both safe and clinically useful. Animal toxicity and human post-mortem studies suggest clinical safety with the long term infusion of intrathecal bupivacaine at the low doses used (Kroin *et al*. 1987; Sjoberg *et al*. 1992). However, there are other reports in both the animal and human clinical literature of potential neural toxicity of local anaesthetic agents when used over long periods. One study showed neurotoxicity after subarachnoid infusions of bupivacaine, lidocaine, and 2-chloroprocaine in a chronic rat model (Li *et al*. 1985). These neurotoxic effects were related to both dose and duration and bupivacaine appeared to have a lesser effect then either lignocaine or tetracaine. There are also reports in the anaesthesia literature of permanent neurological damage, specifically the cauda-equina syndrome, when local anaesthetic (5% lignocaine) was used in concentrations needed for spinal anaesthesia, particularly when delivered through small-bore intrathecal catheters (Rigler *et al*. 1991). It is unclear whether this significant clinical complication was related to the drug, catheter, technique, or a combination of factors. One report suggests that no tachyphylaxis occurred with prolonged continuous spinal infusions of bupivacaine (Raj *et al*. 1986).

Positive analgesic responses with the use of local anaesthetic-opioid intraspinal mixtures for the treatment of cancer and non-cancer related pain have been reported (Coombs *et al*. 1982; Tanelian and Cousins 1989; Berde *et al*. 1990; Nitescu *et al*. 1990; DuPen and Williams 1992; Krames and Lanning 1993). At our institution, when patients no longer receive adequate analgesia with an arbitrary ceiling of 20 mg of intrathecal morphine (or its equivalent with other opioids) we add bupivacaine to the morphine. The usual starting dose is 7 mg bupivacaine per day. The dose of opioid is kept stable at 20 mg morphine or its equivalent and the bupivacaine is increased by 20% per week until analgesia or side-effects occur. According to Van Dongen *et al*. (1993) neurologic side-effects to intrathecal bupivacaine do not occur before 25 mg are infused per 24 hours.

We have been using clonidine in patients who have failed to respond to the addition of bupivacaine to the opioid. Our usual starting dose is 25 ug/day with the dose being titrated upwards by 20% per week until efficacy or side-effects develop. As with the bupivacaine, the clonidine is increased whilst the opioid dose remains constant.

Clonidine, an alpha-2 adrenergic receptor agonist, used intrathecally or epidurally in animal studies and in humans has been shown to provide potent analgesia whether used alone or in combination with intraspinal opioids. Clonidine is experimental and is not approved for clinical use in the USA. Maeyaert and Kupers (1993) reported the use of intrathecal clonidine and morphine in patients with nonmalignant pain syndromes including both neuropathic and nociceptive pain. Their diagnoses included failed back surgery syndrome, ankylosing spondylitis, reflex sympathetic dystrophy, pelvic pain, etc. Twenty four patients were given 20–120 ug/day of intrathecal clonidine for a mean of 14 months. These investigators found that the addition of clonidine to morphine produced significantly better pain relief than the opioid alone. Other authors have found that combining the alpha-2 adrenergic receptor drug, clonidine, with a mu receptor ligand provides more profound analgesia at a lower dose than would be expected if either drug were given alone (Spaulding *et al.* 1979; Wilcox *et al.* 1987; Eisenach *et al.* 1989; Kitahata 1989). This phenomenon of one drug adding to the effect of another is called 'synergy'.

Animal models of neuropathic pain have demonstrated antinociception with treatment by intrathecal clonidine and other alpha 2 agonists (Yaksh and Reddy 1981). Clonidine appears to block substance P release at the presynaptic receptor and blocks the firing of the second order nociceptive neuron. Clonidine acts primarily at the spinal cord level where noradrenaline receptors are found (Spaulding *et al.* 1981) but may also have supraspinal effects at the rostral ventral medulla, especially with oral administration. Clonidine's ability to stimulate alpha-2 adrenoreceptors in the brain stem to reduce sympathetic outflow has been used for years in the treatment of hypertension.

Daily intrathecal dosages in humans have ranged from 3–60 ug/kg. Filos *et al.* (1994) studied the analgesic effect of 150, 300, or 450 ug clonidine given intrathecally after caesarean section to 30 women with general anaesthesia. Good analgesia was noted immediately for up to 80 minutes post-operatively. Currently, a multicentre protocol is being conducted in the US using infusion rates of continuous intrathecal clonidine via implanted infusion devices from 0.7–4 ug/hr. Clonidine in 150 or 500 ug/ml in 20 ml vials will be used to fill the intrathecal pumps (unpublished observations).

Studies in different animals and humans have demonstrated no neuropathology after intraspinal clonidine. The main side-effect of clonidine given intrathecally is hypotension. Humans may also experience decreases in heart rate. Electrolytes, glucose, and cortisol levels were found to be stable in humans after infusion of clonidine (Eisenach *et al.* 1989). Other side-effects include dry mouth, drowsiness, dizziness, and constipation. Sudden withdrawal of clonidine can precipitate agitation and hypertension.

Clonidine may be useful in facilitating a spinal mu receptor holiday in patients who have become tolerant to high doses of opioids (Coombs *et al.* 1985). Clonidine may also be effective in neuropathic pain (Eisenach 1993; DuPen *et al.* 1993) and sympathetically mediated pain syndromes.

Complications relating to intrathecal drug infusion pumps

Complications of intraspinal opioids

The side-effects of opioid infusions include nausea, vomiting, urinary retention, generalized pruritus, constipation, over sedation, confusion, hyperalgesia/myoclonus syndrome, ménière-like symptoms, nystagmus, herpes reactivation, polyarthalgia, amenorrhoea, or peripheral oedema (Malone *et al.* 1985; Levy 1990; Sjoberg *et al.* 1991; Erdine and Yucel 1994). An attempt should be made to manage these symptoms pharmacologically before switching to another spinal agent. Respiratory depression although a known consequence in opioid naïve patients (Von Roenn *et al.* 1991; Coyle and Foley 1991) is rarely seen in patients tolerant to opioids due to extensive prior use. Tolerance to one opioid analgesic does not necessarily mean tolerance to all. Analgesia can be restored by switching to a different opioid at about half the equivalent dose.

Complications of intrathecal pump implantation

Some of the complications associated with the technique of surgical implantation of drug infusion pumps are bleeding leading to epidural haematoma, spinal cord compression, and cauda equina syndrome leading to paresis and/or bowel and bladder dysfunction. Surgical infections can lead to disastrous consequences. Therefore, strict adherence to sterile technique, preoperative antibiotics and intraoperative antibiotic irrigation are mandatory. If infection involves the implant, failure to remove it can lead to persistence and spread of the infection. Intrathecal and epidural infections should be treated aggressively.

Damage to vital tissues such as nerve rootlets, the conus medularis, or spinal cord can lead to complications such as radiculitis, myelitis, paresis, loss of bowel and bladder control, myelopathic pain, even paraplegia. Long term catheter placement close to the substance of the spinal cord may lead to the growth of non-specific expanding sterile masses around the catheter tip with resultant cord compression and myelopathy. Inappropriate tunnelling technique may damage organs in the thoracic or abdominal cavity with associated peritonitis.

Cerebrospinal fluid leaks can occur around the intrathecal catheter. This may lead to a post-dural puncture, headache, and may lead to cerebrospinal spinal fluid hygromas, a subcutaneous collection of cerebrospinal fluid surrounding the catheter. Most of these hygromas last approximately 2–4 weeks. Repeated draining of the fluid is unnecessary and may lead to contamination of the fluid.

The incidence of pump pocket seromas can be reduced by using abdominal binders but, as with hygromas, seromas too are self limiting. Mechanical catheter complications include breaking, movement, kinking, disconnection, and obstruction at the tip. If the pump has a side port, simple injection of non-ionic contrast dye or technetium 84 very carefully into the side port may help in the diagnosis. It is important to remember to aspirate from the side port before injecting because the catheter system may contain highly concentrated drug that, when pushed into the intrathecal space, could lead to unwanted neurologic events.

Complications of pump maintenance

Overfilling, battery failure, pump failure, hybrid failure, and torsion or flipping of a freely movable pump can occur. The normal battery life of a programmable pump depends on the flow rate. Normally, the pump battery should last from 3–5 years. Drug and pump incompatibility such as seen with meperidine, a pH incompatibility problem, can lead to corrosion of the pump's internal mechanical delivery systems. Flipping of a pump makes it impossible to fill. Anchoring of the pump to fascia or placing the pump within a provided-for dacron pouch may prevent its movement within the pocket.

The pump must be refilled through the central fill port, not fill through the side port. Any injection of drug into the catheter side port can lead to overdose, morbidity, and death. Overdose due to intrathecal opioids can cause muscle rigidity, seizures, hypertension, cardiovascular collapse, and severe respiratory depression. Reprogramming errors can be reduced by checking and rechecking the programmer's work before discharging the patient.

Other methods of neuraxial drug administration

Percutaneous temporary epidural catheters are useful for managing pain in patients with a limited prognosis—less than one month (see Fig. 9.11). They are also useful in

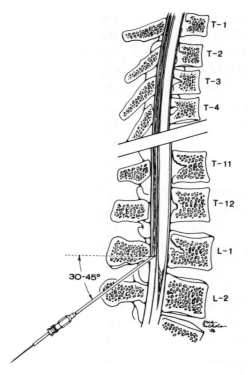

Fig. 9.11 Insertion of catheter and wire-guide stylet. Paramedian epidural needle position facilitates epidural catheter threading. (From Waldman, S.D. *et al.* (1996). *Interventional pain management* (ed. S.D. Waldman and A.P. Winnie) p. 183. W.B. Saunders, Co., Philadelphia, PA.)

the management of perioperative pain. A disadvantage of these methods is associated migration, kinking, dislodgement or other mechanical problems. Chronic use carries with it the risk of infection, especially in immunocompromised patients.

Continuous epidural analgesia with either local anaesthetics, clonidine, or opioids, or combinations of any of the above are indicated only in patients where less invasive therapies fail to provide analgesia or where systemic adminstration of opioids is associated with a high level of intractable side-effects such as dysphoria, severe, intractable nausea and vomiting, hallucinations, or over-sedation. Patients with brachial or lumbo-sacral plexus metastases or patients with tumours involving peripheral nerves might develop pain that is non-opioid responsive. These patients may respond to continuous epidural infusion of local anaesthetics or combinations of opioids with local anaesthetics and or clonidine.

Permanent silicone-rubber epidural catheters have been used as a cost-effective method for neuraxial administration of opioids, clonidine, and local anaesthetics. Implantation of the catheter can be performed under local anaesthesia and intravenous sedation. Drug delivery by bolus injections, continuous infusion, and/or patient controlled administration is left up to the discretion of the physician. The risk of dislodgement and infection is lower with these ports when comparing them to percutaneous temporary catheters (Dejong and Kansen 1994; DuPen *et al.* 1990). However, in patients who only have a few days of life expectancy, temporary epidural catheters that are not tunnelled will suffice.

Subcutaneous implanted injection ports have more stability in the subcutaneous tissue and are less likely to be mechanically dislodged than temporary catheters (Dejong and Kansen 1994). In the US they have only been approved for epidural administration, however they can be used effectively for intrathecal infusion. Because the skin over them comprises a relatively small area, these parts carry the risk of potential infection and subcutaneous fibrosis.

Neurolysis

Neurolysis, or destruction of neural tissue may be performed surgically, chemically using neurodestructive chemical agents, thermally with radio frequency, or by freezing with cryoneurolysis. A careful selection of patients and a thorough understanding of the pathophysiology of the specific malignancy may help determine the appropriate modality of neurolysis.

Chemical neurolytic agents

Several neurolytic agents may be used for neurolysis. Commercially available preparations of absolute ethyl alcohol, phenol, or glycerol are available. Ammonium compounds and hypertonic solutions have been tried in the past but are not used as much as the above mentioned agents. Absolute (100%) alcohol is available in the United States. Alcohol is a clear colourless fluid which absorbs water on exposure to air. It is stable at room temperature. Our practice uses alcohol in this undiluted form. Alcohol acts by precipitation of the proteins in neural tissue and extraction of phospholipids and cholesterol resulting in neural degeneration. If used intrathecally, as in subarachnoid alcohol neurolysis, alcohol is relatively hypobaric and therefore rises in the cerebrospinal fluid after injection (Fig. 9.12); because of this, correct positioning of a patient undergoing alcohol subarachnoid neurolysis is essential. Alcohol may also be used for neurolysis of the trigeminal and glossopharyngeal ganglia as well as coeliac, lumbar, and superior hypogastric sympathetic gangliolysis. Alcohol neurolysis is extremely painful and is usually, except in subarachnoid neurolysis, preceded by injection of local anaesthetic to block the area before the injection of alcohol. Alcohol is known to cause spasm of adjacent vasculature resulting in vasospasm.

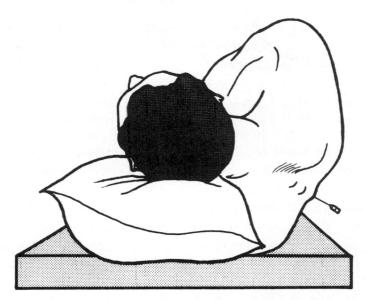

Fig. 9.12 Proper positioning of the patient with left-sided pain for intrathecal injection of phenol in glycerine. (From Waldman, S.D. *et al.* (1996). *Interventional pain management* (ed. S.D. Waldman and A.P. Winnie) p. 183. W.B. Saunders, Co., Philadelphia, PA.)

Phenol is also available in the United States. Phenol is a clear, colourless poorly soluble solution that is unstable at room temperature. In lower concentrations phenol acts as a local anaesthetic, but at higher concentrations it is neurodestructive. Phenol therefore lacks the local algesic properties of alcohol. Commonly used phenol concentrations in our practice vary between 6–10%. Unlike alcohol phenol is hyperbaric relative to the cerebrospinal fluid; when using phenol in subarachnoid phenol neurolysis, patient positioning is also of vital concern (Fig. 9.13). Phenol has an affinity for vascular structures and is therefore a less preferred choice than alcohol when considering transaortic coeliac plexus blocks. Complications relating to phenol include cardiac and liver toxicity. Both phenol and alcohol have been used for neurolysis of peripheral nerves, but both may cause peripheral neuritis. The incidence of peripheral neuritis is greater when alcohol is used (Katz 1974; Cousins *et al.* 1988*b*).

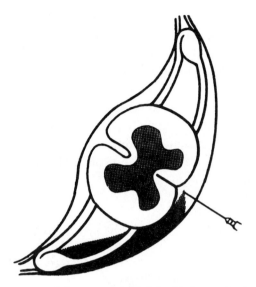

Fig. 9.13 Proper positioning of the patient with left-sided pain for intrathecal injection of phenol in glycerine. (From Waldman, S.D. *et al.* (1996). *Interventional pain management* (ed. S.D. Waldman and A.P. Winnie) p. 183. W.B. Saunders, Co., Philadelphia, PA.)

Glycerol, although not generally conceived as neurotoxic, has been used for trigeminal neurolysis, causing Wallerian degeneration of the ganglion (Hakanson 1981).

Radio-frequency thermocoagulation

Radio-frequency thermocoagulation uses a radio-frequency generator connected to a grounding dispersion pad and radio-frequency probe electrical cables. The radio-frequency generator has the ability to measure the electrode current, voltage, impedance, probe temperature, time of lesioning, and is usually accompanied with a nerve stimulator to locate the desired neural tissue to be destroyed (Fig. 9.14). Radio-frequency current heats tissue surrounding the non-insulated tip which in turn raises the temperature of the electrode tip causing a thermal lesion. The average lesion is ellipsoid and the dimensions may vary from 3–10 mm depending upon the current, the time of use, and the size of the lesioning tip of the probe or needle.

Indications: Radio-frequency thermocoagulation is indicated where neurodestruction of central neural tissues is indicated and when the tissue to be destroyed is accessible to placement of the radio-frequency probe or needle. Radio-frequency thermocoagulation has been used for neurolysis of central neural fibres while cryoneurolysis is a preferred choice for peripheral neural fibres. Radio-frequency thermocoagulation has been used for thermal lesioning of the Gasserian trigeminal ganglion (Sweet and Wepsic 1974; Broggi *et al*. 1990), neural enervation of cervical, thoracic, and lumbar facet joints (Savitz 1991; Sluijter 1990; Mehta and Sluijter 1979; Sluijter and Mehta 1981; Stolker *et al*. 1993), sacroiliac joints (Laslett and Williams 1994), the cervical and thoracic sympathetic chain (Wilkinson 1984a, b; Geurts and Stolker 1993), the lumbar sympathetic chain (Pernak 1995; Noe and Haynesworth 1993), and cervical, thoracic, lumbar, and

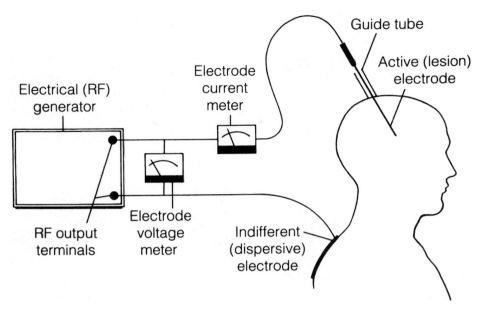

Fig. 9.14 The basic radiofrequency (RF) lesioning circuit. (From Waldman, S.D. *et al.* (1996). *Interventional pain management* (ed. S.D. Waldman and A.P. Winnie) p. 183. W.B. Saunders, Co., Philadelphia, PA.)

sacral dorsal root ganglia (Van Kleef *et al.* 1993, 1995). Most recently, there have been reports of thermal lesioning of the intradiscal nucleus in patients with discogenic pain of cervical and lumbar discs (Troussier *et al.* 1995). Although this approach to disc pain is compelling, as the alternative interventional treatment is fusion, only small numbers of patients have been reported. Much more needs to be known before this treatment can or should be applied to all patients with this disease.

Procedure: Radio-frequency thermocoagulation requires the use of a radio-frequency generator and nerve stimulator and various radio-frequency insulated needles and/or probes. Sterile technique should be meticulously observed throughout the procedure. These procedures are performed under local anaesthesia, intravenous sedation, and fluoroscopic guidance (as described for the various blocks above). Location is everything and therefore, before undertaking these procedures the surgeon must be knowledgeable of appropriate neuroanatomy and fluoroscopic anatomic relationships in all X-ray projections including the anteroposterior, oblique, and lateral projections.

Once the needle tip has been located anatomically and fluoroscopically appropriate sensory and motor testing of the target is mandatory. Sensory testing of the tip of the probe or needle in relationship to the neural target is performed at 50 Hz. If the needle is in the appropriate position and close to the intended target the patient will experience pain at less than 0.5 volts at 50 Hz of stimulation. To guard against destroying vital motor function, the intended target is stimulated at 2 Hz. If motor stimulation occurs at voltage less than 3 × the voltage necessary for sensory stimulation, the needle tip is located too close to vital motor fibres and lesioning might result in motor deficit. If motor stimulation does occur at voltage less than 3 × the voltage necessary for sensory stimulation, the needle must be moved and the sensory and motor testing must be repeated.

Local anaesthetic is injected through the needles prior to the radio-frequency thermo-coagulation. In our practice we use 0.5 ml of 4% lignocaine to block the intended target temporarily before lesioning. Average times and temperatures may vary between patients and the site of neurodestruction intended. For a thorough guide to radio-frequency thermocoagulation it is suggested that the reader read a review of this topic (Ray 1982).

Cryoneurolysis

Equipment: A cryoprobe has an inner and an outer tube. High pressure N_2O or CO_2 is passed via the outer tube to a cooling chamber and returns via the inner tube. This process expands the gas and rapidly cools the tip of the probe to $-70\,°C$. The cryoprobe should be tested prior to use within a patient. When the probe is tested in a cup of sterile water, an ice ball forms at the tip of the probe within seconds (Fig. 9.15).

Indications: Unlike radio-frequency thermal neurolysis cryoneurolysis may be used for neurolysis of peripheral nerves. Cryoneurolysis has been used for temporary cryo-destruction of several spinal pain generators such as those arising from the spinal facet joints. Neuromas of the ilioinguinal and iliohypogastric nerves that arise after surgery can be denervated using cryoanalgesia. Pain arising from damage to the coccyx may be treated with cryoneurolysis of the coccygeal nerve (Trescott 1994). Pain emanating from the branches of the trigeminal nerve can be relieved with cryoneurolysis of these branches (Barnard *et al*. 1978). Duration of relief with cryoneurolysis lasts approximately 3–6 months but may vary in individual cases (Evans 1981; Holden 1975; Lloyd *et al*. 1976).

Procedure: The procedure is carried out under sterile conditions. Appropriate placement of the probe adjacent to the neural target is guided by fluoroscopy if appropriate and by sensory testing. Local anaesthesia after sensory testing and intravenous sedation ensure comfort of the patient. An angiocath, appropriate to the size of the probe used, is passed down through prepped skin toward the intended target. The needle is withdrawn and the angiocath cannula is left in place. A cryoprobe is placed through this cannula and is carefully advanced to make contact with the intended target. The probe tip is supplied with a nerve stimulator and is used to test the nerve at both 50 Hz and 2 Hz similar to the manner described for radio-frequency. Cryolesioning occurs over 2 cycles, each one consisting of 60–120 seconds on and 30–60 seconds off. Pain relief can vary anywhere from 2 weeks to 2 months (Holden 1975; Lloyd *et al*. 1976).

Conclusions

This chapter addresses some of the key issues regarding more complex interventional techniques for the treatment of cancer pain. We have discussed more complex nerve

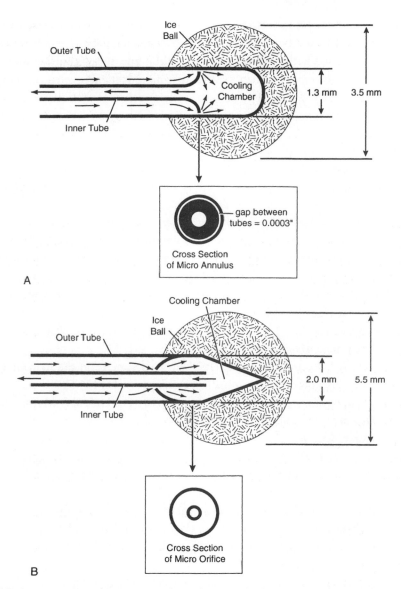

Fig. 9.15 Cross-sections of two commonly used cryoprobe designs. A and B. High-pressure gas goes in through the outer tube at 650–800 lb/in². Low-pressure gas is vented out at 80–100 lb/in². Gas flow is at 7–9 L/min. Test conditions: tip is inserted into water at 36 +/– 1°C; an ice ball is formed within 60 seconds.

blocks and the use of implanted spinal drug delivery systems for the relief of cancer pain not relieved by more conservative therapies recommended by the World Health Organization guidelines. Choosing a treatment for patients suffering cancer-related pain should follow the KISS principle, 'keep it sweet and simple'. The World Health Organization 'ladder approach' obeys this important principle, but fails to offer therapies to patients when the guidelines have failed. It is our firm belief that the therapies discussed within this chapter offer alternatives to physicians and other caregivers treating cancer patients when the WHO guidelines have failed. These therapies, though invasive have been shown to offer pain relief to patients suffering from intractable cancer pain and therefore should be used before abandoning the suffering patient. We hope that the knowledge contained within this chapter will add immeasurably to the 'tools of the trade' for physicians treating patients suffering from cancer pain.

References

Aldrete, J.A., Vascello, L.A., Ghaly, R., and Tomlin, D. (1994). Paraplegia in a patient with an intrathecal catheter and a spinal cord stimulator. *Anesthesiology*, **81**, 1542–5.

Arner, S., and Arner, B. (1989). Differential effects of epidural morphine in the treatment of cancer related pain. *Acta Anesthesiologica Scandinavica*, **29**, 332–6.

Arner, S., and Meyerson, B. (1988). Lack of analgesic effect of opioids on neuropathic and idiopathic forms of pain. *Pain*, **33**, 11–23.

Arter, O., and Racz, G.B. (1990). Pain management of the oncologic patient. *Seminars in Surgical Oncology*, **6**, 162–5.

Auld, A.W., Maki-Jokela, A., and Murdoch, D.M. (1984). Intraspinal narcotic analgesia in the treatment of chronic pain. *Spine*, **10**, 777–81.

Barnard, J., Lloyd, J., and Green, C. (1978–9). Cryosurgery in the management of intractable facial pain. *British Journal of Oral Surgery*, **16**, 135–7.

Barolat, G., Schwartzman, R., and Woo, R. (1989). Epidural spinal cord stimulation in the management of reflex sympathetic dystrophy. *Stereotactic and Functional Neurosurgery*, **53**, 29–31.

Barolat, G., Schwartzman, R.J., and Aries, L. (1988). Chronic intrathecal morphine infusion for intractable pain in reflex sympathetic dystrophy. *Proceedings of the American and Canadian Pain Societies*, **17**.

Bedder, M.D., Burchiel, J.K., and Larson, A. (1989). Cost analysis of two implantable narcotic delivery systems. *Proceedings of the American Pain Society*, **70**, 142.

Behar, M., Magora, F., Olshwang, D., and Davidson, J.T. (1979). Epidural morphine in treatment of pain. *Lancet*, **1**, 527.

Berde, C.B., Sethna, N.F., Conrad, L.S., Hershenson, M.B., and Shillito, J. Jr. (1990). Subarachnoid bupivacaine analgesia for seven months for a patient with a spinal cord tumor. *Anesthesiology*, **72**, 1094–6.

Bonica, J.J. (1990). Cancer pain. In *The management of pain* (ed. Lea and Febiger Malvern), pp. 400–60. Malvern, Pennsylvania.

Boring, C.C., Squire, T.S., and Tong, T. (1994). Cancer statistics 1994. *CA Cancer J Clin*, **44**, 7–26.

Brazenor, G.A. (1987). Long-term intrathecal administration of morphine: a comparison of bolus injection via reservoir with continuous infusion by implanted pump. *Neurosurgery*, **21**, 484–91.

Broggi, G., Franzini, A., Lasio, G., Giorgi, C., and Servello, D. (1990). Long-term results of percutaneous retrogasserian thermorhizotomy for 'essential' trigeminal neurologia. *Insitito Neurologico C. Besta*, 26–8.

Brown, D.L., Bulley, C.K., and Quiel, E.L. (1987). Neurolytic celiac plexus block for pancreatic cancer pain. *Anesthesia and Analgesia*, **66**, 869–73.

Brown, D.L. (1989). A retrospective analysis of neurolytic celiac plexus block for non-pancreatic intra-abdominal cancer pain. *Regional Anesthesia*, **14**, 63–5.

Burkel, W.E., and McPhee, M. (1970). Effect of phenol injection into peripheral nerve of rat: Electron microscope studies. *Archives of Physical Medicine and Rehabilitation*, **51**, 391–5.

Coombs, D.W., Colburn, R.W., DeLeo, J.A., Hoopes, P.J., and Twitchell, B.B. (1994). Comparative spinal neuropathology of hydromorphone and morphine after 9 and 30 day epidural administration in sheep. *Anesthesia and Analgesia*, **78**, 674–81.

Coombs, D.W., Pageau, M.G., Saunders, R.L., and Mroz, W.T. (1982). Intraspinal narcotic tolerance: preliminary experience with continuous bupivacaine HCL infusion via implanted infusion device. *International Journal of Artificial Organs*, **5**, 379–82.

Coombs, D.W., Saunders, R.L., Fratkin, J.D., Jensen, L.E., and Murphy, C.A. (1986). Continuous intrathecal hydromorphone and clonidine for intractable cancer pain. *Journal of Neurosurgery*, **64**, 890–4.

Coombs, D.W., Saunders, R.L., Gaylor, M., and Pageau, M.G. (1981). Epidural narcotic infusion: implantation technique and efficacy. *Anesthesiology*, **55**, 469–75.

Coombs, D.W., Saunders R.L., and Gaylor, M. (1983). Relief of continuous chronic pain by intraspinal narcotics infusion via an implanted reservoir. *Journal of the American Medical Association*, **250**, 2336–9.

Coombs, D.W., Saunders, R.L., Lachance, D., Savage, S., Ragnarsson, T.S., and Jensen, L.E. (1985). Intrathecal morphine tolerance; use of clonidine, DADLE, and intraventricular morphine. *Anesthesiology*, **62**, 358–63.

Cousins, M.J., and Bridenbaugh, P.O., 1987; Patt, 1993; Raj, 1992: Nonpharmacologic interventions: invasive therapies. Clinical practice guideline number 9; In *Management of Cancer Pain*, 95–9.

Cousins, M.J., Cherry, D.A., and Gourlay, G.K. (1988a). Acute and chronic pain: use of spinal opioids. In *Neural blockade in clinical anesthesia and management of pain*, (ed. M.J. Cousins and P.O. Bridenbaugh) (2nd edn), pp. 955–1029. J.B. Lippincott, Philadelphia.

Cousins, M.J., Dwyer, B., and Gibb, D. (1988b). Chronic pain and neurolytic neural blockade. In *Neural blockade* (ed. M.J. Cousins and P.O. Bridenbaugh) (2nd edn), pp. 1053–84. J.B. Lippincott, Philadelphia.

Cousins, M.J., Mather, L.E., Glynn, C.J., Wilson, P.R., and Graham, J.R. (1979). Selective spinal analgesia. *Lancet*, **1**, 1141–2.

Coyle, N., and Foley, K.M. (1991). Alterations in comfort: pain. In *Cancer pain nursing* (ed. S.B. Baird, R. McCorkle, and M. Grant), pp. 782–91. Saunders, Philadelphia.

Davidson, B.J., Hsu, T.C., and Schantz, S.P. (1991). The genetics of tobacco-induced cancer susceptibility. *Cancer Epidemiologic Bio-markers Preview*, **1**, 83–9.

de Leon-Casasola, O.A., Kent, E., and Lema, M.J. (1993). Neurolytic superior hypogastric plexus block for chronic pelvic pain associated with cancer. *Pain*, **54**, 145–51.

DeJong, P.C., and Kansen, P.J. (1994). A comparison of epidural catheters with or without subcutaneous injection ports for treatment of cancer pain. *Regional Anesthesia*, **78**, 94–100.

Dennis, G.C., and DeWitty, R.L. (1987). Management of intractable pain in cancer patients by implantable morphine infusion systems. *Journal of the National Medical Association*, **79**, 939–44.

Du Pen, S.L., Peterson, D.G., Williams, A., and Bogosian, A.J. (1990). Infection during chronic epidural catheterization. Diagnosis and treatment. *Anesthesiology*, **73**, 905–9.

DuPen, S.L., Eisenach, J.C., Allin, D., and Zaccaro, D. (1993). Epidural clonidine for intractable cancer pain. *Regional Anesthesia Supplement*, **18**, (45), 7–8.

DuPen, S.L., and Williams, A.R. (1992). Management of patients receiving combined epidural morphine and bupivacaine for the treatment of cancer pain. *Journal of Pain and Symptom Management*, **27**, 125–7.

Eisenach, J.C., Rauck, R.L., Buzzanell, C., and Lysak, S.Z. (1989). Epidural clonidine analgesia for intractable cancer pain: phase 1. *Anesthesiology*, **71**, 647–52.

Eisenach, J.C. (1993). Overview: First International symposium on alpha-2 adrenergic mechanisms of spinal anesthesia. *Regional Anesthesia*, **18**, 1–4.

Erdine, S., and Yucel, A. (1994). Long-term results of intrathecal morphine in 65 patients. *The Pain Clinic*, **7**, 27–30.

Evans, P. (1981). Cryoanalgesia: The application of low temperatures to nerves to produce anesthesia or analgesia. *Anaesthesia*, **36**, 1003–13.

Filos, K.S., Goudas, L.C., Patroni O., and Polyzoo, V. (1994). Hemodynamic and analgesic profile after intrathecal clonidine in humans. *Anesthesiology*, **81**, 591–601.

Foley, K.M. (1985). Treatment of cancer pain. *The New England Journal of Medicine*, **313**, 84–95.

Galizea, E.J., and Lahiri, S.K. (1974). Paraplegia following coeliac plexus block with phenol. *British Journal of Anaesthesia*, **46**, 539–40.

Geurts, J.W.M., and Stolker, R.J. (1993). Percutaneous radiofrequency lesion of the stellate ganglion in the treatment of pain in upper extremity reflex sympathetic dystrophy. *The Pain Clinic*, **6**, 17–25.

Gissen, A.J., Datta, S., and Lamber, D. (1984). The chloroprocaine controversy. II. Is chloroprocaine neurotoxic? *Regional Anesthesia*, **9**, 135.

Goodman, R.R. (1981). Treatment of lower extremity reflex sympathetic dystrophy with continuous intrathecal morphine infusion. *Applied Neurophysiology*, **50**, 425–6.

Hakanson, S. (1981). Trigeminal neuralgia treated by the injection of glycerol into the trigeminal cistern. *Neurosurgery*, **9**, 638–9.

Hansdottir, V., Hedner, T., Woestenborghs, R., and Nordberg, G. (1991). The CSF and plasma pharmacokinetics of sufentanil after intrathecal administration. *Anesthesiology*, **74**, 264–9.

Hassenbusch, S.J., Stanton-Hicks, M.D., Soukup, J., Covington, E.C., and Boland,

M.B. (1991). Sufentanil citrate and morphine/bupivacaine as alternative agents in chronic epidural infusions for intractable non-cancer pain. *Neurosurgery*, **29**, 76–82.

Haymaker, W., and Woodhall, B. (1945). *Peripheral nerve injuries*, Saunders, Philadelphia.

Hays, R.L., and Palmer, C.M. (1994). Respiratory depression after intrathecal sufentanil during labor. *Anesthesiology*, **81**, 511–2.

Hegedus, V. (1979). Relief of pancreatic pain by radiography guided block. *American Journal of Radiology*, **133**, 1101–2.

Holden, H.B. (1975). *Practical cryosurgery*. Pitman Medical Publishers, London.

Honet, J.E., Arkoosh, V.A., Norris, M.C., Huffnagle, H.J., Silverman, N.S., and Leighton, B.L. (1992). Comparison among intrathecal fentanyl, meperidine and sufentanil for labor analgesia. *Anesthesia and Analgesia*, **75**, 734–9.

Hughes, J., Smith, T.W., Kosterlitz, H.W., Fothergill, L.A., Morgan, B.A., and Morris, H.R. (1975). Isolation of two related pentapeptides from brain with potent opiate activity. *Nature*, **258**, 577–9.

Humphrey, E.W., Ward, H.B., and Perri, R.T. (1995). Lung cancer. In *American Cancer Society Textbook of clinical oncology*, pp. 220–35 (2nd edn).

Ischia, S., Ischia, A., Polati E., and Finco, G. (1992). Three posterior percutaneous celiac plexus block techniques. A prospective randomized study in 61 patients with pancreatic cancer pain. *Anesthesiology*, **76**, 534–40.

Jacobson, L. (1989). Clinical note: relief of persistent postamputation stump and phantom limb pain with intrathecal fentanyl. *Pain*, **37**, 317–22.

Katz, J. (1974). Current role of neurolytic agents. *Advanced Neurology*, **4**, 471.

Kitahata, L.M. (1989). Spinal analgesia with morphine and clonidine. *Anesthesia and Analgesia*, **68**, 191–3.

Krames, E.S., and Lanning, R.M. (1993). Intrathecal infusional analgesia for nonmalignant pain: analgesic efficacy of intrathecal with or without bupivacaine. *Journal of Pain and Symptom Management*, **8**, 539–48.

Krames, E.S., Gershow, J., Glassberg, A., Kenefick, T., Lyons, A., Taylor, P., and Wilkie, D. (1985). Continuous infusion of spinally administered narcotics for the relief of pain due to malignant disorders. *Cancer*, **56**, 696–702.

Kroin, J.S., McCarthy, R.J., Penn, R.D., Kerns, J.M., and Ivankovich, A.D. (1987). The effect of chronic subarachnoid bupivacaine infusion in dogs. *Anesthesiology*, **66**, 737–42.

Lanning, R.M., and Hrushesky, W.J.M. (1990). Cost comparison of wearable and implantable drug delivery systems. *Proceedings of American Society of Clinical Oncology*, **9**, 322.

Laslett, M., and Williams, M. (1994). The reliability of selected pain provocation tests for sacroiliac joint pathology. *Spine*, **19**, 1243–9.

Levy, M.H. (1990). Oral controlled-release morphine: guidelines for clinical use. In *Advances in Pain Research and Therapy*, Vol. 14 (ed. C. Benedetti), p. 285. Raven, New York.

Li, D.F., Bahar, M., Cole, G., and Rosen, M. (1985). Neurological toxicity of the subarachnoid infusion of bupivacaine, lignocaine, or 2-chloroprocaine in the rat. *British Journal of Aneasthesia*, **57**, 424–9.

Lloyd, J., Bernard, J., and Glynn, C. (1976). Cryoanalgesia: A new approach to pain relief. *Lancet*, **2**, 932–4.

Lo, J.N., and Buckley, J.J. (1982). Spinal cord ischemia: A complication of celiac plexus block. *Regional Anaesthesia*, **7**, 66–8.

Long, D.M., Erickson, D., Campbell, J., and North, R. (1981). Electrical stimulation of the spinal cord and peripheral nerves for pain control: A ten year experience. *Applied Neurophysiology*, **44**, 207–15.

Maeyaert, J., and Kupers, R. (1993). Intrathecal drug adminstration in the treatment of persistent non-cancer pain: A three years experience. Presented at *Interventional Pain Management*. Dannemiller Memorial Education Foundation, Aug. 15–19, 1993.

Mahler, P.L., and Forrest, W. (1975). Relative analgesic potencies of morphine and hydromorphone in post operative pain. *Anesthesiology*, **42**, 602–7.

Malone, B.T., Beye, R., and Walker, J. (1985). Management of pain in the terminally ill by administration of epidural narcotics. *Cancer*, **55**, 438–41.

Maurette, P., Tauzin-Fin, P., Vincon, G., and Brachet-Lierman, A. (1989). Arterial and ventricular CSF pharmacokinetics after intrathecal meperidine in humans. *Anesthesiology*, **70**, 961–6.

Meglio, M., Cioni, B., and Rossi, G.F. (1989). Spinal cord stimulation in management of chronic pain: a 9-year experience. *Journal of Neurosurgery*, **70**, 519–23.

Mehta, M., and Sluijter, M.E. (1979). The treatment of chronic back pain: A preliminary survey of the effect of the radiofrequency denervation of the posterior vertebral joints. *Anesthesia*, **34**, 768–75.

Messahel, F.M., and Tomlin, P.J. (1981). Narcotic withdrawal syndrome after intrathecal administration of morphine. *British Medical Journal*, **283**, 471–2.

Miller, D.L. (1985). CT guidance for celiac plexus neurolysis: posterior and anterior approaches. *Regional Anesthesia*, **10**, A47.

Moore, D.C., Spierdijk, J., vanKleef, J.D., Coleman, R.L., and Love, G.F. (1982). Chloroprocaine neurotoxicity: four additional cases. *Anesthesia and Analgesia*, **61**, 155–9.

Myers, D.P., Lema, M.J., and DeLeon-Casasola, O.A. (1993). Interpleural analgesia for treatment of severe cancer pain in terminally ill patients. *Journal of Pain and Symptom Management*, **8**, 505–10.

Nitescu, P., Appelgren, L., Linder, L.E., Sjoberg, M., Hultman, E., and Curelaru, I. (1990). Epidural versus intrathecal morphine-bupivacaine: assessment of consecutive treatments in advanced cancer pain. *Journal of Pain and Symptom Management*, **5**, 18–26.

Noe, C.E., and Haynesworth, R.F. (1993). Lumbar radiofrequency sympatholysis. *Journal of Vascular Surgery*, **17**, 801–6.

North, R.B., Kidd, D.H., Zahurak, M., James, C.S., and Long, D.M. (1993). Spinal cord stimulation for chronic intractable pain: experience over two decades. *Neurosurgery*, **32**, 384–95.

North, R.B., Cutchis, P.N., Epstein, J.A., and Long, D.M. (1991). Spinal cord compression complicating subarachnoid infusion of morphine. *Neurosurgery*, **29**, 778–84.

O'Leary, K.A., and Myers, D.P. (1997). Interpleural analgesia and neurolysis. *In Techniques of regional anesthesia and pain management*, Vol. 1, no. 1, 11–17.

Onofrio, B.M., Yaksh, T.L., and Arnold, P.G. (1981). Continuous low dose intrathecal morphine administration in the treatment of chronic pain of malignant origin. *Mayo Clinic Proceedings*, **55**, 469–74.

Patel, D., Janardhan, Y., Merai, B., Robalino, J., and Shevde, K. (1990). Comparison of intrathecal meperidine and lidocaine in endoscopic urologic procedures. *Canadian Journal of Anaesthesia*, **37**, 567–70.

Penn, R.D., and Paice, J.A. (1987). Chronic intrathecal morphine for intractable pain. *Journal of Neurosurgery*, **67**, 182–6.

Pernak, J. (1995). Percutaneous radiofrequency thermal lumbar sympathetectomy. *The Pain Clinic*, **80**, (1), 99–106.

Pert, C.B., and Snyder, S. (1973). Opiate receptors demonstration in nervous tissue. *Science*, **179**, 1011–3.

Plancarte, R., Amescua, C., Patt, R.B., and Aldrete, J.A. (1990). Superior hypogastric plexus block for pelvic cancer pain. *Anesthesiology*, **73**, 236–9.

Portnoy, R.K. (1993). Inadequate outcome of opioid therapy for cancer pain: Influences on practitioners and patients. In *Cancer Pain* (ed. R.B. Patt) pp. 119–28. Lippincott, Philadelphia.

Raj, P.R., Denson, D.D., and de Jong, R.H. (1986). No tachyphylaxis with prolonged, continuous bupivacaine. In *New aspects in regional anaesthesia 4*: major conduction block: tachyphylaxis, hypotension, and opiates (ed. H.J. Wust and M. Stanton-Hicks) pp. 10–18. Springer-Verlag, Berlin, New York.

Ravidrin, R.S., Bond, V.K., Tasch, M.D., Gupta, C.D., and Luerssen, T.G. (1980). Prolonged neural blockade following regional anesthesia with 2-chloroprocaine. *Anesthesia and Analgesia*, **59**, 447–8.

Ray, C.D. (1982). Percutaneous radiofrequency facet nerve block. In *Radionics procedure technique series*, Burlington, MA Radionics Corporation.

Reiz, S., and Nath, S. (1986). Cardiotoxicity of local anesthetic agents. *British Journal of Anaesthesia*, **58**, 736–8.

Reynolds, F. (1987). Adverse effects of local anesthetics. *British Journal of Anaesthesia*, **59**, 78–9.

Richardson, R.R., Siqueira, E.B., and Cerullo L.J. (1977). Spinal epidural neurostimulation for treatment of acute and chronic intractable pain. *Neurosurgery*, **5**, 344–51.

Rigler, M.L., Drasner, K., Krejcie, T.C., Yelich, S.J., Scholnick, F.T., DeFontes, J., and Bohner, D. (1991). Cauda equina syndrome after continuous spinal anesthesia. *Anesthesia and Analgesia*, **72**, 275–81.

Savitz, M.H. (1991). Percutaneous radiofrequency rhizotomy of the lumbar facets: Ten years' experience. *Mount Sinai Journal of Medicine*, **58**, 177–8.

Shealy, C.N., Mortimer, J.T., and Reswick, J. (1967). Electrical inhibition of pain by stimulation of the dorsal column: Preliminary clinical reports. *Anesthesia and Analgesia*, **46**, 489–93.

Shetter, A.G., Hadley, M.N., and Wilkinson, E. (1986). Administration of intraspinal morphine for the treatment of cancer pain. *Neurosurgery*, **18**, 740–7.

Shulman, M.S., Walkerlin, G., Yamaguchi, L., and Brodsky, J.B. (1987). Experience with epidural hydromorphone for post-thoracotomy pain relief. *Anesthesia and Analgesia*, **66**, 1331–3.

Sjoberg, M., Appelgren, L., Einarsson, S., Hultman, E., Linder, L.E., Nitescu, P., and Curelaru, I. (1991). Long-term intrathecal morphine and bupivacaine in 'refractory' cancer pain. I. Results from the first series of 52 patients. *Acta Anesthesiologica Scandinavica*, **35**, 30–43.

Sjoberg, M., Karlsson, P.A., Nordborg, C., Wallgren, A., Nitescu, P., Appelgren, L., Linder, L.E., and Curelaru, I. (1992). Neuropathologic findings after long-term intrathecal infusion of morphine and bupivacaine for pain treatment in cancer patients. *Anesthesiology*, **76**, 173–86.

Sluijter, M.E., and Mehta, M. (1981). Recent developments in radiofrequency denervation for chronic back and neck pain. [abstract]. *Pain Supplement*, **1**, 290.

Sluijter, M.E. (1990). Radiofrequency lesions in the treatment of cervical pain syndromes. In *Radionics procedure technique series*, Burlington, MS, Radionics.

Spaulding, J.C., Venafro, J.J., Ma, M.G., and Fielding, S. (1981). The dissociation of the antinociceptive effect of clonidine from supraspinal structures. *Neuropharmacology*, **18**, 103–5.

Spaulding, T.C., Fielding, S., Venafro, J.J., and Lal, H. (1979). Anti-nociceptive activity of clonidine and its potentiation of morphine analgesia. *European Journal of Pharmacology*, **58**, 19–25.

Stolker, R.J., Vervest, A.C.M, and Groen, G.J. (1993). Percutaneous facet denervation in chronic thoracic spinal pain. *Acta Neurochirurgica*, (Wien), 82–90.

Sweet, W.H., and Wepsic, J.G. (1974). Controlled thermocoagulation of trigeminal ganglion and rootlets for differential destruction of pain fibers. *Journal of Neurosurgery*, **40**, 143–56.

Tanelian, D.L., and Cousins, M.J. (1989). Failure of epidural opioid to control cancer pain in a patient previously treated with massive doses of intravenous opioid. *Pain*, **36**, 359–62.

Thi, T.V., Orliaguet, G., Liu, N., Delaunay, L., and Bonnet, F. (1992). A dose-range study of intrathecal meperidine combined with bupivacaine. *Acta Anesthesiologica Scandinavica*, **36**, 516–8.

Trescott, A. (1994). Workshop for cryotherapy. Presented at the Sixth International Congress on Pain, Atlanta.

Trivedi, N.S., Halpern, M., Robalino, J., and Shevde, K. (1990). Spinal anaesthesia with low dose meperidine for knee arthroscopy in ambulatory surgical patients. *Regional Anaesthesia*, **15**, 43.

Troussier, B., Lebus, J.D., and Chirossel, J.P. (1995). Percutaneous intradiscal radiofrequency thermocoagulation—A cadaveric study. *Spine*, **20**, 1713–8.

Tung, A.S., Tenicela, R., and Winter, P.M. (1980). Opiate withdrawal syndrome following intrathecal administration of morphine. *Anesthesiology*, **53**, 340.

Van Dongen, RTM, Crul, BJP, and de Bock, M. (1993). Longterm intrathecal infusion of morphine and morphine/bupivacaine mixtures in the treatment of cancer pain: a retrospective analysis of 51 cases. *Pain*, **55**, 107–111.

Van Kleef, M., Barendse, G., and Dingemans, W. (1995). Effects of producing a radiofrequency lesion adjacent to the dorsal root ganglion in patients with thoracic segmental pain. *Clinical Journal of Pain*, **11**, 325–32.

Van Kleef, M., Spaans, F., Dingemans, W., Barendse, G.A., Floor, E., and Sluijter, M.E. (1993). Effects and side effects of a percutaneous thermal lesion of the dorsal root ganglion in patients with cervical pain syndrome. *Pain*, **52**, 49–53.

Varga, C.A. (1989). Chronic administration of intraspinal local anesthetics in the treatment of malignant pain. *Proceedings of the American Pain Society*, 71.

Vecht, C.J. (1989). Nociceptive nerve pain and neuropathic pain. Letter to Editor, *Pain*, **39**, 243–4.

Vokes, E.E., Weischselbaum, R.R., Lippman, S.M., and Hong, W.K. (1993). Head and neck cancer. *New England Journal of Medicine*, **328**, 184–94.

Von Roenn, J.H., Cleeland, C.S., and Gonin, R. (1991). Results of a physician's attitude toward cancer pain management survey by ECOG. *Proceedings of the American Society of Clinical Oncology*, **10**, 326.

Wang, J.F., Nauss, L.A., and Thomas, J.E. (1979). Pain relief by intrathecally applied morphine in man. *Anesthesiology*, **50**, 149–51.

Wang, B.C., Hillamn, D.E., Spielholz, N.I., and Turndorf, H. (1984). Chronic neurologic deficits and nesacaine-CE an effect of the anesthetic 2-chloroprocaine or the antioxidant sodium bisulfite? *Anesthesia and Analgesia*, **63**, 445.

Wilcox, G.L., Carlsson, K.H., Jochim, A., and Jurna, I. (1987). Mutual potentiation of anti-nociceptive effects of morphine and clonidine on motor and sensory responses in rat spinal cord. *Brain Research*, **405**, 84–93.

Wilkinson, H.A. (1984*a*). Percutaneous radiofrequency upper thoracic sympathectomy: A new technique. *Neurosurgery*, **15**, 811–4.

Wilkinson, H.A. (1984*b*). Percutaneous upper thoracic sympathetectomy. *New England Journal of Medicine*, **311**, 34–6.

Wong, G.Y., and Brown, D.L. (1995). Transient paraplegia following alcohol celiac plexus block. *Regional Anesthesia*, **20**, 352–5.

World Health Organization (1989). *Cancer pain relief* (2nd edn). World Health Organization, Geneva.

Wulf, H., Gleim, M., and Mignat, C. (1994). The stability of mixtures of morphine hydrochloride, bupivacaine hydrochloride and clonidine hydrochloride in portable pump reservoirs for the management of chronic pain syndromes. *Journal of Pain and Symptom Management*, **9**, 308–11.

Yaksh, T.L., and Rudy, T.A. (1977). Studies on the direct spinal action of narcotics in the production of analgesia in the rat. *Journal of Pharmacologic Experiments and Therapeutics*, **202**, 411–28.

Yaksh, T.L., and Reddy, SVR. (1981). Studies on the primate on the analgetic effects associated with intrathecal actions of opiates, alpha-adrenergic agonists and baclofen. *Anesthesiology*, **54**, 451–67.

Yaksh, T.L. (1978). Analgetic actions of intrathecal opiates in cat and primates. *Brain Research*, **153**, 205–10.

Zimmerman, C.G., and Burchiel, K.M. (1991). The use of intrathecal opiates for malignant and non-malignant pain: management of thirty-nine patients. *Proceedings of the American Pain Society*, **97**–101.

TEN

Percutaneous cordotomy

J.C.D. WELLS

It is logical to assume that targeted destruction of pain pathways will relieve pain. Unfortunately most neuronal pathways have mixed fibres, and destruction of the pain fibres involves destruction of useful function such as motor and sensory nerve tissue. The most logical way of interrupting pain fibres therefore is to destroy them in the anterolateral quadrant of the spinal cord, where they lie as a distinct pathway. If this area can be targeted and interrupted accurately significant relief of pain can be achieved. Thus the complication of interruption of sensory and motor pathways is avoided. There still remains the difficulty of the dysaesthetic sensation that can occur in a pain denervated area.

History

The realization that pain fibres were localized in the anterolateral quadrant of the spinal cord prompted surgical destruction of this area from the beginning of the century (Spiller and Martin 1912). This has been described as the start of functional neurosurgery. However it is a major operation, and is therefore inappropriate for most patients with terminal cancer.

Mullan et al. (1963) used a needle technique in the upper cervical cord, placing a radioactive tipped electrode near the quadrant, which produced progressive destruction and contralateral analgesia. The technique was modified to use a direct current (Mullan et al. 1965) and later refined to use radio-frequency electrical current (Rosomoff et al. 1965). Levin and Cosman (1980) developed temperature monitoring during the procedure. The procedure as described by them has changed little to this day. The technique enjoyed popularity with a band of skilled operators during the 1970s and 1980s and in experienced hands gives good results. It is used less now, probably appropriately so.

Rationale

The nociceptive pathway is complicated and inconsistent. Most pain fibres (90%) cross the mid-line as they ascend in the spinal cord, usually over three or four spinal segments. It is commonly accepted that nociceptive fibres are arranged towards the surface of the anterolateral column in distinct laminae (Fig. 10.1). Sacral fibres lie nearest to the dentate ligament, then lumbar, thoracic and finally, more anterior and nearer to the anterior horn, there are fibres from the cervical region. Ascending and descending respiratory fibres lie nearby.

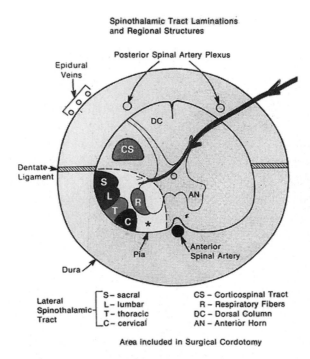

Spinothalamic Tract Laminations and Regional Structures

Lateral Spinothalamic Tract	S – sacral	CS – Corticospinal Tract
	L – lumbar	R – Respiratory Fibers
	T – thoracic	DC – Dorsal Column
	C – cervical	AN – Anterior Horn

Area included in Surgical Cordotomy

Fig. 10.1   Spinothalamic tract laminations and regional structures.

Due to a fortuitous lack of bone at the C1/C2 interspace, and not at any other space, the cervical spinal cord can be approached from its lateral aspect at this level (Mullan *et al*. 1963, Rosomoff *et al*. 1965). Other approaches have been described (Linn *et al*. 1966; Crue *et al*. 1968; Hitchcock and Leece 1967) but have found less popularity. The lateral percutaneous technique is the simplest and even this is difficult enough! The use of CT scanning to locate the anterolateral quadrant has been described. (Fenstermaker *et al*. 1995).

The procedure is carried out in the operating theatre, using a full sterile technique. The patient has to be awake and aware, and so pre-medication is not usually given. It is essential to have complete co-operation and adequate response from the patient when sensory testing is performed. Small doses of intravenous fentanyl or N_2O and oxygen can be given to appropriate patients, to prevent restlessness from pain. Adequate local anaesthesia must be provided. Once local anaesthetic has been infiltrated, a needle is inserted into the cerebrospinal fluid (CSF) via a lateral approach, attempting to introduce the tip anterior to the dentate ligament. This position is confirmed by the use of a suspension of lipiodol in saline, emulsified so that globules deposit on the dentate ligament (Fig. 10.2). Electrical measurements of impedance and stimulation are then made using a lesion generator, whilst the needle is advanced into the spinal cord. When a satisfactory position is obtained, a radio-frequency current is passed through the needle tip, heating the local tissue. This produces a concise and limited lesion to the anterolateral tract. The efficacy of the procedure can be tested immediately by means of pinprick using a sharp stick. The lesion can be enlarged if inadequate analgesia has been achieved.

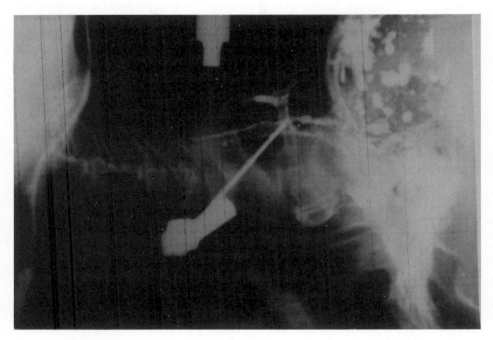

Fig. 10.2   Needle placement for percutaneous cardotomy.

Post-operatively the patient may develop a low pressure cerebrospinal fluid leak headache, and C2 nerve root pain. Analgesia is needed for this. Nonsteroidal drugs (NSAID), paracetamol or tramadol are appropriate. These patients have often been on large and ineffective doses of opioids prior to the procedure. If they are on slow-release morphine this needs to be changed to an immediate-release form 48 hours before cordotomy. This is to prevent a sustained opioid effect following the lesion, leading to postoperative respiratory depression. Ventilation, blood pressure, motor power, and temperature need close and careful monitoring. Inevitably there is a Horner's syndrome on the ipsilateral side which reduces over the next few weeks. Thermo-anaesthesia is present over the analgesic area, and may extend several segments above or below. The patient needs to be informed of this prior to and after the procedure, and avoid insensible heat or cold damage to the affected side.

Selection of patients

Given the significant and long-lasting destruction of the anterolateral quadrant which occurs, it is perhaps surprising that one of the problems with all types of cordotomy is that the analgesia does not last. The effect often wears off in eighteen months to three years (Nathan 1963a; Rosomoff *et al.* 1965). In some patients the effect can last longer (Lipton 1989). This is not a method of pain relief for patients with a normal expectation of life. Cordotomy should be restricted to those patients not expected to survive for more than a year. It is appropriate for many patients with terminal cancer, but not for patients in whom effective therapy might lead to a remission. It can also be used for patients in the terminal stages of other conditions such as AIDS and severe vascular disease.

The treatment is only suitable for patients with pain below the C5 dermatone. This is because of the decussation of fibres, and the fact that the fibres from C5 and above may not cross until above the C1/C2 interspace. A successful lesion can be performed without adequate analgesia. Thus a careful history and examination must be made of any patient with upper quadrant pain, to make sure that the pain does not extend above C5. The technique is most suited for patients with unilateral pain below C5, but particularly pain of an intermittent nature. (A pathological fracture of the femur, giving severe pain on movement or attempted walking, which goes away to virtually nothing with rest is a good indication). Cordotomy is also very useful for difficult neurogenic pain states which cannot be relieved by medication.

Some patients with severe pain from one site also have pain at another site (Bowsher 1988). When the first pain is relieved, the appreciation of the second pain becomes intense. This can occur during the cordotomy procedure itself, so that a patient with, say, right leg pain complains of left leg pain when the lesion is completed, rather than noticing relief of the right leg pain.

Ventilatory depression is a possible and significant complication. Reduced ventilatory function on the side of the pain is a relative contra-indication to cordotomy (Krieger 1973; Rosamoff *et al.* 1965; Lahuerta *et al.* 1992). The lesion is carried out on the opposite side, to the pain, therefore the function of that lung will be compromised. This might lead to severe respiratory problems if it occurs in addition to the already compromised function of the ipsilateral lung (Lipton 1989). There are methods of avoiding this but these are beyond the scope of most operators.

Patients with pelvic problems are more likely to experience problems with micturition.

Results of cordotomy

Results from centres with good experience of carrying out the technique are similar. 80% of cordotomies, in well selected patients, produce complete analgesia and thermo-anaesthesia. In 4% the effect wears off rapidly. In these patients it is assumed that oedema of the cord produced the expected relief, rather than a proper lesion having been made. The treatment can be repeated but a significant number of patients decline. Lipton (1989) reported a total of 86% of patients selected eventually obtain effective unilateral pain relief.

Some patients develop contralateral pain and others develop dysaesthesia. Adequate and complete analgesia in the long term occurs in about 70% of patients, there is partial relief in about 20% and there is no relief at all in 10%. This latter group represents some in whom there is a failure of technique or co-operation by the patient, and some in whom there is severe contralateral pain which is not capable of being controlled with medication (Lahuerta *et al.* 1985).

Reasons for failure of the technique

In some patients it is impossible to carry out the procedure, either because of technical difficulties, or because of patient restlessness. It is better to abandon the procedure than to struggle on and produce an inappropriate lesion with side-effects. However, other failures also occur.

1. There may be a return of pain, correlating with a retraction in the pinprick level. An incomplete lesion has been made and the cord recovers.

2. Painful dysaesthesia occurs at and below the level of the lesion (approximately 5–7% of patients).

3. Pain perceived by the patient as ipsilateral was in fact contralateral, with a major pain on one side masking the perception of a more minor pain on the other side. When a successful lesion is made, the original pain disappears, only to be replaced by the contralateral pain being as bothersome as the initial problem.

Complications

An ipsilateral Horner's syndrome is seen in virtually all patients, and patients and staff should be warned of this. This attenuates with time and is not a problem in practical terms. Weakness of the ipsilateral leg is apparent in over half of the patients as compared with preoperative levels. At one month, weakness is a problem in less than 2% of patients (Lahuerta *et al.* 1985). Patients with a pre-existing motor deficit are warned that this will probably become worse in the postoperative period, but this effect will reduce with time. Other infrequent complications recorded included ataxia, hemiparesis, headache, and hypotension.

Mortality

Mortality from the procedure has to be distinguished from mortality from the underlying condition. Approximately 1–6% of patients are described as dying from complications of the procedure. This is almost universally from ventilatory depression. The rate will vary according to the ventilatory function of the selected patient group. Mortality in bilateral C1/C2 cordotomies is in the region of 20%, with many patients developing an 'Ondine's curse' type syndrome (Hitchcock and Leece 1967). Mortality in patients with mesothelioma or carcinoma of the lung also approaches 20% because of ventilatory problems. A much lesser mortality rate, of under 4%, from new ventilatory depression is seen in other groups of patients.

Micturition and impotence

A unilateral cordotomy in a normal patient does not usually cause problems. In our hands, urinary retention requiring catherization occurred in 20% of patients (Lahuerta *et al*. 1985). All but two of these patients had pre-existing problems, with disease affecting the pelvis or nerve control of micturition. In 17% of patients function was restored within a few days, with 3% requiring permanent catherization, two-thirds of these having undergone bilateral cordotomy. The chance of long-term urinary problems in patients with a unilateral cordotomy, without pre-existing bladder disease or symptoms, is 1% or less. Impotence has been reported, but almost exclusively in young men having cordotomies for non-malignant pain.

Dysaesthesia

Most patients notice disagreeable hypersensitivity to light touch in the affected area, but in only 5–20% is this recorded as being significantly unpleasant or long-standing. Most appreciate the analgesia that the procedure has achieved.

Conclusion

Percutaneous cordotomy can provide excellent pain relief in the management of some otherwise difficult to manage pain syndromes. Careful selection of patients can minimize complications and side-effects. The procedure itself is not simple. It requires expensive and elaborate equipment. It is best undertaken by those who are going to have regular experience in carrying out the technique. It would seem appropriate for perhaps one centre in each regional area of population density approaching one million. A better understanding of the technique with its advantages and disadvantages, appropriate referral to appropriate centres, and the honing of skills developed in these centres, should allow this useful technique to bring relief to distressed patients who might otherwise die with their pain unrelieved.

References

Bowsher, D. (1988). Contralateral mirror-image pain following anterolateral cordotomy. *Pain*, **33**, 63–5.

Crue, B.L., Todd, E.M., and Carregal, E.J.A. (1968). Posterior approach for high cervical percutaneous radiofrequency cordotomy. *Confinia Neurologica*, **30**, 41–52.

Fenstermaker, K.A., Sternau, L.L., Takaoka, Y. (1995). CT-assisted percutaneous arterior cordotomy. *Surgical Neurology*, **43**, 147–9.

Hitchcock, E., and Leece, B. (1967). Somatotropic representation of the respiratory pathways in the cervical cord of man. *Journal of Neurosurgery*, **27**, 320–9.

Krieger, A.J., and Rosomoff, H.L. (1973). Sleep induced apnea. Part 1. A respiratory and autonomic dysfunction syndrome following bilateral percutaneous cervical cordotomy. *Journal of Neurosurgery*, **39**, 168–80.

Lahuerta, J., Buxton, P., Lipton, S. *et al.* (1992). The location and function of respiratory fibres in the second cervical spinal cord segment: respiratory dysfunction syndrome after cervical cordotomy. *Journal of Neurology, Neurosurgery, and Psychiatry*, **55**, 1142–5.

Lahuerta, J., Lipton, S., and Wells, J.C.D. (1985). Percutaneous cervical cordotomy: results and complications in a recent series of 100 patients. *Annals of the Royal College of Surgeons of England*, **67**, 41–4.

Levin, A.B., & Cosman, E.R. (1980). Thermocouple-monitored cordotomy electrode. *Journal of Neurosurgery*, **53**, 266–8.

Linn, P.M., Gildenberg, P.L., and Polakoff, P.P. (1966). An anterior approach to percutaneous lower cervical cordotomy. *Journal of Neurosurgery*, **25**, 553–60.

Lipton, S. (1989). Percutaneous cordotomy. In *A textbook of pain*, (ed. P.D. Wall and R. Melzack) (2nd edn), pp. 832–9. Churchill Livingstone, Edinburgh.

Mullan, S., Harper, P.V., Hekmatpanah, J., Torres, H., and Dobbin, G. (1963). Percutaneous interruption of spinal pain tracts by means of a strontium 90 needle. *Journal of Neurosurgery*, **20**, 931–9.

Mullan, S., Hekmatpanah, J., Dobbin, G., Beckman, F. (1965). Percutaneous intramedullary cordotomy utilising the unipolar anodal electrolytic lesion. *Journal of Neurosurgery*, **22**, 548–53.

Nathan, P.W. (1963). Results of antero-lateral cordotomy for pain in cancer. *Journal of Neurology, Neurosurgery and Psychiatry*, **26**, 353–62.

Rosomoff, H.L., Carroll, F., Brown, J., and Sheptak, P. (1965). Percutaneous radio-frequency cervical cordotomy technique. *Journal of Neurosurgery*, **23**, 639–44.

Spiller, W.G., Martin, E. (1912). The treatment of persistent pain of organic origin in the lower part of the body by division of the antero-lateral column of the spinal cord. *Journal of the American Medical Association*, **58**, 1489–90.

ELEVEN

Neurosurgical pain management

SAMUEL J. HASSENBUSCH AND
MEREDITH DICKENS

Neurosurgical procedures have generally been used relatively late in the overall management of patients; however, earlier use is now suggested. Although many intracranial procedures are old, recent advances have renewed interest in their use. Some of these improvements, such as focused radiotherapy, allow almost non-invasive interventional pain techniques at the intracranial level. The role of spinal ablative procedures, which is relatively low risk, remains stable, in overall pain management. Single procedures, performed under local anaesthesia with short hospital admissions and low morbidity, are now useful.

The relative roles of ablative and augmentative procedures are still controversial in neurosurgical pain management. Some ablative procedures have been available for 40–50 years yet, in many situations, have been replaced by newer augmentative procedures during the past decade. Techniques for intracranial ablative procedures have been improved significantly in the past five years. The use of improved stereotactic equipment and guidance by computerized tomography (CT) and magnetic resonance imaging (MRI), has improved the accuracy of intracranial procedures largely eliminated the need for ventriculography. Procedures can be performed under local anaesthesia, with intravenous sedation, and require only a twist drill hole, rather than a burr hole or a craniotomy.

Indications

Patients must have severe pain that is not relieved adequately by systemic medications or simple neurolytic procedures. Some of the procedures are used for chronic pain from cancer causes. Others, such as thalamotomy and cingulotomy, have been used for pain from non-cancer causes (Foltz 1962; Hurt and Ballantine 1974; Mempel and Dietrich-Rap 1977; Sano 1987; Santo *et al.* 1990). It is not clear whether delayed recurrence of pain represents extension of the underlying tumour to new anatomic areas or late failure of the procedure (Coombs 1988; Yaksh and Onofrio 1987).

Neurosurgical procedures are used for both nociceptive and neuropathic pain. With the exception of thalamotomy, nociceptive pain responds better to intracranial procedures, which cover larger body areas. Neuropathic pain often responds better to spinal procedures that have more limited areas of coverage. The choice of a specific operation needs to be individualized for each patient based upon considerations of the type of pain (severity), the location of pain and its primary cause.

Techniques

The methods to position neurosurgical lesions are relatively standard. Some of the original ablations were placed using open surgical techniques (Lewin 1961, 1972). Now, closed operations using stereotaxis under ventriculogram, CT or MR guidance have become standard. Air or contrast ventriculography was the traditional, accurate method for placing lesions at coordinates defined by the anterior commissure-posterior commissure (AC-PC) line (Spiegel *et al*. 1947; Spiegel 1982). This often required general anaesthesia because of the need for ventriculography. It could not adjust for inter-patient variability in anatomy.

CT and MR for stereotactic guidance eliminate the need for ventriculography and provide an improved ability to correct for individual patient variation in anatomy (Hadley *et al*. 1985; Hassenbusch and Pillay 1992*a*; Fig. 11.1). MR imaging is especially useful in the identification of relevant anatomy, but suffers from a lower accuracy because of magnetic field inhomogeneity (Hassenbusch and Pillay 1993; Pillay and Hassenbusch 1992). The trajectory for the electrode placement, with MR imaging, can be planned in relation to other brain structures. Angled slices that correspond to the trajectory for the electrode placement can be performed and the target site and the actual trajectory through various brain structures can be found on these slices.

Radiosurgery, for example using the Gamma Knife, is increasingly used to create ablative lesions for treatment of chronic pain and functional disorders (Fig. 11.2).

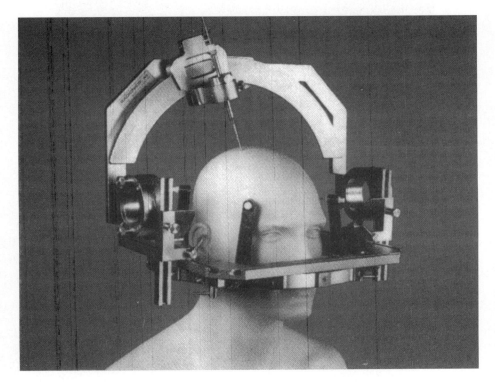

Fig. 11.1 Stereotactic frame used for CT- and MRI-guided neurosurgical stereotactic procedures.

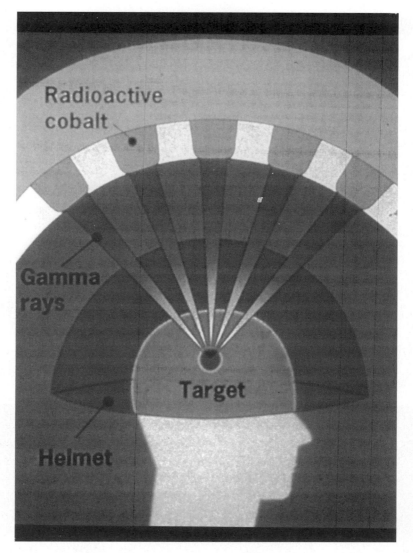

Fig. 11.2 Stereotactic radiosurgery showing cobalt sources emitting gamma rays. The common point is focused at target for ablation (e.g. pituitary gland).

Targets in the thalamus and the anterior limb of the internal capsule have been widely reported (Leskell 1968; Steiner *et al.* 1980; Lindquist *et al.* 1991). The radiosurgical technique for these pain-relieving lesions uses a similar technique to that for focused radiation (radiosurgery) for a brain tumour. Radiosurgery is non-invasive to the brain. It is not clear to what extent the lesions become smaller, and perhaps less effective, over time after the radiation exposure.

   The following procedures are either commonly used at the moment or, based upon past reports, offer significant relief with minimal morbidity. Some treat specific pain areas such as the head or legs, but others treat more generalized areas of pain. These descriptions are based upon an anatomic progression from rostral to caudal sites.

Thalamotomy

In the late 1930s and early 1940s, there were increasing reports of the use of thalamo-tomy in the treatment of patients with Parkinson's disease. Russel Meyers built on these ideas to create a means to preserve involuntary movements through an open pal-lidotomy (Tasker 1990). The thalamotomy procedure was revived and explored when human stereotaxic procedures became popular. If pallidal lesions were effective, it was reasoned that lesions of their thalamic projections in the ventrolateral nucleus of the thalamus would also be effective (Tasker 1990).

Thalamotomy is usually considered for non-cancer pain. It can also be effective for the treatment of cancer pain (Sano 1987; Tasker 1990). The targets have been the basal thalamus, medial thalamus, and dorsomedian thalamus. This affects extralemniscal fibres, fibres terminating in the intralaminar and centromedianum nuclei, and the origin of fibres projecting to the frontal lobe (Gildenberg and Hirsberg 1984). The thalamus contains neurons that respond to light, hair bending, pressure on the skin, and tongue, hand, and lip movements (Tasker 1990). One of the most effective sites appears to be the inferior posteromedial thalamus, containing the intralaminar, cen-tromedianum, and parafascicularis nuclei which might affect the palaeospinothalamic tract (Sweet 1980). Combination lesions, such as centromedianum and parafasicularis lesions with dorsomedial nucleus or the thalamic pulvinar lesions, might provide better long-term results (Sweet 1980).

Although lesion size is an important component of this type of operation, it is diffi-cult to determine the optimal size because many surgeons have their own preferences. Specific cases might dictate the need for a specific lesion size in order to avoid compli-cations (Tasker 1990). Thalamotomy is generally considered for intermittent shooting and hyperpathic or allodynic pain. It is considered very effective for steady, burning, or dysaesthetic components of central or deafferentation pain (Tasker 1990). All other means of treatment must have been thoroughly considered because of the possibility of severe complications or disability after thalamotomy (Tasker 1990). Enthusiasm for the use of thalamotomy, however, has waned over the past few years because of con-cerns of pain recurrence after 6–12 months.

The thalamic procedure is an application of many steps. It consists of stereotactic methods, frame imaging, referencing, selecting target location(s), and the introduction of the probe into the brain, without damaging sensitive motor structures (Tasker 1990). These operative steps are followed by interactive verification of proper target location through physiological testing during the operation and lesion (Tasker 1990). A thala-motomy is performed under local anaesthesia because patient cooperation is required for physiological testing. The testing site should be approximately in the 15 mm sagittal plane or the tactile representation of the contralateral manual digits (Tasker 1990).

There are two types of physiological testing that can be used to distinguish whether or not the targeting is accurate. Macrostimulation is a simple procedure. It requires nominal instrumentation with quick progression and total identification of the brain and the spectrum of structures at variable distances from the probe. This process can be executed simultaneously with deep brain recording and using the same electrode. The second method of physiologic investigation is the microelectrode recording technique. This is able to identify only a limited repertoire of structures. A microelectrode is mounted on the arc of the stereotactic frame. It is usually extruded out of its protective tubing with a hydraulic microdrive (Tasker 1990). Actual stimulation with the microelectrode occurs every 1.0 mm at 300 Hz, 100 mA, 0.1 ms, until responses occur below about 15 mA (Tasker 1990). A bipolar concentric electrode, 1.1 mm in diameter with a 0.5 mm tip separated by a 0.5 mm ring, monitors the stimulation. The stimulation effects are used to minimize any morbidity that might occur from electrode placement at the anticipated anatomic target. Nashold implanted electrodes for physiologic recording as a testing method before he performed the procedure (Shieff and Nashold 1987). The implanted electrodes permitted an accurate direction for the placement of the thalamotomy electrode tip during the actual operation (Shieff and Nashold 1987).

Thalamotomy, for nociceptive pain, has been reported to produce transient loss of all contralateral sensory modalities after the operation and also pseudoparesis in many of the cases. The patients seemed to lose the appreciation of position and vibration sense due to the lesions in the ventrocaudal nucleus (Tasker 1990).

Many complications are possible and include paresis, cognitive disorders, infection and mortality (although rare in nociceptive pain cases), seizures, speech disturbance, and other matters related to specific areas of disease. Due to this significant risk, thalamic stimulation should be carried out before considering the creation of a lesion (Tasker 1990).

Cingulotomy

The creation of lesions in the cingulate gyrus originated when Hugh Cairns at Oxford began to remove a portion of the anterior cingulate gyrus in an open operation (Lewin 1972). The use of the open cingulotomy in the 1940s and 1950s produced significant improvements in psychiatric symptoms in most patients (Lewin 1961). In 1962, Foltz first described the application of stereotaxy to bilateral anterior cingulate lesions for pain relief. Ballantine began to use ventriculogram-guided stereotaxy to create smaller lesions in the anterior cingulate gyrus. With the availability of these closed techniques, there is no role for open surgical techniques for cingulotomy. The specific target is the cingulate gyrus, 20–30 mm posterior to the anterior tip of the lateral ventricles. The target is 1.5 mm lateral to midline and 15 mm superior to the roof of the lateral ventricles (Ballantine 1986; Ballantine *et al.* 1987) (Fig. 11.3). The radio-frequency method is used more commonly. Each lesion is created at 75 °C for 60–90 seconds. The result is a cylindrical lesion approximately 10–20 mm long and 5–7 mm in diameter, centred in each cingulate gyrus.

While a cingulotomy has most often been applied to patients with affective disorders, there are numerous reports of its use for severe pain control (Foltz 1962; Hurt and Ballantine 1974; Mempel and Dietrich-Rap 1977; Faillace *et al.* 1981; Ortiz 1972; Sharma 1973, 1974). The mechanism for pain relief is unclear but it presumably

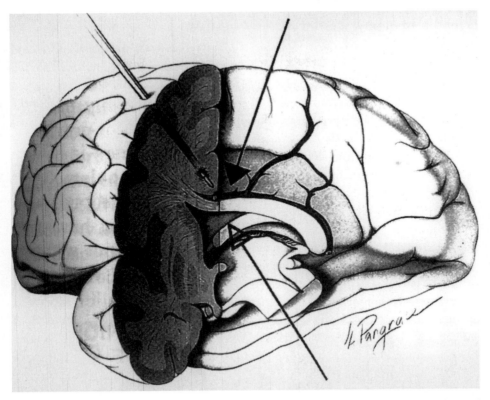

Fig. 11.3 Placement of cingulotomy electrode through cortex. The exposed electrode is located in the left cingulate gyrus near the distal portion of the anterior cerebral arteries (closed arrow) and lateral ventricles (open arrow) (From Hassenbusch 1996).

derives from interruption of the limbic system. This appears to be a very effective procedure for diffuse or multiply-located cancer pain that is mainly nociceptive in character (Pillay 1992; Hassenbusch 1993). Severe pain from diffuse bone metastases is a typical indication.

In many historical series of patients undergoing cingulotomy up to 30% of patients were treated for severe chronic pain. Over half of the patients who were treated with intractable cancer pain had moderate, marked, or complete pain relief at 3 months after the procedure. In patients with severe non-neoplastic pain, 45% had moderate, marked, or complete pain relief more than 3 months afterwards. The procedure is less effective in patients with non-cancer pain, neuropathic pain, or survival times that are longer than 8 months (Pillay and Hassenbusch 1992; Hassenbusch and Pillay 1993).

The main complications with cingulotomy using ventriculogram guidance in the treatment of psychiatric or pain patients have been controllable seizures (9%), transient mania (6%), decreased memory (3%), hemiplegia from intracerebral haematoma (0.3%), and mortality (0.9%) (Ballantine 1986, Ballantine *et al.* 1987; Jenike *et al.* 1991). However, in neuropsychiatric examination, the only abnormalities noted were occasional difficulties in copying complex figures, performing two tapping tests, and rarely memory on an organized serial learning test (Allen and Faillace 1972; Corkin *et al.* 1979; Faillace *et al.* 1981).

Hypothalamotomy

Lesions in the hypothalamus were reported initially for psychoaffective disorders and later cancer pain. Between 1971 and 1982, 28 patients were reported to have received the procedure for pain control (Sano 1962; Fairman 1971). Beta-endorphin concentrations in ventricular cerebrospinal fluid are elevated by electrical stimulation of the hypothalamotomy target prior to ablation of the area. Concentrations remain elevated for at least two days after the hypothalamotomy ablation (Mayanagi *et al.* 1982). After hypothalamotomy, degenerated axon fibres are found ipsilateral in the nucleus ventro-caudalis parvocellularis of Hassler (Vcpc), nucleus parafascicularis, somatosensory cortices, pallidum, and the reticular formation but not in the dorsomedial nucleus of the thalamus (Sano *et al.* 1975). Indications for hypothalamotomy are similar to cingulotomy in terms of cancer pain from rather diffuse sites, especially where there is an emotional or visceral component (Amano *et al.* 1976).

Although initial reports located the target 2 mm below the midpoint and 2 mm lateral to the lateral wall of the third ventricle, more recent reports have suggested that more posterior lesions might be more effective (Sano *et al.* 1975). In one series, 15 of 21 hypothalamotomy procedures were bilateral with 'good' results reported in 62% of patients, cancer pain appeared to respond better than non-cancer pain (Amano *et al.* 1976; Mayanagi *et al.* 1982). There appear to be no significant complications although the published reports are very limited.

Hypophysectomy

Hypophysectomy is generally recommended for patients with severe cancer pain, usually from metastatic breast or prostate carcinoma, with diffuse areas of pain. It can also be effective for hormonally unresponsive tumours (Perrault *et al.* 1952; Katz and Levin 1977; Miles 1979; Williams *et al.* 1980; Levin *et al.* 1983).

For pain relief, open operations for ablation or section of the pituitary gland include the transcranial hypophysectomy (Kudo *et al.* 1968) and the open microsurgical hypophysectomy (Gros *et al.* 1975; Tindall *et al.* 1976; Silverberg 1977; Tindall *et al.* 1979). With the increasing use and improved technology of stereotactic methods, percutaneous stereotactic lesions are being created using radio-frequency thermal techniques, cryotherapy, or interstitial placement of radioactive seeds. The widespread use of focused radiation therapy with the Gamma Knife for pituitary tumours has led to the use of this non-invasive method to create similar lesions.

The analgesic mechanism of action for hypophysectomy remains unclear. It does not act on the limbic system or lessen psychological suffering as its primary mechanism. Evidence exists in favour of hormonal, hypothalamic, and neurotransmitter release mechanisms. A postulated hormonal mechanism entails a humoral substance in the cerebrospinal fluid or hormonal changes via a direct neural mechanism (Miles 1979; Tindall *et al.* 1979). Pain relief is almost immediate and either precedes or does not correlate with tumour regression. In this case, very small amounts of regression cannot be discounted (Levin 1993). Pain relief can occur in the thalamic pain regions and hormonally unresponsive tumors. Analgesia does not seem to correlate with the degree of pituitary ablation experienced (Kapur and Dalton 1969; Zervas 1969; Maddy *et al.* 1971; Silverberg 1977; Levin *et al.* 1983).

Stereotactic instillation of alcohol into the pituitary gland is one of the best described and most common techniques. The use of stereotaxy for chemical hypophysectomy includes injection of 1–5 ml alcohol (Greco *et al.* 1957). The results may be better with alcohol volumes extending to the upper end of this range, that are clearly greater than the volume of the sella (Levin 1993).

After the induction of general anaesthesia and placement of a stereotactic frame, the superoposterior part of the sella is chosen as the initial target. An 18 gauge, 6 inch spinal needle is introduced in a transnasal trajectory that passes through the floor of the sphenoid sinus. This needle is replaced by a 20 gauge spinal needle directed through the sellar wall, with its passage monitored under lateral X-ray fluoroscopy. After the needle tip is placed, 1–2 ml alcohol is injected in aliquots of 0.1 ml. The needle is withdrawn halfway to the floor of the sella and another 1–2 ml is injected (Levin 1993). The needle is withdrawn completely after this last injection. During and after all of the injections, the eyes are monitored for evidence of compression of nerves in the cavernous sinus as evidenced by changes in pupil size or deviation of eyes from the midline.

Intrasellar instillation of alcohol supports a hypothalamic mechanism. Alcohol has been shown to pass to the floor of the third ventricle, hypophyseal portal vessels, and the hypothalamus (Levin 1993). A possible relation to the pain relief properties of the posteromedial hypothalamotomy can be observed. The morphological effects of hypophysectomy, regardless of the method used to perform the ablation, are focused in the anterior hypothalamus, specifically in the supraoptic and paraventricular nuclei (Levin 1993; Daniel and Prichard 1972).

Projections from the paraventricular nucleus of the hypothalamus have been noted to the periaqueductal grey, rostral ventral medulla, and lamina I of dorsal horn. These are important in the descending antinociceptive system (Nilaver *et al.* 1980; Sofroniew 1980; Swanson and Sawchenko 1980; Silverman and Zimmerman 1983). The effects of pituitary ablation on the paraventricular nucleus and the connections of this nucleus to important antinociceptive areas of the brain and spinal cord suggest a mechanism that entails the release of endogenous antinociceptive areas of the brain and spinal cord. It has been observed, that naloxone does not reverse pain relief. Although plasma concentrations of beta-endorphin were elevated in one study, no changes have been found in cerebrospinal fluid concentrations of metenkephalin or beta-endorphin.

Other techniques, such as stereotaxic radio-frequency hypophysectomy, stereotaxic cryohypophysectomy, and interstitial irradiation also use standard stereotactic methods for other intracranial targets (Santo *et al.* 1990; Maddy *et al.* 1971; Yoshii and Fukada 1979; Lipton 1983; Shieff and Nashold 1987). The widespread use of focused radiation with the GammaKnife to treat pituitary tumours suggests its potential use for pain control. Reports are limited concerning focused pituitary radiation for pain control.

In two different series of more than 100 patients each, chemical hypophysectomy appeared to provide significant pain relief. Excellent pain relief was reported in 45–65%

of all patients and 75–85% patients stopped opioid intake. The mean postoperative survival time was 5 months and the mean length of pain relief was 3 months. 50–75% of the patients treated with alcohol injections, suffered from breast or prostate carcinoma, these appeared to have slightly better pain relief than those with other types of tumours (Levin 1993). This length of pain relief was accomplished with one additional alcohol injection in 25–30% patients and with two additional injections in another 3–9% (Madrid 1979; Miles 1979; Levin 1993). Approximately 25% of patients had at least one significant exacerbation of pain after the procedure and one-third of these patients had more than one exacerbation (Levin 1993).

The most common complications were hormonal deficiency, (such as diabetes insipidus) in 5–20% patients, cerebrospinal fluid leak in 1–10% patients, and ocular nerve palsy or temporal field visual loss in 2–10% patients (Levin 1993; Tasker 1993). Most of these changes dissipated or disappeared with time (Levin 1993). Less frequently reported complications included meningitis 0.5–1%, hypothalamic changes, headaches, and carotid artery damage (Tasker 1993). A 2–5% mortality rate was reported in older reports, but mortality seems to be significantly lower with newer percutaneous, stereotactic methods (Lipton 1983; Tasker 1993).

Pulvinotomy

The main indication for pulvinotomy appears to be treatment of intractable cancer pain with qualities and areas of involvement similar to those indicated for cingulotomy or hypothalamotomy (Yoshii *et al.* 1982). In Yoshii and Fukada's (1979) study, pulvinotomy was applied to patients with phantom pain (10 patients), thalamic pain (10), peripheral neuropathy (6), cancer pain (5), herpetic neuralgia (5), and anaesthesia dolorosa (5). Pulvinotomy might be indicated for cancer patients with expected survival times as long as 18 months because of reports of prolonged pain relief in some patients.

In 1966, Kudo *et al.* first described lesions in the pulvinar of the thalamus for pain relief. By 1975, 30 patients were reported to have received this operation. Although the mechanism for pain relief remains unclear, electrophysiologic studies in cats demonstrated that the pulvinar is involved in an indirect route for afferent stimuli (Kudo *et al.* 1968). From the pulvinar, afferent transmission connections have been traced to the temporal lobe and, from there, to the posterior sensory cortex (Laitinen 1977). The oral and medial parts of the pulvinar are involved in pain appreciation (Strenge 1978).

Lesions have been reported in the medial or in both the medial and lateral areas of pulvinar. The lesions have been created in one hemisphere, contralateral to the site of pain, but appear to be more effective with bilateral lesions (Yoshii *et al.* 1982; Yoshii and Fukada 1979; Sweet 1980). The coordinates for pulvinar lesions have been 4 mm superior to the anterior-posterior commissure line, 5 mm posterior to the anterior-posterior commissure line, and lateral to the anterior-posterior commissure line by either 10–11 mm for a medial target or 15–16 mm for a lateral target (Yoshii *et al.* 1982). The resultant lesions, which are 5–6 mm in diameter, are created using ultrasonic probes, with a setting of 75 watts and 2.5 megacycles for 30 seconds, at 2–6 separate sites

(Yoshii *et al.* 1982). Stereotaxis using MR guidance and radio-frequency thermal lesions, has been adapted to create lesions in the pulvinar at the same target coordinates.

Pre-existing pain is most affected by this operation. There is no reported loss of somatic sensation after the procedure (Sweet 1980). Moderate to excellent pain relief has been reported in as many as 25% of patients for periods ranging from one to 2.5 years (Laitinen 1977; Yoshii *et al.* 1982). When the lesions are extended backward to involve the pulvinar, the lesions, especially in the anterior pulvinar, have been more effective than the centrum medianum thalamotomy (Laitinen 1977). Better relief has been noted when the lesions are extended backward to involve the pulvinar and were coupled with thalamotomy lesions in the centrum medianum and parafascicularis (Mayanagi and Bouchard 1976). Analysis of patients after pulvinotomy has shown no apparent changes in speech, intelligence quotient (IQ), or vision. Temporary changes in emotions, such as lachrymoseness, childishness, and excessive excitability and euphoria, have been observed (Yoshii and Fukada 1977, 1979).

Mesencephalotomy

Mesencephalic tractotomy (mesencephalotomy) is the surgical production of lesions in the midbrain. It has been reported to provide significant pain relief in 65–75% of patients on both short-term and long-term (2–4 year) follow-up. It is used especially in the treatment of head and neck cancer. Bosch, in his studies of forty patients suffering from deafferentation pain and cancer pain, used this surgery for possible treatment of thalamic pain, trigeminal neuralgia, postherpetic neuralgia, and phantom-limb pain of the arm (Harris 1985). The target has been at the superior colliculus or inferior colliculus level. It appears that the inferior colliculus target provides a lower incidence of ocular problems, but perhaps with lower success (50–70%). In the studies carried out by Bosch, the target was identified based on intraoperative ventriculography, with water-soluble medium, using the frontal burrhole route (Harris 1985).

The main side effects appear to be difficulties with ocular movement and binocular vision. Mortality rates vary from 1–7% (Frank *et al.* 1989; Shieff and Nashold 1987). Post-operative dysaesthesia has been reported when studying the medial lemniscus after large mesencephalic lesions (Amano *et al.* 1992; Shieff and Nashold 1990). These side-effects could be reduced by using a smaller electrode, neural recording, and more precise electrical stimulation (Amano *et al.* 1992). The area of evoked pain is limited to a very small range (about 2–3 mm of target). It requires the use of a bipolar concentric electrode for extremely precise localized stimulation.

The accuracy of the stereotactic trajectory to the rostral midbrain also reduces morbidity and other risks (Amano *et al.* 1992). The operation should be limited to patients with short life expectancy and lateralized nociceptive pain because of neuropathic side effects. The usual stereotactic techniques are performed under general anaesthesia to standardize the procedure. With a well-defined target, the operation can produce pain relief comparable to other pain relief operations like open anterior cordotomy, midline myelotomy, and dorsal root entry zone (Harris 1985).

The results of this operation vary due to the nature of the particular diseases. The longest duration of pain relief in cancer patients is for pain in the extremities while pain in the chest and abdomen do not respond adequately (Harris 1985). Although nociceptive pain may be sensitive to opioids, mesencephalic surgery and electrical stimulation of grey matter is a successful and viable alternative.

Trigeminal tractotomy

The clinical use of lesions in the descending trigeminal tract and the adjacent nucleus caudalis were prompted historically by the observation that such lesions affected pain and temperature, but not touch sensation (Sjoqvist 1938). The role of the nucleus caudalis in these lesions is based on its probable role as a relay station for pain and temperature transmission from cranial nerves. The nucleus lies on the surface of the medulla, posterior to the dorsal spinocerebellar tract, lateral to the fasciculus cuneatus, and inferior to the restiform body (White 1969).

Trigeminal tractotomy is used to treat intractable pain in the distribution of the trigeminal nerve of patients with head and neck cancer. Since such pain often involves more diffuse areas of the head and neck, mesencephalotomy may be more appropriate (Spiegel 1953). Although trigeminal tractotomy was used in the past for trigeminal and postherpetic neuralgia, it is no longer indicated because of the availability of other percutaneous and open operations.

Both percutaneous and open surgical techniques have been described for this operation. A percutaneous technique has been reported with needle penetration at the C1 foramen magnum area under stereotactic guidance (Nashold *et al*. 1982; Schvarcz 1978). An electrode with a 0.5–0.6 mm diameter is angled 30° cephalad and placed 6 mm lateral to the midline and 4 mm deep in the spinal cord. Electrical stimulation at 50 Hz should provide facial stimulation to low voltage. If the electrode placement is too ventral, stimulation will be felt in contralateral body areas via the spinothalamic tract, and if the placement is too dorsal, stimulation will be felt in ipsilateral areas via the fasciulus cuneatus.

The open operation, based on the procedures described by Sjoqvist (1938), uses a prone position with bone removal from the occiput and C1 unilaterally. After the dura is opened, the nucleus caudalis lesion is created by a transverse knife incision to a depth of 3–5 mm below the surface of the cervicomedullary junction. The incision, which is made 4–8 mm inferior to the obex, extends medially from the fasciculus cuneatus to the rootlets of the spinal accessory nerve. In an attempt to place the lesion as superior as possible, but without injury to the restiform body, an oblique incision angling from superior to inferior as it is made from posterior to anterior can be used. For mouth coverage, extension of the lesion is recommended to involve part of the spinothalamic tract and part of the fasciculus.

Limited published reports of this procedure, either with open or percutaneous techniques, suggest that about 75–85% of patients with head and neck cancer have good pain relief. The tractotomy is often combined with other nerve and/or root sections in the same area. Pain relief in general appears to continue for months, but not years, after the procedure (White 1969). Following tractotomy patients have been documented to have sensory changes in the area of the pain, but not experience significant pain relief. Complications include changes in ipsilateral arm coordination, contralateral leg sensation, and ipsilateral arm and rarely leg proprioception. Most of these deficits are temporary; less frequent complications include Horner's syndrome, dysarthria, gait changes, and hiccoughs. Overall mortality has been estimated at 5–10% in patients with advanced cancer.

Combined procedures

As these intracranial procedures become technically easier to perform, combinations of the techniques become possible. Many of these are based on similar combinations used in the treatment of affective disorders. One reported combination, is the use of cingulotomy and anterior capsulotomy, in which lesions are created in both the cingulate gyrus and the anterior limb of the internal capsule. While this combination has been most reported in the treatment of affective disorders, it has been used for the treatment of severe cancer-related pain. It provides better relief for pain, including neuropathic pain, than cingulotomy alone (Hassenbusch and Pillay 1992*b*). Combinations of targets for thalamotomy also include the pulvinar as an additional target. This improves pain relief as compared to a single site in the thalamus (Mayanagi and Bouchard 1976). Hopefully future research will provide a basis for rational combinations of these procedures and better long-term efficacy in pain control.

Intracerebroventricular (ICV) infusion of opioid

The ICV route is normally a last resort treatment (Siegfried 1998). Morphine is the usual agent. It appears to provide a marked increase in potency as compared to intrathecal or epidural infusions. The mechanism of action may involve supraspinal pathways for analgesia. Daily morphine doses for intracerebroventricular (ICV) delivery range from 50–700 µg/day (Tseng 1984; Dennis and DeWitty 1990; Lazorthes 1988) (Table 11.1).

Table 11.1. Patient characteristics

	Mean	Minimum	Maximum
Age (yr)	57	23	80
Pain duration (mo)	10	0.5	120
Duration of resevoir use (d)	95	1	1362
Morphine dose (mg)	1	0.25	4
Quality of analgesia (%)	78	0	100
Duration of analgesia (h)	22	0	72

(from Karavelis, A., Foroglou, G., Selviaridis, P., and Fountzilas, G. (1996). Intraventricular administration of morphine for control of intractable cancer pain in 90 patients. *Neurosurgery*, **39**, 57–62.)

The opioid can be delivered by an implanted infusion pump. It is placed subcutaneously in the anterior abdominal wall and connected by subcutaneous tubing to an implanted ventricular catheter. The duration of action of the ICV injections appears to be longer than with intraspinal delivery. Some patients can be treated adequately via an implanted ventricular catheter connected to a subcutaneous Ommaya reservoir-type device with 1–2 injections/day (Brazenor 1987).

This form of drug delivery is indicated for head and neck cancer pain. Rarely, it is used for patients with an initial good response to intraspinal infusions of opioids, but with subsequent development of apparent tolerance and very limited (1–3 month) remaining survival time. The safety and side effects of ICV injections or infusions are similar to intraspinal infusions, except that an increased risk of ventilatory depression has been noted in the first three days of the ICV delivery (Dennis and DeWitty 1990; Brazenor 1987).

Several factors determine whether treatment with ICV morphine delivery via a reservoir is feasible in location of the pain, age of the patient, and the history of opioid usage. Lumbar subarachnoid administration of morphine provides better pain relief for the lower limbs, while craniofacial or diffuse pain is responsive to ICV drug delivery (Karavelis *et al.* 1996). The administration of morphine into the ventricle through a catheter-reservoir system was non-destructive and effective for the treatment of nociceptive pain in 20 patients including 18 with cancer (Seiwald *et al.* 1996). Analgesia took a few minutes to begin when low dosses were used. Nociceptive pain was ameliorated in 95% of patients, however, minimal effects were seen in the management of neuropathic pain.

The type of opioid must be considered, for example, in sheep, certain morphine-type drugs, might have problems diffusing through the cerebrospinal fluid to reach distant receptors. Although the obvious anatomical and physiological differences from humans prevent much deeper analysis, the sheep has been shown as a legitimate pre-clinical model (Payne *et al.* 1996). Morphine, hydromorphone, and sucrose can be identified in the lumbar cerebrospinal fluid about 90 minutes after an ICV injection (Siegfried 1998). Hydromorphone is located after 50 minutes. Methadone is not found in the CSF. The ICV administration of lipophilic opioids creates different cerebrospinal fluid distributions compared with hydrophilic drugs (Payne *et al.* 1996).

Deep brain stimulation

The use of deep brain stimulation has been reported in the relief of chronic pain of benign aetiology (Goodman 1990). It is a useful technique for central pain caused by spinal cord lesions, and for patients who have failed to experience adequate pain relief with spinal cord or peripheral nerve stimulation. During this procedure, an electrode implant is carried out under local anaesthesia. A burr hole is made 3 cm from the midline in the coronal structure, with CT and MRI guided stereotaxis. The initial electrode targets are either the periventricular grey/periaqueductal grey (PVG/PAG) area or the ventral posterior lateral thalamus (Goodman 1990). Many surgeons place the electrodes in both areas in each patient, whereas others rely on preliminary stimulation to obtain information about where the electrodes should be sited. The type of pain being experienced and the severity of the situation are determining factors.

Deep brain stimulation of either the PAG region or thalamic sensory nuclei is acutely effective in 61–80% of patients and has an overall success rate of 50–63% for non-cancer pain (Gybels and Kupers 1990; Kumar *et al.* 1990; Young 1990; Young and Rinaldi 1992). Transient complications have included infections, electrode fracture hardware malfunction, implantation site pain, and mild neurologic deficits. Permanent complications occur in 1–2% of patients, these include headache, hemiparesis, intracranial haemorrhage, seizures, and death (Young 1990). In most studies, a higher rate of pain relief is found with spinal stimulation techniques (Goodman 1990). Post-operative results show a 90% success, but long-term benefits are lower ranging from 65–80% (Goodman 1990).

In cancer pain, deep brain stimulation can be indicated for pain not well-treated by ablative procedures. This includes pain from diffuse bone metastases, midline or bilat-eral pain (especially of the lower body), brachial or lumbosacral plexopathy, and recur-rent pain from head and neck cancer (Young 1993). In 31 patients with cancer pain treated with deep brain stimulation, 87% experienced satisfactory relief, with 55% experiencing lasting relief until death (Young 1993).

Complications in both cancer and non-cancer pain are unavoidable, they are greatly influenced by the placement of the electrode. They occur when the electrode is placed in the PAG region. They have been reduced recently with electrode placement in the PVG. Some patients will not benefit from deep brain stimulation, but the possibility of effective pain relief is both promising and realistic to most patients (Goodman 1990).

Dorsal root entry zone lesions

The Dorsal root entry zone (DREZ) operation involves making a series of lesions directed at the substantia gelantinosa and adjoining fibre tracts which will destroy the overactive neurons in the affected segments (Goodman 1990). The goal is to ablate Lis-sauer's tract and laminae I–V in the spinal cord on the side of the pain. The central nuclear groups of the dorsal horn are affected by this ablation. The procedure was first performed for a patient with severe pain secondary to brachial plexis avulsion, who is now completely pain free (Nashold 1988). The pain was from deafferentation. It was believed to have originated from abnormal, active secondary nociceptive neurons in the dorsal horn of the spinal cord (Goodman 1990) (Fig. 11.4). The cord lesions are directed to reduce the cellular hyperactivity seen after deafferentation in central pain syndromes.

The technique involves a laminectomy, either unilateral or bilateral, at the der-matomal level of the area of the pain (Cosmon *et al.* 1984, 1988). The dura mater is opened and an operating microscope used to see the dorsal rootlets entry zone into the spinal cord—the DREZ. An electrode, usually 0.25 mm in diameter with 2 mm exposed metal tip, is then inserted about 2–3 mm into this zone. The lesion is made using a

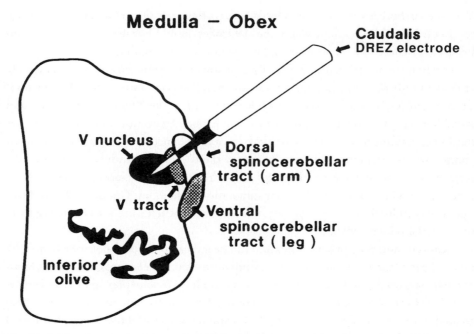

Fig. 11.4 The placement of electrode for DREZ treatment and its relationship with the spinio-cerebellar tract and nucleus caudalis (From Moore and Burchiel 1996).

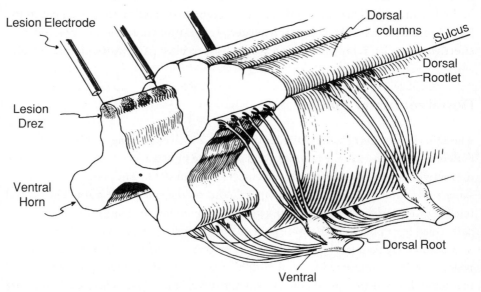

Fig. 11.5 Drawing of the anatomic location of the dorsal root entry zone and the area for the DREZ lesions (From Nashold, 1988).

radio-frequency thermal technique with a tip temperature of 75 °C for 15–20 seconds. A series of such lesions are made along the vertical line of the rootlets, spanning 2–3 dermatomal levels (Fig. 11.5). The lesions are separated by about 1 mm 20–50 lesions are created, depending upon the number of dermatomes involved. The longest series may extend over 5 cm. Laser and ultrasound can be used to create the lesions (Young 1990; Dreval 1992). DREZ has been used for deafferentated or central pain caused by damage to the nervous system.

DREZ is typically considered for the treatment of chronic pain that cannot be treated adequately by medico-pharmacological options. Some of the most suitable candidates for this procedure are those experiencing pain secondary to nerve root avulsion from, for example, brachial plexus injury (Goodman 1990).

For other non-cancer pain, especially central pain from an injury or damage to the central nervous system, creation of lesions in the DREZ may be helpful although the success rate is lower. The most common applications are for brachial plexus avulsion pain, spinal cord injury pain, phantom limb or stump pain, or postherpetic pain (Iskandar 1998).

For brachial plexus avulsion pain, good pain relief at follow-up intervals of 12–48 months, has ranged from 65–80%, although the success rate is more typically 60–65% in series with longer follow-up periods (Iskandar 1998). Phantom limb or stump pain success rates appear to be lower (50–60%) in smaller series with follow-up periods to 60 or 79 months. These lesions have also been applied to pain from trauma to the conus medullaris or cauda equina. In 39 patients with a mean follow-up of 3 years, pain relief was noted in 74% of patients, although the degree of relief varied (Iskandar 1998). Use of DREZ lesioning for intercostal postherpetic neuralgia has shown significantly lower success rates.

For spinal cord injury, this procedure is most useful for the radicular or segmental pain that occurs at or just below the level of the injury. The success rate for good pain control has been reported at 70–75% for this type of pain (Edgar *et al.* 1993; Friedman and Nashold 1986). The diffuse, burning pain over the lower body or phantom pain in the same areas appears to not respond as well to DREZ lesioning. Permanent sensory changes are found in about 10–13% of patients. Permanent motor changes are found in about the same number of patients. Transient sensory or motor changes are seen in about 5% of patients. Infection or cerebrospinal fluid leaks occur in about 5–7% of patients.

Midline myelotomy

The midline myelotomy procedure was first conceived as a way of treating a patient with tabetic abdominal pain (Armour 1927) and first performed by Putnam in 1934. The procedure has undergone many mechanical and functional adjustments for new applications. Midline myelotomy can be performed with mechanical ablation, radiofrequency techniques, or carbon dioxide laser (Fink 1984) to section midline fibres posterior to the central canal of the spinal cord.

The lesions are usually created at the lower thoracic spinal cord level, although Gildenberg and Hirsberg (1984) and others also have reported lesions at C1. The effectiveness in moderate to marked pain relief has been approximately 70%, with only rare complications or side effects. This procedure appears to be effective for lower body pain, especially midline or bilateral pain for which cordotomy or other ablative lesions might not be useful. Furthermore, analgesia from hyperpathia and background pain has been obtained without sensory loss, but with preserved ability to localize and discriminate between sharp and dull stimuli (Schvarcz 1976).

The main goal of performing a commissural myelotomy on the spinal cord is to interrupt all decussating second-order spinothalamic fibres that are contributing to pain perception on both sides of the body through an anterior commissure of the spinal cord. There have only been about 425 cases reported (Sundar-Plassmann and Grumert 1976; Hitchcock 1974; Schvarcz 1976, 1984; Gildenberg and Hirsberg 1984; Broager 1974; Cook and Kawakami 1977; Lippert and Hosobuchi 1974; Papo and Luongo 1976; King 1977; Payne 1984; Fink 1984; Sweet 1984; Adams *et al.* 1988).

Although many different methods have been described there is a lack of knowledge about myelotomy, particularly regarding the mechanism of pain relief. There is also evidence for a tract in the anterior part of the medial borders of the posterior columns mediating both pelvic and more proximal epigastric visceral pain (Hirshberg *et al.* 1996; Al Chaer *et al.* 1996*a, b*).

Two midline myelotomy procedures are presently available for patients: open and closed. The open operation requires an incision in the spinal cord down the exact midline between the two gracilis tracts and ventrally configured down until completely divided. Through this transection, the two sides of the posterior half of the spinal cord are disconnected, independent of each other, and can no longer communicate dorsally. The closed operation involves placement, with a CT-guided technique, of a radio-frequency electrode between the two gracilis tracts.

Summary

A number of neurosurgical procedures for the treatment of intractable pain have been described. Improved stereotactic technology, especially using magnetic resonance guidance, has improved the accuracy and ease of application of intracranial procedures. Information is still not complete concerning the best application of many of these procedures. For the most part, these techniques are applied only to patients with severe pain, since many of the non-surgical options will adequately manage milder pain.

Selection of a specific technique can be based upon expected survival time, pain type and location, preference for ablative or augmentative options and experience available. Although each of these procedures has been championed and found effective by different clinical groups, information is lacking concerning the best procedure for specific pain syndromes. Hopefully, the role of these neurosurgical procedures in the overall management of patients experiencing severe pain will be clarified as more information becomes available.

References

Adams, J.E., and Hosobuchi, Y. (1988). Commissural myelotomy. In *Current techniques in operative neurosurgery*, S.H. (ed. W.H. Sweet), pp. 1185–9. Grune and Stratton, New York.

Al-Chaer, E.D., Lawland, W.B., Westlund, K.N., and Willis, W.D. (1996*a*). Visceral nodiceptive input into the ventral posterolateral nucleus of the thalamus: A new function for the dorsal column pathway. *Journal of Neurophysiology*, **76**, 2661–74.

Al-Chaer, E.D., Lawland, W.B., Westlund, K.N., and Willis, W.D. (1996*b*). Pelvic visceral input into the nucleus gracillis is largely mediated by the postsynaptic dorsal column pathway. *Journal of Neurophysiology*, **76**, 2675–90.

Allen, R.P., and Faillace, L.A. (1972). A clinical test for detecting defects of cingulate lesions in man. *Journal of Clinical Psychology*, **28**, 63–5.

Amano, K., Kitamura, K., Sano, K., Sedino, H. (1976). Relief of intractable pain from neurosurgical point of view with reference to present limits and clinical indications: a review of 100 consecutive cases. *Neurol Med Chir(Tokyo)*, **16**, 141–53.

Amano, K., Kawamura, H., Tanikawa, T., Kawabatake, H., Iseki, H., Taira, T. (1992). Stereotactic mesencephalotomy for pain relief. *Stereotactic and Functional Neurosurgery*, **59**, 25–32.

Armour, D. (1927). Surgery of the spinal cord and its membranes. *Lancet*, **1**, 691.

Ballantine, H.T. (1986). A critical assessment of psychiatric surgery: past, present, and future. In *American handbook of psychiatry*. (ed. P.A. Berger), pp. 1029–45. Basic Books: New York.

Ballantine, H.T., Bouckoms, A.J., Thomas E.K., *et al*. (1987). Treatment of psychiatric illness by stereotactic cingulotomy. *Biological Psychiatry*, **22**, 807–19.

Benabid, A.L., S.R., De Rougemont, J., *et al*., Clinical evaluation of stereotactic isotope hypophysectomy in advanced breast cancer. *Rev Endocrine Rel Cancers* (Suppl), 1978: p. 111–117.

Brazenor, G.A. (1987). Long-term intrathecal administration of morphine: a comparison of bolus injection via reservoir with continuous infusion by implanted pump. *Neurosurgery*, **21**, 484–91.

Broager, B. (1974). Commissural myelotomy. *Surgical Neurology*, **2**, 71.

Cook, A.W., Kawakami, Y. (1977). Commissural myelotomy. *Journal of Neurosurgery*, **47**, 1.

Coombs, D.W. (1988). Intraspinal analgesic infusion by implanted pump. *Annals of the New York Academy of Science*, **531**, 108–22.

Corkin, S., Sullivan, E.V. (1979). Safety and efficacy of cingulotomy for pain and psychiatric disorder. *In Modern concepts in psychiatric surgery* (ed. E.R. Hitchcock, H.T. Ballantine, and B.A. Myerson), pp. 253–272. Elsevier North-Holland, New York.

Cosman, E.R., Nashold, B.J., and Ovelmen-Levitt, J. (1984). Theoretical aspects of radio-frequency lesions in the dorsal root entry zone. *Neurosurgery*, **15**, pp. 945–50.

Cosmon E.R., Rittman, W.J., Nashold, B.S. Jr., *et al*. (1988). Radiofrequency lesion generation and its effect on tissue impedance. *Applied Neurophysiology*, **51**, 230–42.

Daniel, P.M., and Prichard, M.M. (1972). The human hypothalamus and pituitary stalk after hypophysectomy of pituitary stalk section. *Brain*, **95**, 813–24.

Dennis, G.C., DeWitty, R.L. (1990). Long-term intraventricular infusion of morphine for intractable pain in cancer of the head and neck. *Neurosurgery*, **26**, 404–8.

Deshpande, N., Moricca, G. (1981). Saullo, F., *et al.*, Some aspects of pituitary function after neuro-adenolysis in patients with metastatic cancer. *Tumori*, 1981. **67**: p. 355–359.

Dreval, O.N. (1992). Ultrasonice DREZ-operations for treatment of pain due to brachial plexus avulsion. *Acta Neurochirurgica*, **122**, 76–81.

Edgar, R.E., Best, L.G., Quail, P.A., *et al.* (1993). Computer-assisted DREZ microcoagulation: posttraumatic spinal deafferentation pain. *Journal of Spinal Disorders*, **6**, 48–56.

Faillace, L.A., McQueen, J.B., Northrup, B. *et al.* (1981). Cognitive deficits from bilateral cingulotomy for intractable pain in man. *Diseases of the Nervous System*, **32**, 171–5.

Fairman, D. (1971). Hypothalamotomy as a new perspective for alleviation of intractable pain and regression of metastatic malignant tumors. In *Present limits of neurosurgery* (ed. K. Fusek), pp. 525–8. Avicenum Czechoslovakian Medical Press, Prague.

Fink, R.A. (1984). Neurosurgical treatment of non-malignant intractable rectal pain: Microsurgical commissural myelotomy with the carbon dioxide laser. *Neurosurgery*, **14**, 64.

Foltz, E.L. (1962). Pain 'relief' by frontal cingulumotomy. *Journal of Neurosurgery*, **19**, 89–100.

Frank, F., Fabrizi, A.P., Gaist, G. (1989). Stereotactic mesencephalic tractotomy in the treatment of chronic pain. *Acta Neurochirurgica(Wein)*, **99**, 38–40.

Friedman, A.H., Nashold, B.J. (1986). DREZ lesions for the relief of pain related to spinal cord injury. *Journal of Neurosurgery*, **65**, 465–9.

Gildenberg, P.L., Hirsberg, R.M. (1984). Limited myelotomy for the treatment of intractable cancer pain. *Journal of Neurology, Neurosurgery and Psychiatry*, **47**, 94–6.

Goodman, R.R. (1990). Surgical management of pain. *Neurosurgery Clinics of North America*, **1**(3), 701–17.

Greco, T., Cammilli, L., *et al.* (1957). L'alcolizzazione della ipofisi per via transfenoidal nella terapia di particoloari tumori maligni. *Settim Med*, **45**, 355–6.

Gros, C., Privat, J.M., *et al.* (1975). Place of hypophysectomy in the neurosurgical treatment of pain. *Advances in Neurosurgery*, **3**, 264–72.

Gybels, J., Kupers, R. (1990). Deep brain stimulation in the treatment of chronic pain in man: where and why? *Neurosurgery*, **21**, 484–91.

Hadley, M.N., Shetter, A.G., Amos, M.R. (1985). Use of the Brown-Roberts-Wells stereotactic frame for functional neurosurgery. *Applied Neurophysiology*, **48**, 61–8.

Harris, B. (1985). Dorsal rhizotomy. In *Neurosurgery* (ed. R.H. Wilkins), pp. 2430–7. McGraw-Hill, New York.

Hassenbusch, S.J., Pillay, P.K., Barnett, G.H. (1990). Radiofrequency cingulotomy for intractable cancer pain using stereotaxis guided by magnetic resonance imaging. *Neurosurgery*, **27**, 220–3.

Hassenbusch, S.J., Pillay, P.K. (1992*a*). Cingulotomy for intractable pain using stereotaxis guided by magnetic resonance imaging. In *Neurosurgical operative atlas* (ed. S.S. Rengachary and R.H. Wilkins), pp. 449–58. Williams & Wilkins, Baltimore.

Hassenbusch, S.J., Pillay, P.K. (1992*b*). Ablative intracranial neurosurgery for cancer pain: three-year experience and modification of techniques. *Journal of Neurosurgery*, **76**, p. 396A (abstract).

Hassenbusch, S.J., Pillay, P.K. (1993). Cingulotomy for treatment of cancer-related pain. Mt. Kisco, NY: *Futura*, pp. 297–312.

Hassenbusch, S.J. (1996). Surgical management of behavioural and affective disorders. In *The practice of neurosurgery* (ed. G.T. Tindall and D.L. Barrow), pp. 3257–69. Williams & Wilkins, Baltimore.

Hirshberg, R.M., Al-Chaer, E.D., Lawand, N.B., Westlund, K.N., and Willis, W.D. (1996). Is there a pathway in the posterior funiculus that signals visceral pain? *Pain*, **67**, 291–305.

Hitchcock, E. (1970). Stereotactic cervical myelotomy. *Journal of Neurology, Neurosurgery and Psychiatry*, **33**, 224.

Hitchcock, E. (1974). Stereotactic myelotomy. *Proceedings of the Royal Society of Medicine*, **67**, 771.

Hurt, R.W., Ballantine, H.T. Jr. (1974). Stereotactic anterior cingulate lesions for persistent pain: a report on 68 cases. *Clinical Neurosurgery*, **21**, 334–51.

Iskandar, B.J. (1998). Spinal and trigeminal DREZ lesions. In *Textbook of stereotactic and functional neurosurgery* (ed. P.L. Gildenberg), pp. 1573–83. McGraw-Hill, New York.

Jenike, M.A., Baer, L., Ballantine, T., *et al.* (1991). Cingulotomy for refractory obsessive-compulsive disorder. *Archives of General Psychiatry*, **48**, 548–55.

Kanpolat, Y., Akyar, S., Caglar, S., Unlu, A., and Bilgic, S. (1993). CT-guided percutaneous selective cordotomy. In *Acta Neurochirurgica* (ed. F. Loew), pp. 92–6. Springer-Verlag, New York.

Kapur, T.R. Dalton, G.A. (1969). Trans-sphenoidal hypophysectomy for metastatic carcin-oma of the breast. *British Journal of Surgery*, **56**, 332–7.

Karavelis, A., Foroglas, G., Selviaridis, P., Fountzilas, G. (1996). Intraventricular administration of morphine for control of intractable cancer pain in 90 patients. *Neurosurgery*, **39**, 57–62.

Katz, S., Levin, A.B. (1977). Treatment of diffuse metastatic pain by instillation of alcohol in to the sella turcia. *Anesthesiology*, **46**, 115–21.

King, R.B. (1977). Anterior commissurotomy for intractable pain. *Journal of Neurosurgery*, **47**, 7.

Kudo, T., Yoshii, N., Shimizu, S., *et al.* (1966). Effects of stereotactic thalamotomy to intractable pain and numbness. *Keio Journal of Medicine*, **15**, 191–5.

Kudo, T., Yoshii, N., Shimizu, S., *et al.* (1968). Stereotactic thalamotomy for pain relief. *Tohoku Journal of Experimental Medicine*, **96**, 219–30.

Kumar, K., Wyant, G.M., Nath, R. (1990). Deep brain stimulation for control of intractable pain in humans, present and future: A ten-year follow-up. *Neurosurgery*, **26**, 774–82.

Laitinen, L.V. (1977). Anterior pulvinotomy in the treatment of intractable pain. In

Neurosurgical treatment in psychiatry, pain, and epilepsy (ed. W.H. Sweet and J.G. Martin-Rodriguez), pp. 669–72. University Park Press: Baltimore.

Lazorthes, Y. (1988). Intracerebroventricular administration of morphine for control of irreducible cancer pain. *Annals of the New York Academy of Science*, **531**, 123–32.

Leskell, L. (1968). Cerebral radiosurgery: gammathalamotomy in two cases of intractable pain. *Acta Chirurgica Scandinavica*, **134**, 585–95.

Levin, A.B., Katz, J., Benson, R.C., *et al.* (1980). Treatment of pain of diffuse metastatic cancer by stereotactic chemical hypophysectomy: long-term results and observations on mechanism of action. *Neurosurgery*, **6**, 258–62.

Levin, A.B., Ramirez, G., Katz, J. (1983). The use of stereotaxic chemical hypophysectomy in the treatment of thalamic pain syndrome. *Journal of Neurosurgery*, **59**, 1002–6.

Levin, A.B. (1993). Hypophysectomy in the treatment of cancer pain. In *Management of cancer-related pain* (ed. E. Arbit), pp. 281–95. Futura: Mt. Kisco, NY.

Lewin, W. (1961). Observations on selective leucotomy. *Journal of Neurology, Neurosurgery, Psychiatry*, **24**, 69–73.

Lewin, W. (1972). Selective leucotomy: a review. In *Surgical approaches in psychiatry* (ed. L.V. Laitinen), pp. 69–73. University Park Press, Baltimore.

Lindquist, C., Kihlstrom, L., and Hellstrand, E. (1991). Functional neurosurgery: a future for the gamma knife? *Stereotactic and Functional Neurosurgery*, **57**, 72–81.

Lippert, R.G., Hosobuchi, Y., Nielsen, S.L. (1974). Spinal commissurotomy. *Surgical Neurology*, **2**, 373.

Lipton, S. (1983). Percutaneous cervical cordotomy and pituitary injection of alcohol, In *Relief of intractable pain* (ed. M. Swerdlow), pp. 269–304). Elsevier, Amsterdam.

Maddy, J.A., Winternitz, W.W., and Norrell, H. (1971). Cryohypophysectomy in the management of advanced prostatic cancer. *Cancer*, **28**, 322–8.

Madrid, J.L. (1979). Chemical hypophysectomy. *Advances in Pain Research and Therapy*, **2**, 381–91.

Martinez, R., Vaquero, J. (1991). Image-directed functional neurosurgery with the Cosman-Roberts-Wells stereotactic instrument. *Acta Neurochirurgica (Wein)*, **113**, 1769.

Mayanagi, Y., Bouchard, G. (1976). Evaluation of stereotactic thalamotomies for pain relief with reference to pulvinar intervention. *Applied Neurophysiology*, **39**, 154–7.

Mayanagi, Y., Sano, K., Suzuki, I. *et al.* (1982). Stimulation and coagulation of the posteromedial hypothalamus for intractable pain, with reference to beta-endorphins. *Applied Neurophysiology*, **45**, 136–42.

Mempel, E., Dietrich-Rap, Z. (1977). Favorable effect of cingulotomy on gastric crisis pain. *Neurol Neurochirurgica Pol*, **11**, 611–13.

Miles, J. (1979). Chemical hypophysectomy. *Advances in Pain Research and Therapy*, **2**, 373–80.

Moore, K.R., and Burchiel, K. (1996). Surgical management of trigeminal neuralgia. In *The practice of neurosurgery* (ed. G.T. Tindall and D.L. Barrow), pp. 3043–64. Williams & Wilkins: Baltimore.

Nashold, B.S., Jr. (1982). Stereotaxic mesencephalotomy and trigeminal tractotomy, In *Neurological surgery* (ed. J.R. Youmans, 2nd edn), pp. 3702–16, Saunders, Philadelphia.

Nashold, B.S., Jr. (1988). Introduction to second international symposium on dorsal root entry zone (DREZ) lesions. *Applied Neurophysiology*, 51, 76–7.

Nilaver, G., Zimmerman, E.A., Wilkins, J., *et al*. (1980). Magnocellular hypothalamic projections to the lower brain stem and spinal cord of the rat: immunocytochemical evidence for predominance fo the oxytocin-neurophysin system compared to a vaso-pressin-neurophysin system. *Neuroendocrinology*, 30, 150–8.

Ortiz, A. (1972). The role of the limbic lobe in central pain mechanisms: an hypo-thesis relating to the gate control theory of pain. In *Surgical approaches in psychiatry* (ed. L.V. Laitinen and K.E. Livingston), pp. 59–64. University Park Press, Baltimore.

Papo, I., Luongo, A. (1976). High cervical commissural myelotomy in the treatment of pain. *Journal of Neurology, Neurosurgery and Psychiatry*, 39, 105.

Payne, N.S. (1984). Dorsal longitudinal myelotomy for the control of perineal and lower body pain. *Pain*, Suppl 2, S320.

Payne, R., Gradert, T.L., Inturris, C. (1996). Cerebrospinal fluid distribution of opioids after intraventricular and lumbar subarachnoid administration in sheep. *Life Sciences*, 59, 1307–21.

Perrault, M., Klotz, B. *et al*. (1952). L'hypophysectomie totale dans le traite-ment du cancer sein: premier cas francais: avenir de la methode. *Therapie*, 7, 290–300.

Pillay, P.K., Hassenbusch, S.J. (1992). Bilateral MRI-guided stereotactic for intractable pain. *Stereotactic and Functional Neurosurgery*, 59, 33–8.

Putnam, T.J. (1934). Myelotomy of the commissure. *Archives of Neurology and Psychiatry*, 32, 1189.

Rand, R.W. (1964). Stereotactic transsphenoidal cryohypophysectomy. *Bull L A Neurol Soc*. 29, 40–8.

Rezai, A.R., Lozano, A.M., Crawley, A.P., Joy, M.L.G., Davis, K.D., Kwan, C.L., Dosterovsky, J.O., Tasker, R.R., and Mikulis, D.J. (1999). Thalamic stimulation and functional magnetic resonance imaging: localization of cortical and subcortical activation with implanted electrodes. *Journal of Neurosurgery*, 90, 583–90.

Sano, K. (1962). Sedative neurosurgery with reference to posteromedial hypothalamo-tomy. *Neurol Medicochirurgica*, 4, 112–42.

Sano, K., Sekino, H., Hashimoto, I., *et al*. (1975). Posteromedial hypothalamotomy in the treatment of intractable pain. *Confinia Neurol*, 37, 285–90.

Sano, K. (1977). Intralaminar thalamotomy and posteromedial hypothalamotomy in the treatment of intractable pain. *Prog Neurol Surg*, 8, 50–103.

Sano, K. (1987). Neurosurgical treatments of pain: a general survey. *Acta Neuro-chirurgica Suppl*, 38, 86–96.

Santo, J.L., Arias, L.M., Barolat, G., *et al*. (1990). Bilateral cingulumotomy in the treatment of reflex sympathetic dystrophy. *Pain*, 41, 55–9.

Schvarcz, J.R. (1976). Stereotactic extralemniscal myelotomy. *Journal of Neurology, Neurosurgery and Psychiatry*, 39, 53–7.

Schvarcz, J.R. (1978). Spinal cord stereotactic techniques re trigeminal nucleotomy and extralemniscal myelotomy. *Applied Neurophysiology*, 41, 99–112.

Schvarcz, J.R. (1984). Stereotactic high cervical extralemniscal myelotomy for pelvic cancer pain. *Acta Neurochirurgica*, Suppl 33, 431.

Seiwald, M., Alesch, F., and Kofler, A. (1996). Intraventricular morphine administration as a treatment possibility for patients with intractable pain. *Wiener Klinische Wochenschrift*, **108**, 5–8.

Sharma, T. (1973). Absence of cognitive deficits from bilateral cingulotomy for intractable pain in humans. *Tex Med*, **69**, 79–82.

Sharma, T. (1974). Abolition of opiate hunger in humans following bilateral anterior cingulotomy. *Tex Med*, **70**, 49–52.

Shieff, C., Nashold, B.S. (1987). Stereotactic mesencephalic tractotomy for thalamic pain. *Neuro-Science Research*, **9**, 101–4.

Shieff, C., Nashold, B.S. (1990). Stereotactic mesencephalotomy. *Neurosurgery Clinics of North America*, **1**, 825–39.

Siegfried, J. (1998). Intracerebral neurosurgery in the treatment of chronic pain. *Schweizerische Rundschau for Medizin Praxis*, **87**, 314–17.

Silverberg, G.D. (1977). Hypophysectomy in the treatment of disseminated prostate carcinoma. *Cancer*, **39**, 1727–31.

Silverman, A.J., Zimmerman, E.A. (1983). Magnocellular neurosecretory system. *Annual Review of Neuroscience*, **6**, 357–80.

Sjoqvist, O. (1938). Studies on pain conduction in trigeminal nerve: a contribution to the surgical treatment of facial pain. *Acta Psychiatrica and Neurologica*, Suppl. 1–139.

Sofroniew, M.V. (1980). Projections from vasopressin, oxytocin, and neurophysin neurons to neural targets in the rat and human. *Journal of Histochemistry and Cytochemistry*, **28**, 475–8.

Spiegel, E.A., Wycis, H.T., Marks, M. *et al.* (1947). Stereotactic apparatus for operations on the human brain. *Science*, **106**, 349–50.

Spiegel, E.A., Wycis, H.T. (1953). Mesencephalotomy in the treatment of 'intractable' facial pain. *Archives of Neurology*, **69**, 1.

Spiegel, E.A. (1982). Guided brain operations. Karger, Basel.

Steiner, L., Forster, D., Leksell, L. *et al.* (1980). Gammathalamotomy in intractable pain. *Acta Neurochirurgica*, **52**, 173–84.

Strenge, H. (1978). The functional significance of the pulvinar thalami. *Fortschrift Neurol Psychiat*, **46**, 491–507.

Sunder-Plassmann, M., Grumert, V. (1976). Commissural myelotomy for drug resistant pain, In *Clinical neurosurgery* (ed. W.T. Koos and R.F. Spetzler), pp. 165–70. Georg. Thiem Verlag.: Stuttgart.

Swanson, L.W., Sawchenko, P.E. (1980). Paraventricular nucleus: a site for the integration of neuroendocrine and autonomic mechanism. *Neuroendocrinology*, **31**, 410–17.

Sweet, W.H. (1980). Central mechanisms of chronic pain (neuralgias and certain other neurogenic pain). *Res Publ Assoc Res Nerv Ment Dis*, **58**, 287–303.

Sweet, W.H. P. (1984). Operations in the brain stem and spinal canal, with an appendix on open cordotomy. In *Textbook of pain*. (ed. P.D. Wall), pp. 615–31. Churchill Livingstone, Edinburgh.

Talairach, J., Tournoux, P. *et al.* (1956). Technique sterotaxique de la chirurgie hypophysaire par voie nasale: suites operatoires: indications therapeutiques. *Neurochirurgie*, **2**, 3–20.

Tasker, R. (1990). Neurosurgical and neuroaugmentative intervention. In *Cancer pain*, (ed. pp. 471–500). Lippincott, Philadelphia.

Tasker, R.R. (1990). Thalamotomy. *Neurosurgery Clinics of North America*, **1**(4), 841–66.

Tindall, G.T., Ambrose, S.S., Christy, J.H. *et al.* (1976). Hypophysectomy in the treatment of disseminated carcinoma of the breast and prostate gland. *South Med J*, **69**, 579–83.

Tindall, G.T., Payne, N.S., and Nixon, D.W. (1979). Transsphenoidal hypophysectomy for disseminated carcinoma of the prostate gland. *Journal of Neurosurgery*, **50**, 275–82.

Tseng, L.F., Fujimoto, J.M. (1984). Differential actions of intrathecal naloxone on blocking the tail flick inhibition induced by intraventricular beta-endorphin and morphine in rats. *Journal of Pharmacology and Experimental Therapeutics*, **232**, 74–9.

West, C.R., Avellarosa, A.M., Bremer, A.M. *et al.* (1979). Hypophysectomy for relief of pain in disseminated carcinoma of the prostate. *Advances in Pain Research and Therapy*, **2**, 393–400.

White, J.C. (1969). *Pain and the neurosurgeon: a forty-year experience* (ed. C.C. Thomas), pp. 232–51, 314–20. Springfield, IL.

Williams, N.E., Miles, J.B., Lipton, S. *et al.* (1980). Pain relief and pituitary function following injection of alcohol into the pituitary fossa. *Annals of the Royal College of Surgeons of England*, **62**, 203–7.

Yaksh, T.L., Onofrio, B.M. (1987). Restrospective consideration of the doses of morphine given intrathecally by chronic infusion in 163 patients by 19 physicians. *Pain*, **31**, 211–23.

Yoshii, N., Fukada, S. (1977). Several clinical aspects of thalamic pulvinotomy. *Applied Neurophysiology*, **39**, 162–4.

Yoshii, N., Fukada, S. (1979). Effects of unilateral and bilateral invasion of thalamic pulvinar for pain relief. *Tohoku Journal of Experimental Medicine*, **127**, 81–4.

Yoshii, N., Mizokami, T., Ushikubo, Y. *et al.* (1982). Comparative study between size of lesioned area and operative effects after pulvinotomy. *Applied Neurophysiology*, **45**, 492–7.

Young, R.F. (1990). Brain stimulation. *Neurosurgery Clinics of North America*, **1**, 865–79.

Young, R.F. (1990). Clinical experience with radiofrequency and laser DREZ lesions. *Journal of Neurosurgery*, **72**, 715–20.

Young, R.F., Tronnier, V., Rinaldi, P.C. (1992). Chronic stimulation of the Kolliker-Fuse nucleus region for relief of intractable pain in humans. *Journal of Neurosurgery*, **76**, 979–85.

Young, R.F. (1993). Electrical stimulation of the brain for the treatment of intractable cancer pain. In *Management of cancer-related pain* (ed. E. Arbit), pp. 257–69. Futura: Mt. Kisco, NY.

Zervas, N.T. (1969). Stereotaxic radiofrequency surgery of the normal and abnormal pituitary gland. *New England Journal of Medicine*, **280**, 429–37.

TWELVE

Selected surgical approaches

GEOFFREY DUNN

Diagnosis and treatment of pain is an appropriate reason for referral to a general surgeon at any time in the course of a malignant disease. The surgeon has many tasks in the
palliation of cancer including: staging of disease, control of disease, control of pain and
symptoms, reconstruction, and rehabilitation. The preparation of the patient for possible surgical intervention begins with the referring physician. The chances of a helpful
surgical encounter are enhanced by offering realistic expectations before the referral is
made. This requires knowledge on the part of the non-surgeon concerning prerequis-
ites and principles of surgical intervention. The surgeon has a valuable opportunity to
assess non-physical components of 'total pain' (Saunders and Sykes 1993). A surgeon
should be selected for the ability to appreciate the complexity of pain in addition to the
usual considerations of operative prowess or repertoire. The referring physician may
be surprised at the variety and intensity of responses of a patient referred or scheduled
for an operative procedure, even when the prospects of improvement are excellent.
Fears include vulnerability, loss of control or function, helplessness, and fear of complications of anaesthesia or surgery (Strain and Grossman 1975). These anxieties are
present in all those undergoing surgery but are even greater in cancer patients (Gottesman and Lewis 1982; Jacobsen *et al*. 1998). Minimizing or trivializing these concerns
only worsens distress by isolating the patient.

Any patient interested in or capable of tolerating a palliative procedure should be
considered for surgical referral, even if non-surgical approaches to the problem are
available. The patient and carers should understand the reason for surgical referral.
Even if no intervention is recommended, the consultation can at least make that fact a
matter of record and closure. About 30% of the work of a general surgeon involves
cancer (Ball *et al*. 1998). The surgeon can be valuable in validating previous operative
decisions, even after their benefit may have passed. Surgeons have training in wound
management and complicated nutrition problems and can offer valuable opinions,
particularly with progressive disease. They are well qualified to respond to inquiries
about the future course of disease, especially if confined to the abdomen. The timing of
referral to a surgeon is rarely too early, but is commonly too late.

Patients with cancer may have received chemotherapy and/or radiation therapy, as
well as previous surgical therapy. The sequels and complications of these treatments
must be assessed and corrected when possible. The most important supportive preoperative measure is reassurance to the patient that preparation is thorough, so that there
are few surprises at surgery and afterwards. A close partnership with the anaesthesia
team is critical. Considerations for postoperative analgesia may influence selection of

spinal rather than general anaesthetic. The incidence of phantom limb pain following amputation may be lower in patients with short term preoperative pain and patients without limb pain the day before surgery (Bessler *et al.* 1955; Fredericks 1985). Pre-operative epidural blockade reduces the incidence of phantom limb pain in the first year following amputation (Foley 1998). The operative anaesthetic encounter may become the basis for ongoing chronic pain management. Obtaining consent for surgery and anaesthesia provides a valuable opportunity to assess the patient's understanding and reactions to disease and its treatment. Explanation of the procedure, necessary for an informed consent, is another chance to demonstrate interest in the patient's pain. Surgical nurses can be very helpful during this process, serving as the patient's advocate as well as providing a less intimidating opportunity for discussion.

The repertoire of operations available for cancer pain management is a long one. There are no 'standard' procedures, since there is no standard cancer or standard patient. Pain is a subjective phenomenon. The appropriate remedy will vary as much as individuals vary. Commonly other distressing symptoms of disease will be present. The choice of operation should remedy or anticipate as many of these as possible, without unfavourably altering the benefit/risk ratio. The more symptoms that can be relieved, the more justified one is in considering increased risk. Confusion may result when 'palliative' is used to describe lessening of disease rather than symptoms. The term should only be used for procedures where the objective is symptom relief satisfactory to the patient. The ultimate goal of palliative surgery is both decreased symptom burden and enhanced existential satisfaction.

Anatomic resections and bypass procedures

Anatomic resection entails removal of an organ or part of an organ with or without its associated lymphatic and vascular drainages. Cancers presenting with pain are more likely to be advanced. Resection for pain, even in the presence of uncontrollable but relatively asymptomatic distant disease, is a reasonable consideration when disease is resectable or partially resectable, and if the sequelae do not add to the symptom burden of the patient. Anatomic resections are standardized operations with much accumulated, collective experience. Resection provides tissue for pathological evaluation, useful in the event of any subsequent adjuvent treatments. There is little data from prospective trials comparing the efficacy of resection with non-operative approaches.

The first 'successful' gastrectomy, performed by Billroth in 1881 was palliative for a patient who presented with a highly symptomatic and palpable lesion in the epigastrium (Zimmerman and Veith 1967). The original series of radical mastectomies described by Halstead all for advanced, symptomatic disease is another example of palliation (Halstead 1907). The degree of symptom relief the operation offered was good compared to any existing alternatives at the time, and in some cases surgery turned out to be curative. There are still some situations that justify resection of the breast for control of pain, as well as odour, and drainage, even in the face of distant disease unresponsive to treatment or for which no treatment is elected.

Anatomical resection may be used for painful splenomegaly in myeloproliferative disease. Splenectomy does not alter the course of the disease but can reduce transfusion requirements, provide pain relief, reduce dyspnoea and lessen anorexia secondary to stomach compression. The high complication rate following this operation should be considered when offering this choice, for example thrombosis of the splenic vein. Thrombosis can propogate into the portal and superior mesenteric venous systems, resulting in pain, anaemia, intractable ascites, and hepato-renal failure. Preoperative use of antiplatelet and anti-coagulant drugs can lessen the risk (Schwartz 1998). Laporoscopic splenectomy is now an option. It has the advantages of reducing postoperative hospitalization (Philips *et al.* 1994; Friedman *et al.* 1996), decreasing complications, including atelectasis, pancreatitis, ileus, and wound infection (Unger and Rosenbaum 1995) and increasing patient satisfaction (Stoldt *et al.* 1998).

Oesophageal procedures

Oesophageal carcinoma usually presents with dysphagia, but chest pain and odynophagia are also common symptoms. The five year survival following treatment, is approximately 15%. Therefore clear goals for palliation are important. The primary goal of staging oesophageal carcinoma is to determine whether surgical treatment should attempt to cure or palliate symptoms. Curative procedures require a more extensive resection including lymphatic drainages and tumour free margins.

A functional scale of dysphagia can be used as a basis for offering incurable patients palliative resection. In a scale described by Takita *et al.* (1977), dysphagia is graded from eating normally (Grade I) to inability to swallow saliva (Grade VI). Ability to take liquids only (Grade IV) is the point at which palliative resection is indicated. Dysphagia from oesophageal carcinoma has been shown to correlate highly with decreased physical and psychological well-being (Loizou *et al.* 1991). Palliative resection can restore swallowing for the remainder of the patient's life in 90% of cases. The presence of malignant effusion, widespread disease, gross mediastinal disease, local invasion of aorta, tracheobronchial tree, or vertebra, phrenic or recurrent laryngeal nerve paralysis, and Horner's syndrome are contraindications to palliative resection. Poor surgical candidates include patients with advanced age, poor pulmonary function, low serum albumin, reduced ejection fraction, and other significant co-morbid illness.

The two most common operations for oesophageal resection for tumours of the thoracic oesophagus and cardia include: transthoracic approach (Ivor-Lewis) and transhiatal approach (Orringer 1998). Although the idea of laparoscopic resection of the oesophagus sounds appealing, it offers no advantage at this time over open procedures (Robertson *et al.* 1996).

Bypass procedures or stents offer an alternative palliation for non-resectable cancers. Several options for restoration of patency of the lumen are available for lesions of the oesophagus. The most time-tested is bouginage of a stricture with dilators or a hydrostatic balloon. The safety of these procedures is enhanced by endoscopic guidance. The endoscope can also used to deliver a neodymium-YAG laser beam to intraluminal tumour (Kiefhaber 1987; Fleischer 1984), placement of a plastic conduit for brachtherapy isotopes (Greene *et al*. 1995), or placement of an intraluminal stent. The newer self-expanding metallic Wallstent has the advantage of increased comfort and safety over rigid plastic stents. The lumen allows passage of a soft diet. A non-fenestrated stent can be used to block fistulous communication between trachea and oesophagus, preventing aspiration (Do *et al*. 1993). Expandable stents are not retrievable. Tumour growing through the interstices of the stent can be removed by laser. If necessary, a second stent can be placed in tandem through the lumen of the first stent. Perforation and bleeding are the main risks of all intraluminal procedures directed towards the relief of stricture.

Gastric procedures

Resection of the stomach for a painful or bleeding, advanced cancer is the prototype operation for employment of an anatomical resection when palliation of symptoms is the only consideration. There is consensus among surgeons that resection is preferable for the management of symptoms than non-resective approaches such as bypass with gastrojejeunostomy. Life expectancy is also prolonged even though this may not have been the primary goal of therapy. In some cases total gastrectomy may be the best procedure for palliation, but mortality and complication rate is higher. Although re-establishment of intestinal continuity following total gastrectomy is easiest using oesophagojejeunostomy, formation of a Roux-en-Y with a 'j' pouch is associated with fewer post-prandial symptoms, improved postoperative nutritional parameters, and a better quality of life (Bozzetti *et al*. 1996; Nakane *et al*. 1995). A feeding jejeunostomy tube is routinely placed following total gastrectomy. Mortality for gastric resection parallels the extent of resection with a 10% mortality for total gastrectomy. Life expectancy following gastric resections for incurable cancer is several months to a year.

In cases of non-resectable disease, available options include: gastroenterostomy (anastomosis of the proximal jejeunum to the greater curvature of the stomach), stenting, intra-luminal laser ablation, and gastrostomy. Gastrostomy can be performed as an open, laparoscopic, or percutaneous endoscopic procedure (PEG). PEG is best performed under local anaesthesia with sedation. Relative contra-indications to PEG include ascites, coagulopathy, and conditions that preclude apposition of the stomach against the abdominal wall such as extensive tumour or previous gastric or extensive upper abdominal surgery.

Pancreatic procedures

Pancreatic, periampullary and distal common bile duct tumours are all capable of producing pain due to pancreatic ductal obstruction, intestinal obstruction, and nerve infiltration by tumour. Prior to more accurate preoperative imaging and laporoscopic staging many of the symptomatic patients explored were found to have incurable disease. Then attempts to resect the disease were abandoned and a biliary bypass and/or gastric bypass procedure was performed. In many cases open operation can now be substituted with a minimally invasive procedure when palliation of symptoms is the goal of therapy. There is debate about the extent to which open procedures for staging and palliation can be replaced by endoscopic and laporoscopic technique (Espat *et al.* 1999; Sohn *et al.* 1999). There is some precedent for considering resection for the palliation of symptoms from periampullary tumours (Johnson 1995; Lillemoe *et al.* 1996). Resections for cancers of the head of the pancreas, distal common bile duct, and the periampullary region (pancreaticoduodenectomy or 'Whipple' operation) include: the distal common bile duct, the head of the pancreas, the duodenum, and the gastric antrum. Some surgeons prefer to preserve the pylorus. In cases of antrectomy, a vagotomy procedure is performed. Delayed gastric emptying is the most common complication following pancreaticoduodenectomy. This problem will often respond to prokinetics such as metoclopropamide. Another potential complication is development of a pancreatic fistula which is managed by suction closed drainage. The use of octreotide can decrease the volume of fistula losses. The operative mortality for the procedure is 3% and as low as 1% in some centres. Successful palliation of symptomatic tumours of the ampulla by local excision has been described (Branum *et al.* 1996) and provides an alternative for patients unsuitable for pancreaticoduodenectomy. Distal pancreatic resection and splenectomy can be considered for lesions of the body and tail of the pancreas. This operation is spared the potential anastomotic complications associated with pancreaticoduodenectomy.

Any of the procedures can be complemented with intraoperative coeliac ganglion block for the relief of pain, as part of an open surgical procedure (Copping *et al.* 1978). Intraoperative splanchnicectomy, compared to a saline placebo, significantly reduced tumour related pain and delayed onset of pain when not present preoperatively (Lillemoe *et al.* 1993). There were no differences in hospital mortality or morbidity between the two groups. There was increased survival in the treated group in patients with pre-operative pain. Complications of coeliac plexus block include diarrhoea, postural hypotension, and haematoma.

Surgical controversies include the choice of pre-emptive palliation versus palliation of existing symptoms, the selection of endoscopic versus operative intervention, and the choice of open versus laparoscopic operation. Better preoperative staging and laparoscopic staging techniques are lessening the need for open laparotomy to determine resectability for cure. Unresectable, symptomatic patients can be managed by stenting and pharmacologic measures. Only 3% of these patients may ultimately require an open procedure for palliation (Sohn *et al.* 1999). However surgical palliation is effective and lasting, and in high-volume centres, can be accomplished with low morbidity an mortality. Risk factors for perioperative morbidity and mortality in patients undergoing surgical palliation for pancreatic cancer include: poor Karnofsky status, diabetes, and liver metastases (Bakkevold and Kambestad 1993). Pre-emptive surgical palliation addresses multiple symptoms (jaundice, pain, and duodenal obstruction) at one time under one anaesthetic. Surgery also affords the opportunity to assess resectability for cure, which cannot always be determined by preoperative staging.

Endoscopic stenting procedures for relief of jaundice are associated with low morbidity, brief hospital stay, and good patient satisfaction. Several prospective studies have shown that nonoperative biliary stenting is comparable to surgery for the short term relief of malignant obstructive jaundice with a success rate in excess of 90% (Watanapa and Wiliamson 1992). Endoscopic stenting has a lower procedure related complication rate, but a much higher rate of recurrent jaundice. The necessity for secondary procedures for stent replacement because of clogging can occur in up to 30% within three months of insertion. Other complications include cholangitis (25–46%), pancreatitis, acute cholecystitis, and stent displacement (10%). Endoscopic stent placement is the preferred initial approach in frail patients, those with advanced disease with life expectancy of less than three months, and patients not electing surgery. There is no proven advantage to percutaneous biliary stenting procedures in anticipation of curative or palliative operations for malignant obstruction of the bile ducts.

For patients undergoing open operative therapy, the recommended procedures for biliary obstruction include cholodochojejeunostomy or hepaticojejeunostomy. Bypass procedures to the duodenum are discouraged due to the increased incidence of re-obstruction from local disease and the potential problems of combined duodenal and biliary secretions in the event of anastomotic leak. Simple T-tube drainage of the obstructed common duct substitutes the problems of jaundice with the equally problematic loss of fluid and electrolytes. With the current state of radiologic and endoscopic capability, there is no reason to resort to this measure.

For endoscopic treatment of duodenal obstruction, the two main options include laser ablation and stent placement. Both have advantages and limitations. Both procedures are associated with an incidence of perforation (5%), important in lesions requiring multiple re-treatments. The self-expanding metal stent is replacing rigid conduits which were more dangerous and uncomfortable.

Open surgical treatment for unresectable duodenal obstruction has traditionally been bypass by means of an antecolic gastrojejeunostomy. Delayed gastric emptying is a frustrating postoperative complication. A gastrostomy tube is sometimes placed in case this occurs to allow gastric drainage, thus avoiding a nasogastric tube insertion. Positioning of the jejeunal loop in the retrocolic position, instead of the usual antecolic position, may be associated with a lower incidence of this problem (Lillemoe 1998). Some advocate antrectomy with gastrojejeunostomy as the procedure of choice for duodenal obstruction (Lucas *et al.* 1991). Patients bypassed by gastrojejeunostomy should be treated with a histamine (H_2) blocking agent to prevent marginal (stomal) ulceration.

Laparoscopic techniques are increasingly being performed for the relief of biliary and gastric outlet obstruction, but are dependent on local expertise. The results are comparable to open procedures, but the overall benefit when compared to open procedures has not yet been scrutinized in a prospective randomized study. No patient who could not tolerate an open procedure should be referred for a laparoscopic procedure.

Bowel procedures

Mechanical bowel obstruction can be expected in as many as 3–15% of cancer patients (Mercadante 1997). Pain associated with this syndrome is related to the level of obstruction, the nature of the neoplasm, and the degree of bowel distention. When pain is continuous it is usually related to tumour compression of a viscus. When the diagnosis of mechanical bowel obstruction is made in a cancer patient, surgery should be considered. In up to one third of cases that have surgery for suspected malignant obstruction, the cause proves to be benign (Osteen *et al.* 1980; Walsh and Schofield 1984). In obstructions caused by malignancy, over two thirds will be relieved with restored bowel patency (Rubin *et al.* 1989), though subsequent survival is determined by the origin of the disease (Turnbull *et al.* 1989). Up to two years survival following surgery for malignant obstruction has been reported (Beattie *et al.* 1989). Evaluation and relief of obstruction should be concurrent undertakings, beginning with physical examination and decompression. An upright abdominal film may demonstrate air-fluid levels, as well as the presence or absence of air in the colon. Plain abdominal films may be unremarkable in high intestinal obstruction or with extensive encasement of bowel by tumour or radiation fibrosis. A thinned barium study can be helpful in determining the level and degree of obstruction. Delayed transit of contrast due to mesenteric infiltration is a predictor of surgical failure (Turnbull *et al.* 1989). An oral gastrograffin study may resolve some obstructive episodes (Assalia *et al.* 1994). Barium enema or colonoscopy should be used to demonstrate the presence and level of a suspected colonic obstruction.

Considerations for operability are based on the general performance status of the patient and the characteristics of the tumour. Favourable candidates for surgery have good performance status, recent onset of symptoms and no previous abdominal cancer surgery, except primary resection. Absolute contraindications for surgery include re-obstruction following recent laparotomy for obstruction, obstruction following surgery documenting disease unresponsive to treatment, diffuse intra-abdominal disease (miliary studding or multiple palpable masses), rapidly re-accumulating ascites, and poor performance status. Relative contra-indications to surgery include cachexia, low serum albumin, low lymphocyte count, previous radiotherapy to the abdomen or pelvis, age over 65 years, existence of liver or distant metastases, multiple levels of obstruction and significant co-morbid illness.

Initial management of mechanical or functional obstruction in malignant disease includes nasogastric decompression with correction of acute fluid and volume derangements. A brief trial of nasogastric decompression in the absence of clinical or laboratory evidence of bowel ischaemia is safe and may result in spontaneous resolution of the obstruction. Strangulation is rare from carcinomatosis (Gallick *et al.* 1986). Trials of longer than five days rarely benefit. Delay in management decisions risks new complications such as aspiration, intravenous therapy related problems, and prolonged hospitalization. Nasogastric decompression should be used only as a temporary measure while a decision is made for operative versus non-operative management. There is no advantage for long intestinal drainage tubes over nasogastric drainage. Pharmacologic measures for the relief of obstructive symptoms can be initiated during decompression. Octreotide may be beneficial for surgically managed cases. It reduces bowel secretions, making the bowel less distended, therefore less ischaemic and more manageable in the hands of the surgeon (Mercadante 1997).

The period of initial decompression allows the opportunity to clarify the goals of surgery and to provide information about expected outcomes. Discussion about tube and stoma placement, anticipated postoperative care requirements, expected physiological and anatomic changes, possible complications, and survival data all support a truly informed decision about surgery. Equally important is reassurance of a non-operative plan for symptom relief if surgery fails.

Surgery for malignant obstruction is dangerous. Mortality can be as high as 40%. This reflects underlying disease, since similar findings are not seen with the same operations for benign disease. Symptom burden may not decrease with surgery. It may become greater due to complications such as wound dehiscence or enterocutaneous fistula. Baines (1998) makes two critical philosophical points when considering surgery:

- operation should not be undertaken solely based on fear of dying a miserable death from obstruction, since effective pharmacologic remedies are available; and,

- surgery should not be withheld because of knowledge of those same remedies.

The selection of procedure is determined by the level(s) of obstruction, the nature of the pathological processes, and the tolerances of the patient. Patients should be advised of the possibility of an ostomy before surgery for obstruction. Obstructed, unprepared bowel can preclude a safe anastomosis, especially if the bowel has been irradiated. Colonic obstruction is more likely to be relieved by surgery. Unless the obstruction is due to a benign cause or very limited oncologic disease, a gastrostomy tube placed at the time of surgery may be useful if slow or uncertain postoperative recovery of bowel function is anticipated. If the bowel is completely encased with tumour, the safest course of action may be placement of a gastrostomy tube only. A tumour biopsy should be carried out if histologic proof of disease is needed. Definitive operation choices include: lysis of adhesions with repair of bowel wall where serosa is denuded or focally devascularized, resection of obstructing segment with primary anastomosis, resection with formation of an ostomy from proximal bowel and formation of a mucous fistula from the de-functionalized limb. These can be brought out side by side or at separate abdominal wall sites. The mucous fistula can be useful for administration of suppositories. In cases of extensive disease or where there is evidence of radiation enteritis, bypass of the obstruction with enteroenterostomy or entero-colostomy should be used. A proximally placed diverting ileostomy or colostomy, is another choice for unresectable disease. In some cases, a proximal diverting stoma above an anastomosis will be performed. Delayed closure of this type of stoma can be done if patency and healing of the anastomosis is demonstrated. The decision to perform a primary anastomosis must consider relief of symptoms with minimum risk of increasing symptom burden.

If open operation is not pursued, colonic obstruction can be relieved by intraluminal laser ablation of tumour. Extrinsically compressing tumours are not suitable for this due to risk of perforation. Even a small lumen created by laser or a stent can allow passage of air or liquid stool. Adjuvent pharmacologic therapy should then keep stool liquid enough to pass through the stenotic area.

Pseudo-obstruction of the colon (Ogilvie's syndrome) as a consequence of malignancy or its treatment may prompt referral to a surgeon in cases refractory to pharmacologic manipulation. When the caecum is dilated on plain abdominal film, or where vascular compromise of the bowel is suspected, surgical decompression should be considered. Colonoscopic decompression will relieve the distention in the majority of cases, though repeated decompression may be necessary. Success was 88% in one series (Geller *et al*. 1996). Colonoscopy can also determine if mechanical obstruction is present. Epidural anaesthesia has been used to treat this problem, possibly due to the sympathetic blockade it confers (Lee *et al*. 1988). Surgical options include placement of a caecostomy tube or formation of a loop colostomy. Laporoscopic evaluation and placement of a caecostomy tube has also been used (Duh and Way 1993).

Breast procedures

Few problems are more distressing than a painful, ulcerated, bleeding, and malodorous breast mass. Two well recognized pain syndromes are post-mastectomy syndrome and phantom breast syndrome. Surgical palliation of a locally advanced breast tumour should first address the preoperative role, if any, of radiotherapy and chemotherapy. A partial response to these can make a non-resectable lesion resectable and capable of primary closure. Grafting can be done with split-thickness skin, a myocutaneous flap, or omental graft covered with a split-thickness skin graft for breast resections that cannot be primarily closed. Delayed closure can be performed in cases of grossly infected or heavily colonized wounds. If palpable secondary disease of the axilla is present, breast resection should include this to pre-empt ulceration, pain, and arm lymphoedema. Palliation of breast disease is not complete without addressing breast reconstruction. Acknowledgement of the importance of body image is necessary even if the circumstances suggest reconstruction would not be performed. Reconstruction options include the use of tissue expanders, rotational, and free flaps. The only reason to delay reconstruction is a functional status that would make a more prolonged anaesthetic unsafe.

Genito-urinary tract procedures

Organ resection for relief of symptoms can occasionally be justified with carcinoma of the kidney. The decision to operate can be difficult since it is bulkier lesions with adjacent vascular and organ involvement that are more likely to be symptomatic. Even in the presence of distant metastases, operation can be justified for relief of pain, haematuria, and constitutional symptoms (Fowler 1987). In some cases nephrectomy may be considered in anticipation of these symptoms. This should be balanced with the knowledge that survival of patients with distant metastases can be as high as 68% at one year (Couillard and White 1993). Bleeding from advanced kidney carcinoma, which is probably the most pressing reason for palliative nephrectomy, can be managed by selective arterial embolization.

   In patients with good performance status, total or partial organ resection for relief of symptoms can be considered for bulky tumours of the bladder when symptoms are resistant to less invasive means, even with distant disease for which no further therapy is anticipated. If inguinal nodes are grossly involved, their removal should be considered to pre-empt sepsis from fungating, painful, malodorous wounds, or sudden, massive exsanguination. Transurethral resection should be considered first. It can be performed repeatedly for relief of obstruction, bleeding, and strangury.

Partial or total penectomy is an option for pain control in ulcerated and secondarily infected lesions for locally advanced, carcinoma of the penis. If the patient's priorities are preservation of the organ, a combination of techniques may be necessary. For example, an incontinent patient with a painful, malodorous lesion, who desires organ preservation may be managed with topical antibiotics, systemic analgesics, and either an incontinence pad or urinary drainage catheter.

Pain can be caused by malignant ureteral obstruction, usually due to tumours of the prostate, cervix, bladder, and colon (Resnick and Kursh 1992). This is typically flank pain. Fever and symptoms related to uraemia may also be present. There has been controversy about the appropriateness of urological intervention for malignant ureteral obstruction in advanced disease. Recent improvements in endoscopy and stents resulting in substantially lower morbidity and mortality have favoured more active intervention. Tumour type is more predictive of success than degree of renal failure, age, or grade and stage of tumour (Zadra *et al.* 1987). Tumour type is also predictive of the likelihood of technical difficulty for some procedures. Bladder and prostate tumours are more likely to distort landmarks such as the ureteral orifices, making retrograde stent placement more difficult. In more than half the cases of malignant ureteral obstruction, retrograde stenting is not possible (Gasparini *et al.* 1991). In these cases an anterograde or a combination of anterograde and retrograde stenting approaches can be tried. For obstruction not amenable to stenting or where suitable endoscopic equipment and stents are not available, a percutaneous nephrostomy done under radiological or ultrasound guidance will satisfactorily divert the urinary stream. The traditional 'open' operative approach to nephrostomy was associated with an unacceptably high morbidity and mortality (Culkin *et al.* 1987). The disadvantages of urinary tract infection and displacement that attend a percutaneous nephrostomy can be circumvented by a subcutaneous stenting approach (Ahmadzadeh 1991). Self-expanding metal stents have shown promise in lessening stent related complications without sacrificing patency rates.

Resection of malignant masses

'De-bulking' or 'cytoreduction' is best known for its role in the treatment of ovarian carcinoma in conjunction with chemotherapy. It is a non-standardized form of resection that may or may not include an anatomic resection of an organ or organ system. It can be used for the irradiation of symptoms instead of irradiation of disease which is usually disseminated when selecting this therapy. An example is excision of a painful, ulcerated cutaneous implant of metastatic melanoma. Indications for excision can include cosmetically distressing and function compromising lesions. Consent should reflect an understanding of degree of risk and difficulty, together with likelihood of meeting patient-defined goals. Lessening of symptoms rather than disease burden is the desired outcome. In some situations relief of symptoms can be accompanied by prolonged survival, for example re-resection of a slow growing sarcoma with margins that can not be cleared without prohibitive morbidity. If maximum tolerable radiation has been given previously, and surgical excision is not feasible or desired, cryotherapy or devascularization of tumour can be considered. Complications of metabolic acidosis, hyperkalaemia, hypothermia, acute renal failure from tissue lysis, sepsis, and unintended infarct (stroke) following devascularizations should be anticipated. Cryosurgery shows promise for palliative surgery. It has been used for ablation of recurrent head and neck cancer in previously irradiated areas, as well as for ablation of metastatic liver lesions not considered resectable by conventional criteria (Thompson *et al.* 1998).

Resection for control of humorally influenced symptoms

These procedures include orchidectomy for androgen suppression in the treatment of bone metastases from prostate carcinoma, and oophorectomy for oestrogen ablation in the treatment of metastatic breast carcinoma. Oophorectomy is still an option despite the availability of anti-oestrogen and progestational agents. It can be performed laparoscopically. Organ resection may be an alternative to pharmacologic anti-oestrogen therapy in cases where thrombotic risk is high. Completion total thyroidectomy should be performed to enhance radioactive iodine (I^{131}) identification and treatment of bone metastases from papillary and follicular carcinoma. Hepatic resection or debulking of functional metastases from carcinoid tumours can be done to palliate symptoms of flushing and diarrhoea, sometimes with benefit of over a year (McEntee *et al.* 1990). Other approaches include hepatic artery ligation or embolization. Debulking procedures have been used for metastatic gastrinoma and glucagonoma (Norton *et al.* 1985; Montenegro *et al.* 1980). The aggressive palliative surgical approach to palliation can only be justified in an institution demonstrating low morbidity and mortality following liver resection.

Amputations and orthopaedic procedures

The prevalence of skeletal metastases with pain and pathological fracture makes the orthopaedic specialist one of the most commonly called upon surgical consultants in the management of advanced malignancy. The four problems for which orthopaedic consultation should be sought include: bone pain with impending pathological fracture, existing pathological fracture, extremity amputation for control of symptoms and spine stabilization.

Amputations for the purpose of debulking of disease or intractable pain in a functionless extremity may be considered. The trend in management of extremity sarcoma has been to maximize limb preservation and function. There are situations when a well planned amputation is welcomed, for example with an ulcerated, painful and functionally useless extremity, even if mobility is compromised. Prophylaxis against stump pain and phantom limb pain should be considered with involvement of the anaesthetist and prosthetist. Stump pain is a neuropathic pain resulting from a traumatic neuroma at the site of the amputation. Prophylaxis includes measures that spare the transected nerve repetitive trauma (padding with adequate amount of tissue and avoidance of electrocautery when transecting nerves). When the syndrome is established, it can be treated by local injections or medication. In selected cases, the neuroma can be identified and transposed locally into a bed of muscle tissue. This approach can sometimes be used in post-mastectomy syndrome, which can result from neuroma formation of the sensory branches of T1 and T2. Preoperative analgesia in the extremity to be amputated may help to control phantom limb pain that is notoriously refractory to treatment. Preparation prior to amputation should include acknowledgement and readiness for potential adverse psychological reactions to the planned loss of an extremity, or a breast. In some cultures the disposition of the amputated part may be the most critical point of consent. Ambivalence of the patient about the need or the timing for the procedure is an indicator that preparation is not complete. Factors influencing the choice of amputation level include healing and rehabilitation potential. For rehabilitation, 'the longer the easier' applies, though the risk of non-healing is greater at more distal sites, especially in individuals with peripheral vascular disease.

Pain is the most common presentation of skeletal metastasis. Pain is present in approximately two-thirds of radiographically evident bone metastasis (Galasko 1972), and it can precede detection by X-ray. Any bone can develop metastases, and almost any tumour can metastasize to bone, but the distribution favours the axial skeleton. Breast carcinoma accounts for about half of the pathological fractures reported in one series (Galasko 1998). When skeletal metastases are present, investigations such as biopsy and treatment with radiation therapy can precipitate a pathological fracture. Radiation and drug management are the primary treatment of pain due to skeletal metastasis, however, orthopaedic consultation is needed in cases of impending fracture. Factors that predict fracture include: site, and size of the lesion, radiographic appearance of the lesion, and degree of pain. The risk of pathologic fracture increases with the degree of cortical destruction. If more than 50% of the cortex of a long bone is involved, the risk of spontaneous fracture is over 50% (Fidler 1981). Habermann and Lopez (1989) have suggested the following criteria for surgical management of impending pathologic fracture: (1) a painful lytic destructive lesion of 2.5 cm of the cortex; (2) a painful intramedullary lytic lesion greater than 50% of the cross-sectional diameter of the bone; and (3) a progressively painful lesion not relieved by radiation therapy. Routine radiographs and scans have not been reliable predictors (Hipp *et al*. 1995). Scoring systems based on radiographic and clinical features have been devised (Mirels 1989). Stabilization of an impending fracture is less of a problem than repairing one that has occurred. Definitive management of an impending or existing pathological fracture depends on the site and type of fracture, the nature of the underlying disease(s), and the patient's preferences with regard to pain control and preservation of function. Experienced judgement may be necessary to resolve the question of 'How late in the course of disease is operative intervention justified?'. The above management considerations must be weighed against non-operative alternatives which are often of limited value because of the difficult nature of incident pain secondary to fracture. Even in anticipated absence of functional recovery, operative fixation for relief of pain from a femoral shaft fracture can be justified in some individuals with a life expectancy of a few weeks.

Operative intervention is not complete without a course of radiation therapy for radiosensitive tumours. Systemic therapy should be considered as part of the overall plan. Failure to irradiate the fracture site surrenders local control of disease, resulting in pain and loosening of the prosthesis. Radiation therapy can be delayed until there is wound healing, but this is not mandatory. In cases of highly vascular metastases pre-operative embolization may be necessary. Scintography should be performed to rule out other areas of concurrent bone disease prior to proceeding with definitive operative treatment. The use of methyl methacrylate as an artificial matrix has enhanced the possibilities of operative fixation (Harrington 1981; Yablon and Paul 1976). Experience in biomechanical engineering supported by computerized tomography have allowed individualized treatments for complicated fractures where weight bearing potential is a consideration. Depending on the site, prosthetic replacement, intra-medullary fixation with rods, nailing, or some combination of these can be used. Biopsy of the lesion can be obtained during the procedure. Successful results of operative management of lower extremity fractures has encouraged increased use of surgery for upper extremity fractures.

Although many metastatic bone lesions remain occult, back pain is a frequent symptom in this population. Spinal instability accounts for back pain in approximately 10% of patients with disseminated cancer (Galasko and Sylvester 1978). Many parallels can be drawn from the proactive and aggressive surgical approach used for pathological fractures of the appendicular skeleton. Pain from spinal instability is due to mechanical factors precipitating both somatic nociceptive and neuropathic pain, not intrinsically painful metastases. The evaluation of disease is best accomplished by MRI. Scintography should be used to identify non-symptomatic disease. Radiation therapy is an integral part of treatment in radiosensitive tumours. Operative treatment includes anterior and/or posterior approaches to the spine. Decompression is followed by stabilization using implanted hardware. Methylmethacrylate is used for reconstruction of curetted or resected vertebral bodies performed during an anterior approach. Bone grafting may be used with a fixation device for a posterior approach. The adequacy of alignment can be assessed intraoperatively radiographically. Ultrasonography can determine the patency of the spinal canal when evaluating the decompression. Laminectomy alone is contra-indicated in spinal instability. It decompresses inadequately and worsens the instability.

Back pain is virtually always the presentation of spinal cord and cauda equina compression. This devastating complication should always be considered in the assessment of back pain. Permanent paresis or paralysis may be more feared by the patient, and of greater consequence, than pain. If neurologic compromise is present initially it lessens the chance of full recovery of function (Shapiro and Posner 1983). The syndrome commences with localized pain and progresses to loss of motor function. Urinary retention, paraesthesia, and anaesthesia are late signs. Pharmacologic management for back pain in these patients may mask this problem. Failure to control back pain with opioids or a precipitous rise in dose requirement should heighten suspicion of cord compression.

Management of spinal cord compression is similar to that of spinal instability, only it is carried out on an urgent basis. A brief course of high dose steroids is used as an adjunct to the primary treatment, whether operative decompression or radiation therapy. The decision to operate or irradiate in cases not associated with spinal instability should consider: the rapidity of onset of the neurologic deficit, the severity of the symptoms, the number of spinal segments involved, the degree of presumed radiosensitivity of the neoplasm, and the life expectancy of the patient. Urgent surgical intervention should be offered to patients evolving paraplegia or urinary retention in less than 24 hours. Recovery has been reported for longer delays. Rapid neurological deterioration generally portends a poor outcome. Rapid decompression may be the only chance for return of function.

Drainage and shunting procedures for ascites

Ascites develops in up to half cancer patients (Runyon 1993). The cause of ascites is not always malignancy. Problems associated with ascites include: bloating, diffuse abdominal pain, dyspnoea, nausea, early satiety, and gastric reflux. The symptoms, and not the ascites dictate treatment. Operative intervention beyond drugs and paracentesis should be considered for patients with persistent ascites requesting ongoing symptom treatment. The most common surgical approach involves internal drainage of ascites from the peritoneal cavity into the central venous circulation using a shunt. Shunt occlusion is the most common complication of these procedures with up to 50% at six months. Disseminated intravascular coagulation can uncommonly occur within hours of insertion. It is corrected by emergency shunt ligation and correction of the clotting abnormality. Heart failure due to volume overload can occur. It is best treated with diuretic and inotrope therapy carried out in a monitored setting. Infection and leakage at the abdominal insertion site are other complications. Contra-indications to peritoneo-venous shunting include active or recent bacterial peritonitis, viscous or bloody ascites, heart failure, renal failure, hyperbilirubinaemia, oesophageal varices, and coagulopathy. Removal of 50–70% of ascites at the time of insertion, with or without replacement with peritoneal normal saline, has been shown to decrease complications and mortality. Occlusion of the hepatic veins (Budd-Chiarri syndrome) is an important cause of massive and painful ascites associated with primary liver tumours and renal cell carcinoma. Relief has been reported following transjugular intrahepatic portosystemic shunt (TIPS). The procedure is technically demanding and results are operator dependant (Rossle *et al*. 1998).

Miscellaneous procedures

Some painful ulcers, whether directly from malignancy or due to the debilitating systemic effects of progressive neoplasm may be remedied by excision and primary closure. When primary closure is not feasible, grafting is performed. Surgeons with expertise in burns would be a wise choice of consultant for this particular problem because of their familiarity with wound healing difficulties.

Surgery can promote comfort, as well as eliminate pain. An example of this is formation of a tracheostomy for palliation for dyspnoea due to decreased ventilatory reserve. The procedure can be done under local infiltration anaesthesia as well as a general anaesthetic. Delayed complications include sepsis, tracheal obstruction due to granulation, stenosis of the trachea, crusting of the tracheostomy tube with secretions and haemorrhage due to vascular erosion. The use of low pressure, high volume tracheal tube cuffs and lightweight connections have prevented complications (Andrews and Pearson 1971; Grillo *et al.* 1971). A fenestrated tube allows speech, particularly important from a palliative point of view. Occasionally malodorous drainage from the tracheostomy can be a problem. Application of antibiotic powder to the site and cleansing of the tracheostomy tube in dilute acetic acid are helpful for this.

Vascular access can promote comfort if appropriately selected and expeditiously carried out. If long term venous access for administration of medication for pain and non-pain symptoms is anticipated, the individual is probably better served by elective placement of central venous access, than repetitive venepunctures at unpredictable times, for peripheral access. This decision should be made with the occasional, but often serious complications of central venous access in mind. These complications include sepsis, pneumothorax, haemothorax, hydrothorax, air embolism, thrombosis, malposition, infection, catheter occlusion, and nerve injury. Central venous access also requires ongoing surveillance by trained personnel to assess patency and presence of infection. Subcutaneously tunnelled catheters such as the Hickmann or Broviac are best inserted at the subclavian position for reasons of patient comfort and ease of dressing. These are silicone rubber catheters that require daily heparin flushing. The Groschong catheter is a silastic catheter with a three-way pressure sensitive valve and requires only weekly saline flushing when not in use. Other advantages of this system include reduced risk of reflux of blood which predisposes to clotting and infection as well as less risk of air embolism.

Conclusion

The surgeon has much to offer the patient with cancer related pain in terms of counsel, procedures and re-assurance. Reassurance will steadily increase with the satisfactory relief of pain in all its dimensions.

References

Ahmadzadeh, M. (1991). Clinical experience with subcutaneous urinary diversion: new approach using a double pigtail stent. *British Journal of Urology*, **67**, 596–99.

Andrews, M.J., and Pearson, F.G. (1971). The incidence and pathogenesis of tracheal injury following cuffed tube tracheostomy and assisted ventilation: an analysis of a two year prospective study. *Annals of Surgery*, **173**, 249.

Assalia, A., Schein, M., Kopelman, D., Hirshberg, A., and Hashmonai, M. (1994). Therapeutic effect of oral gastrograffin in adhesive, partial small bowel obstruction: a prospective randomized trial. *Surgery*, **115**, 433–7.

Baines, M.J. (1998). The pathophysiology and management of malignant intestinal obstruction. In *Oxford textbook of palliative medicine* (ed. D. Doyle, G. Hanks, and N. MacDonald), pp. 526–34. Oxford University Press.

Bakkevold, K.E., and Kambestad, B. (1993). Morbidity and mortality after radical and palliative pancreatic surgery. *Annals of Surgery*, **217**, 356–68.

Ball, A.B.S., Baum, M., Breach, N.M., Shepherd, J.H., Shearer, R.J., Thomas, J.M., *et al*. (1998). Surgical Palliation. In *Oxford textbook of palliative medicine* (ed. D. Doyle, G. Hanks, and N. MacDonald), pp. 282–97. Oxford University Press.

Beattie, G.J., Leonard, R.C.F., and Smyth, J.F. (1989). Bowel obstruction in ovarian cancer: a retrospective study and review of the literature. *Palliative Medicine*, **3**, 275–80.

Bessler, B., Cohen, S.J., and Magnussen, S. (1955). The problem of phantom breast and phantom limb pain. *Journal of Nervous and Mental Disorders*, **123**, 181–7.

Bozetti, F., Bonfanti, G., Castellani, R., Maffioli, L., Rubino, A., Diazzi, G., *et al*. (1996). Comparing reconstruction with Roux-en-Y to a pouch following total gastrectomy. *Journal of the American College of Surgeons*, **183**, 243–8.

Boxer, C.C., Waisman, J., Lieber, M.M., Mampuso, F.M., and Skinner, D.G. (1979). Renal carcinoma: computor analysis of 96 patients treated by nephrectomy. *Journal of Urology*, **122**, 598–601.

Branum, G.D., Pappas, T.N., and Meyers, W.C. (1996). The management of tumours of the ampulla of Vater by local resection. *Annals of Surgery*, **224**, 621–7.

Copping, J., Willix, R., and Kraft, R. (1978). Palliative chemical splanchnicectomy. *Archives of Surgery*, **98**, 418–20.

Couillard, D.R., and deVere White, R.W. (1993). Surgery of renal cell carcinoma. In *Kidney Tumours*, Urologic Clinics of North America, Vol. 20(2), (ed. C.A. Olsson and I.S. Sawczuk), pp. 263–75. W.B. Saunders, Philadelphia.

Culkin, D.J., Wheeler, J.S., Marsans, R.E., Nam, S.I., and Canning, J.R. (1987). Percutaneous nephrostomy for palliation for metastatic ureteral obstruction. *Urology*, **30**, 229–31.

Do, Y.S., Song, H.Y., Lee, B.H., Chin, S.Y., and Park, J.H. (1993). Esophagorespiratory fistula associated with esophageal cancer: Treatment with a Gianturco stent tube. *Radiology*, **187**, 673–77.

Duh, Q.Y., and Way, L.W. (1993). Diagnostic laparoscopy and laparoscopic cecostomy for colonic pseudo-obstruction. *Diseases of the Colon and Rectum*, **36**, 65–70.

Epstein, M. (1980). The LeVeen shunt for ascites and hepatorenal syndrome. *New England Journal of Medicine*, **302**, 628–30.

Espat, N.J., Brennan, M.F., and Conlon, K.C. (1999). Patients with laparoscopically staged unresectable pancreatic adenocarcinoma do not require subsequent surgical biliary or gastric bypass. *Journal of the American College of Surgeons*, **188**, 649–57.

Fleischer, D. (1984). Endoscopic laser therapy for carcinoma of the esophagus. *Endoscopy Review*, **1**, 37–49.

Fidler, M. (1981). Incidence of fracture through metastases in long bones. *Acta Orthopaedica Scandinavica*, **52**, 623–27.

Foley, K.M. (1998). Pain assessment and cancer pain syndromes. In *Oxford textbook of palliative medicine* (ed. D. Doyle, G. Hanks, and N. MacDonald), pp. 310–28. Oxford University Press.

Fowler, J.E. (1987). Nephrectomy in renal cell carcinoma. In *Controversies in urologic oncology*, Urology Clinics of North America, Vol. 14 (ed. J.P. Donohue), pp. 749–56.

Fredericks, J.A.M. (1985). Phantom limb and phantom limb pain. In *Handbook of clinical neurology*, Vol. 1, pp. 395–404. Elsevier Science Publishers, New York.

Friedman, R.L., Fallas, M.J., Carroll, B.J., Hiatt, J.R., and Phillipos, E.H. (1996). Laparoscopic splenectomy for ITP. *Surgical Endoscopy*, **10**, 991–5.

Galasko, C.S.B. (1998). Orthopaedic principles and management. In *Oxford textbook of palliative medicine* (ed. D. Doyle, G. Hanks, and N. MacDonald), pp. 477–87. Oxford University Press.

Galasko, C.S.B. (1972). Skeletal metastases and mammary cancer. *Annals of the Royal College of Surgeons*, **50**, 3–28.

Galasko, C.S.B., and Sylvester, B.S. (1978). Back pain in patients treated for malignant tumours. *Clinical Oncology*, **4**, 273–83.

Gallick, H.J., Weaver, D.W., Sachs, R.J., and Bouwman, D.L. (1986). Intestinal obstruction in cancer patients. *The American Surgeon*, **52**, 434–7.

Gasparini, M., Carroll, P., and Stoller, M. (1991). Palliative percutaneous and endoscopic urinary diversion for malignant ureteral obstruction. *Urology*, **38**, 408–12.

Geller, A., Petersen, B.T., and Gostout, C.J. (1996). Endoscopic decompression for acute colonic pseudo-obstruction. *Gastrointestinal Endoscopy*, **44**, 144–50.

Gottesman, J., and Lewis, M.S. (1982). Differences in crisis reactions among cancer and surgery patients. *Journal of Consulting Clinical Psychology*, **50**, 381–8.

Greene, F.L., Bouleware, R.J., and Bianco, J. (1995). Role of esophago-gastroscopy in application and follow-up of high-dose rate brachytherapy for treatment of esophageal carcinoma. *Surgical Laparoscopy and Endoscopy*, **5**, 425–30.

Grillo, H., Cooper, J.D., Geffin, B., and Pontoppidan, H. (1971). A low pressure cuff for tracheostomy tubes to minimize tracheal injury: A comparative clinical trial. *Journal of Thoracic and Cardiovascular Surgery*, **62**, 898.

Habermann, E.T., and Lopez, R.A. (1989). Metastatic disease of bone and treatment of pathological fractures. In *Bone tumors: evaluation and treatment*, Orthopedic Clinics of North America, Vol. 20, (ed. M.M. Lewis), pp. 469–86. W.B. Saunders, Philadelphia.

Halstead, W.J. (1907). The results of radical operations for the cure of cancer of the breast. *Annals of Surgery*, **46**, 1–27.

Harrington, K.D. (1981). The use of methylmethacrylate for vertebral-body replacement and anterior stabilization of pathological fracture-dislocations of the spine due to metastatic malignant disease. *Journal of Bone and Joint Surgery*, **63A**, 36–46.

Hipp, J.A., Springfield, D.S., and Hayes, W.C. (1995). Predicting pathologic fracture risk in the management of metastatic bone defects. *Clinical Orthopedics and Related Research*, **312**, 120–35.

Holm, A., Halpern, N.B., and Aldrete, J.S. (1989). Peritoneovenous shunt for intractable ascites of hepatic, nephrogenic, and malignant causes. *The American Journal of Surgery*, **158**, 162–6.

Jacobson, P.B., Roth, A.J., and Holland, J. (1998). Surgery. In *Psycho-oncology* (ed. J. Holland), pp. 257–66. Oxford University Press.

Johnson, C.D. (1995). Palliative resection of pancreatic adenocarcinoma. A survey of British surgeons. *HPB Surgery*, **8**, 181–3.

Kiefhaber, P. (1987). Indications for endoscopic Neodymium-YAG laser treatment in the gastrointestinal tract. Twelve years experience. *Scandanavian Journal of Gastroenterology*, **139**, 53.

Lee, J.T., Taylor, B.M., Singleton, B.C. (1988). Epidural anaesthesia for acute pseudo-obstruction of the colon (Ogilvie's syndrome). *Diseases of the Colon and Rectum*, **31**, 686–91.

Lillemoe, K.D. (1998). Palliative therapy for pancreatic cancer. In *Pancreatic cancer*, The Surgical Oncology Clinics of North America, Vol. 7 (ed. H.A. Pitt), pp. 199–216.

Lillemoe, K.D., Cameron, J.L., Kaufman, H.S., Yeo, C.J., Pitt, H.A., and Sauter, P.K. (1993). Chemical splanchnicectomy in patients with unresectable pancreatic cancer. A prospective randomized trial. *Annals of Surgery*, **217**, 447–57.

Lillemoe, K.D., Cameron, J.L., Yeo, C.J., Sohn, T.A., Nakeeb, A., Sauter, P.K. *et al.* (1996). Pancreaticoduodenectomy. Does it have a role in the palliation of pancreatic cancer? *Annals of Surgery*, **223**, 718–28.

Loizou, L.A., Grigg, D., Atkinson, M., Robertson, C., and Brown, S. (1991). A prospective comparison of laser therapy and intubation in endoscopic palliation for malignant dysphagia. *Gastroenterology*, **100**, 1303–10.

Lucas, C.E., Ledgerwood, A.M., and Bender, J.S. (1991). Antrectomy with gastro-jejeunostomy for unresectable pancreatic cancer causing duodenal obstruction. *Surgery*, **110**, 583.

McEntee, G.P., Nagorney, D.M., Kvols, K.L., Moertel, C.G., and Grant, C.S. (1990). Cytoreductive hepatic surgery for neuroendocrine tumors. *Surgery*, **108**, 1091–6.

Mercadante, S. (1997). Assessment and management of mechanical bowel obstruction. In *Topics in palliative care*, Vol. 1 (ed. R. Portnoy and E. Bruera), pp. 113–28.

Mirels, H. (1989). Metastatic disease in long bones: proposed scoring system for diagnosing impending pathologic fractures. *Clinical Orthopedics and Related Research*, **249**, 256–64.

Montenegro, F., Lawrence, G.D., Macon, W., and Pass, C. (1980). Metastatic glucagonoma. *The American Journal of Surgery*, **139**, 424–7.

Mulvaney, D. (1955). Vesico-coelomic drainage for the relief of ascites. *Lancet*, Oct. 8, 748–9.

Nakane, Y., Okumura, S., Akehira, K., Okamura, S., Boku, T., Okusa, T., *et al.* (1995). Jejeunal pouch reconstruction after total gastrectomy. *Annals of Surgery*, **222**, 27–35.

Norton, J.A., Sugarbaker, P.H., Doppman, J.L., Wesley, R.A., Maton, P.N., Gardner, J.D., *et al.* (1985). Aggressive resection of metastatic disease in selected patients with malignant gastrinoma. *Annals of Surgery*, **203**, 352–9.

Orringer, M.B. (1998). Esophageal tumors. In *Current surgical therapy* (6th edn), (ed. J.L. Cameron), pp. 59–62. Mosby, St. Louis.

Osteen, R.T., Guyton, S., Steele, G. Jr., and Wilson, R.E. (1980). Malignant intestinal obstruction. *Surgery*, **87**, 611–5.

Phillips, E.H., Carroll, B.J., and Fallas, M.J. (1994). Laparoscopic splenectomy. *Surgical Endoscopy*, **8**, 931–3.

Resnick, M.I., and Kursh, E.D. (1992). Extrinsic compression of the ureter. In *Campbell's urology* (6th edn), (ed. P.C. Walsh, A.B. Retik, T.A. Stamey, and E.D. Vaughn), pp. 533–69. W.B. Saunders, Philadelphia.

Robertson, G.S.M., Lloyd, D.M., Wicks, A.C.B., and Veitch, P.S. (1996). No obvious advantages for thoracoscopic two-stage oesophagectomy. *British Journal of Surgery*, **83**, 675–8.

Rossle, M., Siegerstetter, V., Huber, M., and Ochs, A. (1998). The first decade of the transjugular intrahepatic portosystemic shunt (TIPS): state of the art. *Liver*, **18**, 73–89.

Rubin, S.C., Hoskins, W.J., Benjamin, I., and Lewis, J.L. Jr. (1989). Palliative surgery for intestinal obstruction in advanced ovarian cancer. *Gynecologic Oncology*, **34**, 16–9.

Runyon, B.A. (1993). Ascites. In *Diseases of the liver* (7th edn.), (ed. L. Schiff and E.R. Schiff), pp. 990–1015. Lippincott, Philadelphia.

Saunders, C., and Sykes, N. (1993). *The management of terminal malignant disease*, (3rd edn). Edward Arnold, London.

Shapiro, W.R., and Posner, J.B. (1983). Medical versus surgical treatment of metastatic spinal cord tumours. In *Controversies in neurology*, (ed. R.A. Thompson and J.R. Green), pp. 57–65. Raven Press, New York.

Schwartz, S.I. (1998). Splenectomy for hematologic disorders. In *Current surgical therapy*, (6th edn). (ed. J.L. Cameron), pp. 545–8. Mosby, St. Louis.

Sohn, T.A., Lillemoe, K.D., Cameron, J.L., Huang, J.J., Pitt, H.A., and Yeo, C.J. (1999). Surgical palliation of unresectable periampullary adenocarcinoma in the 1990s. *Journal of the American College of Surgeons*, **188**, 658–69.

Stoldt, H.S., Audisio, R.A., Halverson, A.L., and Sackler, J.M. (1998). Application of minimal access surgery in the management of diverse malignancies. In *Minimal access surgery in oncology* (ed. J.G. Geraghty, J.M. Sackier, and H.L. Young), pp. 137–42. Greenwich Medical Media Ltd., London.

Strain, J., and Grossman, S. (1975). *Psychological care of the medically ill*. Appleton-Century-Crofts, New York.

Takita, H., Vincent, R.G., Caicido, V., and Gutierrez, A.C. (1977). Squamous cell carcinoma of the esophagus: A study of 153 cases. *Journal of Surgical Oncology*, **9**, 547–54.

Thompson, D.M., Tetik, C., and Arregui, M.I. (1998). Laparoscopy and other minimally invasive techniques in patients with advanced intraperitoneal disease.

In *Minimal access surgery in oncology* (ed. J.G. Geraghty, J.M. Sackier, and H.L. Young), pp. 109–20.

Turnbull, A.D.M., Guerra, J., and Starnes, H.F. (1989). Results of surgery for obstructing carcinomatosis of gastrointestinal, pancreatic, or biliary origin. *Journal of Clinical Oncology*, **7**, 381–6.

Unger, S.W., and Rosenbaum, G.J. (1995). Laparoscopic splenectomy. In *Principles of laparoscopic surgery* (ed. M.E. Arrugui, R.J. Fitzgibbon, N. Katkhouda, J.B. Mcernan, and H. Reich), pp. 356–65. Springer-Verlag, New York.

Wagner, F., Nasseri, R., Laucke U., and Hetzer, R. (1998). Percutaneous dilatational tracheostomy: results and long-term outcome in critically ill patients following cardiac surgery. *Thoracic and Cardiovascular Surgery*, **46**, 352–6.

Walsh, H.P.J., and Schofield, P.F. (1984). Is laparotomy for small bowel obstruction justified in patients with previously treated malignancy? *British Journal of Surgery*, **71**, 933–5.

Watanapa, P., and Williamson, R.C.N. (1992). Surgical palliation for pancreatic cancer: developments during the past two decades. *British Journal of Surgery*, **79**, 8–20.

Yablon, I.G., and Paul, G.R. (1976). The augmentive use of methylmethacrylate in the management of pathologic fractures. *Surgery, Gynecolgy, and Obstetrics*, **143**, 177–83.

Zadra, J.A., Jewett, M.A.S., Keresteci, A.G., Rankin, J.T., St. Louis, E., Grey, R.R. *et al.* (1987). Non-operative urinary diversion for malignant ureteral obstruction. *Cancer*, **60**, 1353–7.

Zimmerman, L.M., and Veith, I. (1967). *Great ideas in the history of Surgery*, pp. 488–98. Dover Publications, Inc., New York.

Zucker, K.A., and Miscall, B.G. (1998). Laparoscopic splenectomy. In *Current surgical therapy* (6th edn), (ed. J.L. Cameron), pp. 1222–7. Mosby, St. Louis.

THIRTEEN

Acupuncture and TENS

JACQUELINE FILSHIE AND JOHN W. THOMPSON

Melzack (1994) described many historical ways in which sensory stimulation and modulation have been used to reduce pain throughout history. These include the more aggressive forms of counterirritation or stimulation, scarification, cauterization and cupping and lesser stimulating therapies, acupuncture and transcutaneous electrical nerve stimulation (TENS).

Traditional Chinese acupuncture

Acupuncture

Classic acupuncture texts by Veith (1972) translating the *Yellow Emperor's classic of internal medicine* and *Celestial lancets* by Lu and Needham (1980) provide an invaluable source of historical and traditional information. There is still much debate over the exact historical origins of acupuncture (Beyens 1998) and the origins may have been as long ago as the 21st century BC (Ma 1992) or as recently as 100 AD (Lim 1989). The Chinese saw an intimate correspondence between man and his environment and an inherent conformity with a natural law or Tao. Yin and Yang represent forces of opposite polarity, negative and positive, feminine and masculine, receptive and creative, dark and light which should be in balance for healthy function. They acknowledged a dualism of approach integrating the life essence 'Jing' with 'Shen' the spirit. They describe the circulation of Qi (pronounced Chi) or vital energy which is partly innate and present at birth 'where Qi agglomerates there is life' and 'when Qi disperses then there is death' possibly representing the spirit and also the body where the Qi is fuelled by food and respiration during life.

The Qi circulates both deeply and superficially in a series of meridians which are invisible lines joining a series of invisible acupuncture points on the surface of the body. There are 12 paired, 2 unpaired, and several extra meridians. The meridians and their associated organs (for example spleen and pericardium) do not necessarily bear a meaningful relationship to each other when studying Western anatomy and physiology. Bearing in mind that it was not until the 20th century that anatomy was formally studied in the east, it is not surprising that leaps of imagination occurred to elaborate theories to give meaning to their concepts. Beyens (1998) has said 'The ancientness of acupuncture does not justify a systematic acceptance of the Chinese vision of this particular technique'. Traditional eastern acupuncture diagnosis utilizes numerous other laws. The law of the five elements wood, fire, earth, metal, and water and an intricate pulse diagnosis assessing the 'quality' of pulse in three superficial and three deep areas of the radial artery at each wrist were of considerable diagnostic value. However, some doubt has been cast on the validity of the pulse diagnosis, (Vincent 1992). Also, important note was taken of the colour, texture, and consistency of the tongue (Maciocia 1997).

After using the many 'laws' to diagnose a condition and an excess or deficiency of energy in a meridian, specific acupuncture points are stimulated with a needle to tonify or sedate as appropriate. Sometimes moxa (the pith of Artemesia Japonica) is burned close to the skin or applied to the needle itself—moxibustion, as another method to achieve stimulation of acupuncture points.

Many important acupuncture points are tender in health and many more become tender in disease states. Acupuncture point 'recipes' which are decried by purists but used extensively by most acupuncturists usually include needling of strong points such as large intestine 4 (LI4) Fig. 13.1. When an acupuncture point is stimulated, an extremely small minority of patients experience a propagated sensation in a line which partly coincides with the pathway of a meridian (Macdonald 1989). To date there is neither proof nor convincing disproof of the existence of meridians. Traditional acupuncture point stimulation produces a sensation known as De Qi or 'Teh Chi', which is a feeling of aching, numbness, heaviness, and paraesthesia around the point. Some feel that this sensation is essential for an acupuncture effect to occur but an increasing minority of western acupuncturists challenge this point of view (Vincent *et al.* 1989; Mann 1992; Baldry 1993). Some aspects of traditional chinese acupuncture are summarized in Table 13.1.

Table 13.1. Traditional chinese acupuncture

Qi	Concept of Vital energy, pivotal to understanding Innate Qi/spirit Acquired Qi nourished by food/respiration
Yin and Yang	Forms of opposite polarities, must be in harmony for health Yin negative, feminine, receptive, dark Yang positive, masculine, creative, light
Five elements	Wood, fire, earth, metal, water.
Tongue diagnosis	Colour, consistency, surface.
Meridians	12 paired: lungs, large intestine, stomach, spleen, heart, small intestine, bladder, kidneys, pericardium (circulation), triple energiser (metabolism), gall bladder, liver. 2 unpaired: conception vessel, governor vessel Extra points and meridians
De Qi	Needling sensation, aching, numbness, tingling, heaviness, fullness, soreness. Rarely patients describe propagated sensation or lightening flash along meridian
Moxa moxibustion	Pith of artemesia Japonica heated near acupuncture points or thermal stimulation to needle.
Excess or deficiency states	Difficult concepts for western trained physicians to assimilate such as blocked or stagnating Qi due to external and internal causes.
Acupuncture recipes	Decried by purists but used extensively with extra points

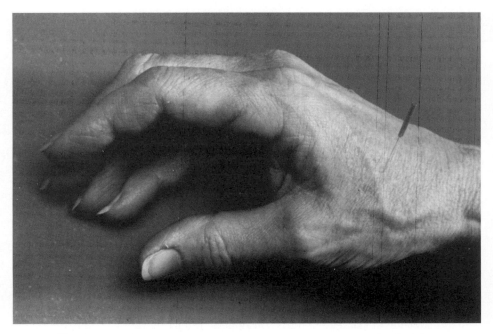

Fig. 13.1 LI4 (large intestine 4) acupuncture point—a strong analgesic point.

Modern acupuncture

Most doctors trained in both the west and the east, take a conventional medical history from a patient, perform a clinical examination and order any special investigations before making a diagnosis. The rather charming and philosophical concepts of traditional Chinese acupuncture with Qi and Yin and Yang can fit in with a modern medical approach if a circulation of blood, hormones and nutriments represent some concept of Qi and if Yin and Yang represents homeostasis. A new polarity has appeared between acupuncturists, with some fiercely attached to the traditional approach and who may oppose and dismiss the neurophysiological approach, and others who hold traditional concepts in disdain and with scepticism. The unfortunate dualism has probably delayed progress in scientific clinical research and validation of both forms of treatment.

The authors of this chapter feel that most of the effects of acupuncture are due to neurophysiological modulation of multiple homeostatic mechanisms both known and unknown and that metaphysical components should be debated in philosophical circles. The increasing and fascinating area of psychoneuroimmunomodulation could go part way to explain how acupuncture works on both the body and the mind (for example Ding *et al.* 1983; Bianchi *et al.* 1991; Jonsdottir 1999).

In many pain clinics around the world, acupuncture has now become standard therapy amongst orthodox treatments. Less emphasis is placed on the metaphysical or phenomenological approach and more on physical signs, a segmental approach to point selection, trigger point therapy plus a selection of traditional strong extrasegmental

Table 13.2. Modern acupuncture

Manual acupuncture	needle size :	36–30 g. NB disposable
	with/without introducer	
	depth needle :	subcutaneously
		intramuscularly
		periosteal stimulation
	time :	1–3 seconds–20 minutes
	stimulation	minimal
		vigorous twirling of needles
Electrical acupuncture	2–4 Hz	low frequency
	100 Hz	high frequency
Needle placement	segmental,	
	combined segmental and traditional points	
	tender points,	
	trigger points,	
	surrounding techniques	
	recipe points	
Acupuncture analgesia	electroacupuncture with analgesia and sedation	
	electroacupuncture with conventional anaesthesia	
Auricular therapy	'tender' points or 'recipe' points needled	
Laser therapy	not strictly acupuncture	
Acupressure	less effective	
Ryoduraku	electrical treatment of reduced skin impedence	
Veterinary	± electroacupuncture—animals possibly less likely to be placebo responders!	

points (Table 13.2 summarizes modern acupuncture). Not all practitioners endeavour to elicit the sensation of De Qi, some use minimal stimulation for up to 20 minutes and some use vigorous stimulation for up to 20 minutes. Disposable needles are mandatory to prevent transmission of infection. Personal inclination largely determines the size of needles preferred, whether an introducer is employed, needle depth, duration of needling, and quality of stimulation used.

Some patients are more sensitive to acupuncture than others and have been called 'strong reactors' by Felix Mann (1992). Indeed cancer patients appear to react more strongly to acupuncture than non-cancer patients although this has not been formally studied. Brockhaus and Elger (1990) have described a population distribution of analgesic response on normal volunteers ranging from non-responders to high responders. It would be interesting to repeat this in a cancer population, many of whom require shorter, more gentle treatments. There appears to be a shift of a population distribution with more cancer patients being extra sensitive to treatment and more patients, particularly those with extensive disease, being resistant to treatment. It is prudent to give a gentle treatment on the first consultation following which treatment can be intensified or reduced, based on an individual's response.

Electroacupuncture

This was introduced initially as a substitute for the vigorous manual acupuncture used perioperatively and described as 'acupuncture analgesia'. Despite wide publicity it is now used for less than 8% operations in China and then usually with supplemental analgesia. It is also used in conjunction with conventional anaesthesia to augment analgesia and for chronic pain conditions in particular. The use of electroacupuncture (EA) has been well reviewed by White (1998). Various frequencies and intensities of stimulation are used which have differing effects on the release of neurotransmitters. High intensity EA is more likely to release dynorphins and serotonin and low intensity EA releases enkephalins, endorphins, endogenous steroids and oxytocin. Much work remains to be done on the choice of optimal stimulation for selected pain problems in cancer patients.

Auricular acupuncture

Nogier (1972) developed a 'micro' point system on the external helix of the ear. An upside down foetus is represented on the pinna. Although this idea seems somewhat far fetched, the Chinese also have developed a similar 'microsystem' with points on the ear representing body parts. A study of 40 patients showed that tenderness, found by a physician examining the ears with no prior knowledge of the patients medical condition, corresponded with distant painful areas of the body in 75% of cases (Oleson *et al.* 1980). They supported the hypothesis of somatotopic organization of the body on the ear. The specificity of point location on the ear may be of lesser importance in treatment of addictions (Lewith and Vincent 1998) and possibly other clinical problems, as the ear is richly innervated. Auriculoacupuncture has the advantage of being readily accessible in immobile patients and has distinct practical advantages in the overdressed patient!

Laser therapy

Though not strictly acupuncture, the application of low power lasers to acupuncture points has been shown to help pain of rheumatoid arthritis (Bliddal *et al.* 1987; Colov *et al.* 1987; Seichert 1991), trigeminal neuralgia (Walker *et al.* 1987), and post herpetic neuralgia (Moore *et al.* 1988). But there are greatly conflicting results as reviewed by Baldry (1998) and Baxter (1989) and minimal evidence to date on peripheral neuro-activity. Naturally a non-invasive form of treatment is appealing, were it to be effective, especially for paediatric use. It is eminently suitable for double blind studies.

Acupressure

Acupressure is more popular with lay acupuncture practitioners but has less effect than acupuncture with needles. It is commonly used on children in China and called 'tui na'. It has been shown to be effective for nausea and vomiting associated with morning sickness of pregnancy (de Aloysio and Penacchioni 1992; Belluomini *et al.* (1994).

Ryodoraku

Ryodoraku is practised in Japan, when treatment is given after electrical detection of areas of low impedence on the body (Yoshino and Kumio 1977; Hyodo 1990). Nakatani and Yamashita (1977) show Ryodoraku acupuncture points in areas of skin containing sweat glands. Modern Ryodoraku theory attributes the heterosegmental effects of acupuncture to interactions between the sympathetic and somatic nervous systems (Bowsher 1998).

Veterinary acupuncture

There is increasing interest in the subject of veterinary acupuncture for domestic, farm, and racing animals. Acupuncture, electroacupuncture, and transcutaneous spinal analgesia (TSE) are all used with varying degrees of success. It is widely felt that animals are less likely to be placebo responders!

Principles of treatment

Non-cancer pain

Acupuncture remains first line treatment for hundreds of painful and non-painful conditions in China. *Essentials of Chinese acupuncture* (1980) outlines traditional treatment and *Medical acupuncture* (Filshie and White 1998) summarizes scientific studies and theories for many conditions, particularly pain problems.

Acupuncture has been used for a variety of chronic pain problems with 40–80% symptomatic improvement in primary care. More variable success has been reported in the chronic pain clinic setting (Hester 1998). Trigger point therapy is the mainstay treatment for a wide variety of musculoskeletal and visceral disorders and treatment is elegantly summarized by Baldry (1993). Trigger points are hyperirritable loci within a taut band of skeletal muscle or its associated fascia. They are painful on compression and can exhibit a characteristic referral pattern of pain or autonomic dysfunction (Travell and Simons 1983). Trigger points may also exhibit a jump sign and a twitch response. Gerwin *et al.* (1997) have established inter-observer reliability in finding trigger points following a training period. Pressure sensitive devices can also aid their identification (Reeves *et al.* 1986; Delaney and McKee 1993). Trigger points can be active or latent. Hubbard and Berkoff (1993) have demonstrated increased electromyographic activity in trigger points, which was made more prominent by a psychological stressor (McNulty *et al.* 1994). They may also coincide with some acupuncture points (Ward 1996). A segmental approach to treatment, relevant to the affected dermatomes, myotomes, and sclerotomes giving rise to pain, makes good sense. This method is widely used in treatment, as are strong traditional analgesic points such as LI4 (Fig. 13.1) which have been shown to increase pain thresholds in numerous experimental pain studies (for example Stacher *et al*. 1975; Chapman *et al*. 1976). Lundeberg *et al*. (1988) found a combination of segmental and strong extra segmental points most efficacious for chronic non-cancer pain.

Cancer pain

Tremendous advances have been made in cancer pain management in recent years. Pharmacological and psychological support have become the mainstay of conventional treatment. Nevertheless, 10–20% of patients remain inadequately controlled by drug treatment. In late stage disease these figures are often higher–over 50% (Von Roenn *et al*. 1993). Three groups of patients can be identified who are the principal non-responders to conventional therapy:

- those who are extremely sensitive to medication:
- those who are in significant pain despite high doses of analgesics and coanalgesics;
- those who have a mixture of pain and emotional problems. This is a particular problem in patients who are either angry about their diagnosis or who deny it.

Additional formal emotional support, counselling, cognitive behavioural approaches, or psychiatric help may be needed.

Acupuncture can be useful for all these groups of patients. Gentle stimulation, using a mixture of segmental points appropriate to the affected segments, trigger points and strong analgesic extrasegmental points, e.g. LI4 are the most likely to be effective. Recent neurophysiological work (Lundeberg 1998, personal communication) has shown that up to six treatments are required to facilitate analgesia in acupuncture; this may occur via 'switching on' preprodynorphin and preprometenkephalin genes. The ideal initial treatment timing schedule would be twice weekly for 3 weeks or weekly for 4–6 weeks with an initial treatment interval of not more than 1 week. The treatment intervals could then be increased based on the longevity of response.

The earliest report of the use of acupuncture for cancer pain described short lived relief for 3–72 hours in 8 patients, accompanied by a sense of relaxation and mental alertness following treatment (Mann in Bowsher *et al*. 1973). Wen (1977) described the use of acupuncture for 29 cancer patients poorly controlled by conventional medication in late stage disease. They were given an intensive treatment schedule with several electroacupuncture sessions on the first day, followed by 3 treatments a day reducing to one treatment a day, pain relief permitting. Pain medication could be reduced with this regimen.

Filshie and Redman (1985) and Filshie (1990) summarized their results in 339 patients with a heterogeneous group of conditions. These patients had drug intolerance or failure of conventional treatment when attending a pain clinic in a cancer hospital. Patients had been investigated appropriately and staged in the specialist cancer centre. Analgesic medication was reduced if acupuncture treatment was successful. Three weekly acupuncture treatments were given with minimal stimulation to assess suitability

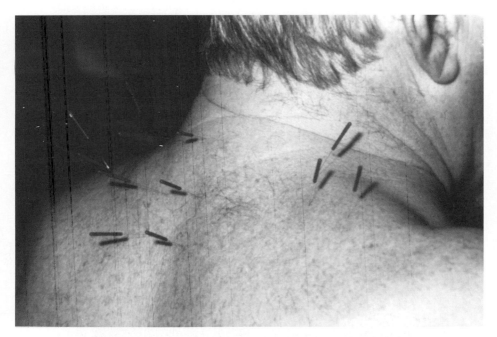

Fig. 13.2 Segmental acupuncture and trigger point treatment for head, neck, and upper arm pain.

for treatment on an outpatient basis. After 3 treatments 52% and 56% of patients obtained worthwhile lasting analgesia. Generally, after three or four treatments, the response was sufficient to permit intervals between treatments to be increased. A further 30% and 22% had analgesia for 2 days or less and may have benefited from multiple treatments per week. It was noticed that the greater the tumour burden the shorter the length of relief from the treatment. Eighteen per cent and 20% respectively had no pain relief. Many patients had a significant improvement in mobility. In contrast with many non-malignant pain problems, cancer patients' pains tend to need more frequent top-ups of treatment, even when they are in remission from the disease. Patients with cancer treatment related pain such as post-surgical pain syndromes and post-irradiation pain derived much more prolonged benefit than patients with metastatic disease. Filshie *et al.* (1997) reported a detailed psychological profile and audit of 67 patients with breast cancer who had pain associated with the surgery, radiotherapy, and tumour in the chest, axilla, and arm. There was a statistically significant drop in average pain, worst pain, interference with lifestyle, distress, pain behaviour, and depression after one month of treatment.

The main principles of treatment include the use of paravertebral segmental points appropriate to the affected pain dermatomes, myotomes, and sclerotomes. Paravertebral needling at C7, T1, and T2 plus any trigger points in the suprascapular areas are especially useful for pains relating to the head and neck region and upper arm and chest (Fig. 13.2). Needling is sometimes interchangeable with sympathetic blockade with accompanying improvement of skin discoloration in the hand and enhanced healing of ulcerated areas, even radionecrotic ulcers (Filshie 1988). Strong upper limb traditional

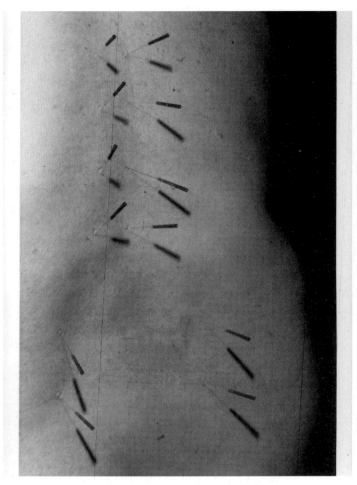

Fig. 13.3 Segmental acupuncture and sacro-iliac points for low back and lower limb pain.

points like L14 can also be used. Paravertebral needling of Lumbar 1 to Lumbar 4 (Fig. 13.3) is particularly useful for pain and vascular problems affecting the lower limb and low back areas. Sacroiliac joint points and the addition of sacral points bilaterally over the exit sites of the sacral nerves are useful for intrapelvic pain problems. The addition of trigger points and selected strong analgesic traditional points such as ST36, LR3, and SP6 may augment pain control. Painful ulcers, or scars and areas of post herpetic neuralgia (PHN) are loosely surrounded by needles 'surrounding the dragon', in addition to appropriate paravertebral needling. Medication may be needed in addition for post herpetic neuralgia when 25–75 mg dothiepin and small doses of methadone e.g. 5 mg nocte initially, may work synergistically with acupuncture in resistant cases.

Muscle spasm is particularly helped by trigger point acupuncture. Visceral problems are helped by a mixture of paravertebral segmental points relating to the affected segments plus selected traditional points. Phantom limb pain can also be helped by acupuncture, using paravertebral needling on the ipsilateral side and contralateral needling on the opposite limb. Acupuncture has been shown to elicit phantom limb sensations as well as to alleviate pain (Xue 1986). However, based on personal experience, it can significantly relieve symptoms in the majority of patients.

Tolerance

Tolerance to treatment may be due to a recurrence of metastatic disease. Therefore a general acupuncturist who fails to increase analgesia after 3 or 4 acupuncture treatments may need to refer the patient for further investigations. Patients who have had long lived relief from acupuncture and who then develop less than two days' relief are often found to have developed new metastatic disease. Once treated, these patients may revert back to being acupuncture responsive again. There are several ways to try to increase the length of action of analgesia in cancer patients. These include increasing the frequency of treatments as Wen showed (1977). It is not practical to treat outpatients so frequently and indwelling semi-permanent needles may be used.

Dillon & Lucas (1999) have shown a statistically significant reduction in pain in 28 patients in a hospice using semipermanent needles inserted in the ear. The needles were placed in areas of tenderness found using a spring loaded probe which the patients could massage if the pain became intense. In a study on advanced cancer related breathlessness, Filshie *et al.* (1996) extended the beneficial results of treatment on breathlessness by using two small indwelling semipermanent needles at the top of the sternum. These could be rubbed in the event of panic attacks and severe shortness of breath. These may be useful for multiple symptom control such as pain control, relief of anxiety, and nausea. Tolerance to acupuncture may be in part due to an increase of cholecystokinin, an endogenous opioid antagonist which is also released by acupuncture (Han *et al.* 1986a). If cholecystokinin has an antalgesic effect in cancer patients, it may be possible, with more specific targeted therapy, to manipulate these effects pharmacologically in future. It is frequently possible to use TENS as a backup for acupuncture when the effects of acupuncture wear off between outpatient appointments. Paravertebral segmental placements with or without distal electrode placement points can be used. However, TENS and acupuncture are not interchangeable.

Relief of symptoms is not restricted to pain control. Dyspnoea has already been mentioned. Acupuncture is also useful for nausea and vomiting (Vickers 1996), rehabilitation after stroke (Johansson *et al.* 1993) radiation induced xerostomia (Lundeberg 1999), hiccough, radiation rectitis, itch, and depression (Thompson and Filshie 1998).

Evidence of efficacy

Many variables are involved in acupuncture treatments (Table 13.2). There is no strict consensus on treatment for any condition. Thus the 'dose' and quality of acupuncture may be widely different from study to study. Many clinical studies use electro-acupuncture (EA) but much clinical practice does not include this. Therefore the results of trials may not necessarily represent the results in clinical practice. One problem with acupuncture research is the choice of a credible, preferably needleless, placebo.

A range of designs have emerged and have been reviewed by Hammerschlag (1998):

1. Comparing acupuncture with no treatment, or waiting list delayed treatment groups (Christensen *et al.* 1992).

2. Comparing acupuncture with a non-invasive placebo control e.g. Mock TENS (MacDonald *et al.* 1983) or a blunt cocktail stick (White *et al.* 1996) or tapping an introducer onto the skin (Lao *et al.* 1995) or a novel needle with a retractable handle (Streitberger and Kleinhenz 1998).

3. Comparing acupuncture with minimal needling or standard needling at differing sites (Hansen and Hansen 1983 and Jobst *et al.* 1986).

4. Acupuncture has also been compared with standard care such as medication (Loh *et al.* 1984) or physiotherapy (Ahonen *et al.* 1983).

5. Acupuncture has been added to standard care and compared with its results (Aglietti *et al.* 1990; Gunn *et al.* 1980).

It does not help that both acupuncture and the placebo effect are mediated to some extent by endogenous opioids (Ter Riet *et al.* 1998). The difficulty in separating the active from the 'non-specific' effects of the treatment remains. It has been shown that both real and minimal acupuncture and diazepam had a greater effect on pain reduction than placebo diazepam (Thomas *et al* (1991). The numbers studied precluded a distinction being made between the two 'doses' of acupuncture.

Both traditional and western trained doctors will undoubtedly induce some degree of a 'non specific' or placebo response. This will have an additional effect on the actual needling. Therefore acupuncture is the sum of the specific effect of needling, plus a variable degree of placebo or non-specific effect depending on the dynamics between the patient, therapist, and context of therapy.

Recent systematic reviews and meta-analyses on efficacy of acupuncture for antiemesis (Vickers 1996), back pain (Ernst and White 1998), and dental pain (Ernst and Pitler 1998) have addressed many of the weaknesses outlined in the early meta-analyses on pain (Ter Riet *et al.* 1990; Patel *et al.* 1989). Heterogeneous data with widely differing methodologies were quite rightly criticized for their methodological weaknesses. Collective collaboration is underway for developing acceptable methods for future trials. When available, prospective randomized controlled studies for control of pain and many other symptoms can begin in earnest.

Side effects

Acupuncture is widely thought to be a harmless treatment as long as general precautions are taken and it is thought to incur fewer side-effects than medication. A large study to identify minor and major side-effects of treatment is underway in 30000 acupuncture treatments (White *et al.* 1997). Side-effects range from minor ones with bleeding, bruising, post needling pain to sleepiness and euphoria (which is seldom a problem!). Syncope, vertigo, and dizziness can also occur in a minority of cases. More serious side-effects include pneumothorax, hepatitis, septicaemia, cardiovascular trauma and trauma to the spinal cord, endocarditis, pericarditis, retained needles and burns from moxibustion (Rampes and James 1995; Rampes 1998). Knowledge of anatomy, compulsory use of sterile disposable needles and commonsense could have probably prevented the majority of these incidents. Deep needling techniques are inappropriate and could be dangerous in the cachectic patient. Death has been caused by perforation of a congenital malformation of the lower sternum (Halavorsen *et al.* 1995).

There are still clinics in both East and West which do not use adequate sterilization techniques and the single use of disposable needles is mandatory. Drugs are between the 4th and 6th cause of death in the USA (Lazarou *et al.* 1998). This is 'dimensions' greater than acupuncture side-effects (Ernst—personal communication 1998). Acupuncture, by giving symptomatic relief, can mask disease or its progression. Unexpected short lived relief in a patient merits further investigation. There is one report of an indwelling gold needle which caused an artefact in a scan, similar to that of a metastasis (Otusaka *et al.* 1990). Finally, numerous patients describe coincidental improvement whilst undergoing treatment, e.g. prostatism, migraine, psoriasis, hay fever, and dumping syndrome—a welcome contrast!

Contraindications

Needling should not be performed around the area of an unstable spine in patients with good neurological function below that level. This is because there is a serious, theoretical danger of removing protective muscle spasm around an unstable area, with the real danger of further compression and transection, (Filshie 1990). If this problem arises TENS can be used as a substitute. This is a safe alternative as it has less effect on muscle spasm. Acupuncture can be given to the legs below the lesion with impunity. It is commonsense not to needle a patient with gross clotting dysfunction, but gentle superficial needling in a patient with platelets over 20000 units and a slightly prolonged prothrombin time is acceptable. Acupuncture should never be used on patients who bruise spontaneously. Needles should not be inserted directly into superficial sites of tumour or in the limbs of patients affected with moderate to severe lymphoedema. Contralateral needling can be used for patients with lymphoedema combined with ipsilateral paravertebral stimulation. Minimal superficial needling may not be completely contra-indicated for ipsilateral mild lymphoedema. Electroacupuncture should not be used for patients who have a pacemaker. Most practitioners are cautious about needling patients in pregnancy in case of inducing a miscarriage.

Training and facilities needed

In view of the potential complications and contra-indications to acupuncture. It is vital an acupuncturist should have adequate training. In the UK there are doctors, physiotherapists, osteopaths, chiropractors, nurse practitioners and non-medically qualified practitioners who practice acupuncture.

There is a major advantage for medical practitioners to train in acupuncture. They will already have attained diagnostic skills, will know the natural history of the different types of cancer and are able to anticipate and diagnose early signs of relapse. In the UK, several courses are approved by the British Medical Acupuncture Society (BMAS) which can lead to accreditation. The BMAS uses a neurophysiological approach to training. Less emphasis is placed on traditional concepts and diagnostics but great emphasis on safe use of acupuncture for pain and symptom control.

Paramedical practitioners

Physiotherapists, osteopaths, and chiropractic practitioners are trained in diagnostic techniques. They are theoretically capable of treating cancer patients. Nurses, apart from midwives, are rarely given practitioner status in their own right. The training programmes are variable in length and quality. Some have a particular traditional Chinese acupuncture bias which is unpalatable to some doctors. It is desirable to give acupuncture with the blessing and under joint control with the oncology team, so that potential masking of malignant disease or its progression is unlikely and that patients are not treated inappropriately for an unstable spine for example.

Non-medical practitioners

There are numerous training courses for non-medical practitioners. Some are university based with detailed instruction on anatomy and physiology in the early years, but are usually traditionally based without the western diagnostic skills. In these cases, it is vital that any treatment is supervised by the general practitioner or oncologist so that there is minimal danger of masking complaints or causing harm.

Transcutaneous electrical nerve stimulation

Electrical stimulation of the human body for therapeutic purposes, particularly for the relief of pain, has been employed since early times. Evidence from cave drawings suggest that the Egyptians of the Fifth Dynasty (2500 BC) used the electric fish *Malapterurus electricus* to relieve pain. Hippocrates in 400 BC referred to the use of the electric torpedo for the treatment of headache and arthritis; and the Roman physician Scribonius Largus almost certainly used the electrical ray fish *Torpedo marmorata* for the treatment of gout.

A critical turning point in the history of electrotherapy was the advent of the gate control theory of pain proposed by Melzack and Wall (1965). This hypothesis was immediately verifiable and was quickly put to the test by Wall and Sweet who showed that high-frequency (50–100 Hz) percutaneous electrical nerve stimulation relieved chronic neurogenic pain (Wall and Sweet 1967). Further corroboration came when

Table 13.3. Clinical pain conditions that have been treated successfully with TENS

- Peripheral nerve disorders
- Peripheral nerve injury
- Complex regional pain syndrome
- Amputation pain
- Phantom limb pain
- Post-herpetic neuralgia

Spinal cord and spinal root disorders
- Dorsal root compression and spinal nerve compression

Pain associated with neoplastic lesions
- Metastatic bone pain

Muscle pain
- Secondary muscle spasm
- Musculoskeletal disorders

Joint pain
- Rheumatoid arthritis
- Osteoarthritis

Acute pain
- Acute orofacial pain
- Postoperative pain

Based on Woolf (1989)

Shealy and his colleagues (1967) showed that electrical stimulation of the dorsal column was also effective for the relief of chronic pain. In 1973 Long reported the results of transcutaneous electrical nerve stimulation (TENS) which, until then, had been used to select patients for spinal cord stimulator implantation. It was soon realized that TENS alone was effective, thus obviating the need for spinal cord stimulator implantation. Following the development of solid-state electronics which made it possible to manufacture small battery-operated stimulators the use of TENS evolved rapidly.

More recent developments of TENS have involved the use of different patterns of electrical stimulation which include pulsed ('burst'), modulation (ramped), random, and complex waveforms all designed with the aim of improving the efficacy of TENS. Examples of clinical pain conditions that are now commonly treated with TENS are listed in Table 13.3.

Techniques

Several forms of TENS are in common use. These are classified in Table 13.4.

Table 13.4. Forms of TENS in common use

Form	Features Pulse pattern and duration [μsec]	Amplitude [=volts] and current [mA]	Frequency [Hz]	Effects
1. Continuous TENS = Conventional	Continuous 150–200 μsec	Low 10–30 mA	High: 40–150 Hz	'Strong but comfortable' sensation of pins and needles (paraesthesiae) directed into area supplied by stimulated nerve(s). Effect due to stimulation of Aβ [group 2] nerve fibres. Muscle contractions should not occur unless electrodes have been placed over muscle belly or especially if over a motor point.
2. Pulsed Tens = 'burst'	Bursts 150–200 μsec	Low 10–30 mA	Low: bursts of 100 Hz at 1–2Hz	'Strong but comfortable' sensation of bursts of pins and needles. Muscle contractions should not occur unless electrodes have been placed over muscle belly or especially if over a motor point.
3. Acupuncture-like TENS = high intensity pulsed	Bursts 150–200 μsec or > 200 μsec	High 15–50 mA	Low: bursts of 100 Hz at 1–2 Hz	Strong sensation of bursts of pins and needles accompanied by non-painful phasic twitching of muscles in the myotomes stimulated.

Note:
(i) On some stimulators **modulated** outputs are available. **Frequency modulation:** the frequency of the continuous output is varied between preset limits in a regular pattern, for example, between 90–55 Hz over 90 msec, 1.3 times a second (Tulgar *et al.* 1991). **Amplitude modulation:** the amplitudes of each group of shocks which make up each pulse or burst are unequal and form a rising staircase of increasing amplitude. This pattern of amplitude modulation produces a stroking sensation under the electrodes which is more comfortable for the patient.
(ii) On some stimulators a **randomized continuous output** is available, the purpose of which is to reduce the development of tolerance to TENS which may occur more readily with a regular pattern of stimulation due to habituation of the nervous system.
(iii) Stimulators are now available that produce **complex wave forms** designed to operate with a single pair of electrodes (Likon *et al.* 1992) or multiple electrodes activated randomly (Codetron *et al.* 1988), although their role in TENS therapy, especially for palliative care, remains unclear. Other developments include H-wave stimulation, microcurrent electrical stimulation (MES) and Transcutaneous spinal electroanalgesia (TSE) (Macdonald and Coates 1995) which uses very high frequency stimulation (2000 Hz) with very short pulses (4μs) of high voltage (>120 v).
(iv) So-called Brief Intense TENS (continuous pattern with high frequency/high intensity) is occasionally used for short periods when maximum analgesia of quick onset is required to cover some minor surgical procedure (Mannheimer and Lampe 1984).

Equipment

TENS equipment comprises the stimulator (including connecting leads) and electrodes. During the past fifteen years, the number of stimulators designed specifically for TENS therapy has increased steadily worldwide. Stamp and Wood have published two comparative evaluations of the transcutaneous stimulators available (Stamp and Wood 1981; Stamp and Rose 1984) (Table 13.5). Since this is a profitable market, new models appear frequently. Before making a purchase, the potential buyer should check that any stimulator under consideration has as a minimum the following features:

- Compact, lightweight, conveniently shaped, sturdily built and easily attachable to belt or pocket.
- On-off/amplitude (strength) and frequency controls of convenient size and shape, easily accessible and adjustable; sufficiently protected from accidental knocking or disturbance.
- Availability of pulse patterns, continuous (conventional) and pulsed ('burst') patterns essential, modulation (ramped) and random patterns desirable.
- Connecting lead(s) should be lightweight, flexible and able to connect to all standard types of electrodes.
- Low battery drain. Where necessary able to be used with rechargeable batteries and supplied with a simple, compact mains battery charger.
- Simple, lucid instruction manual.
- Minimum 2 year guarantee.
- Reliable and rapid maintenance service.

pain clinics should have two or three standard models of stimulator which have been found by patients and staff to be effective, reliable, and economical. This is a more satisfactory arrangement than purchasing a mixture of stimulators of different design

Table 13.5. Main characteristics of stimulators for transcutaneous electrical nerve stimulation

---

Country of Origin: Finland, Israel, Japan, UK, USA

Dimensions: $6 \times 4.9 \times 1.78$ cm (smallest)–$12 \times 8.5 \times 3.6$ cm (largest)

Weight (inc. battery): 55–220g.

Pulse width: 200 μsec fixed or 10–500 μsec adjustable

Pulse frequency: 1.5–100 Hz adjustable; rarely fixed.

In some instruments 'packets' or 'bursts' of pulses available at 2Hz

Channels: 1 or 2

Battery type (with or without optional rechargeable kit)

PP3, $2 \times$ AA or special.

Battery Life: 40–120 hrs (occasionally 4–16 hrs)

Guarantee: 0.5–2 years

(Stamp and Wood 1981; Stamp and Rose 1984).

and manufacture, each with its own idiosyncrasies and electrical incompatibilities with respect to the others. In many pain clinics it is the normal practice for stimulators to be loaned out to a patient for an initial trial period of, say, one month. If the trial of TENS proves successful then the stimulator can be supplied to the patient with the aid of public or private support.

Practical use

Standard electrode positions have been worked out for many pain conditions on a dermatomal basis combined with trial and error. When starting a patient on a trial of TENS therapy it is important to check that the electrode positions used initially are appropriate to the pain condition being treated (Fig. 13.4). Nevertheless, it is also important to establish that the electrode positions employed are optimum. This can only be achieved by encouraging the patient to alter the sites of application within reasonable limits. Where there are no standard electrode positions the following procedure should be adopted:

• Initially place electrodes over painful site and stimulate.
• If initial placement brings inadequate relief, relocate electrodes over next largest nerve which innervates the affected area and restimulate.

For all electrode positions continue as follows:

• The stimulus sensation should be directed into the painful area.
• The tingling sensation produced by TENS should be 'strong but comfortable' and *not* just tolerable.
• Neither continuous (conventional) TENS nor pulsed (burst) TENS should be permitted to produce muscle twitching or spasm. By contrast, acupuncture-like TENS (Acu-TENS) is deliberately adjusted to a strength that evokes muscle twitching (Table 13.4).
• to treat large areas of pain, multiple electrodes may be needed.

Use of electrodes

TENS electrodes are either reusable or disposable and can be classified as follows:

Reusable electrodes: are either (a) conducting rubber pads used with electrode jelly and tape or (b) self-adhesive conductive polymer pads which do not require jelly or tape. They are available in various sizes (mm): 40 × 40 (small), 93 × 42 (large), 210 × 40 (post-operative), 28 or 50 circular (for face). The anticipated life of these electrodes varies, for (a) is 3–6 months but for (b) is usually about 10–14 days. However, in practice and with care, the useful life can be substantially longer.

Disposable electrodes: are self-adhesive conductive polymer pads available in the same range of sizes as above. Each electrode has an anticipated life of about 2–4 days.

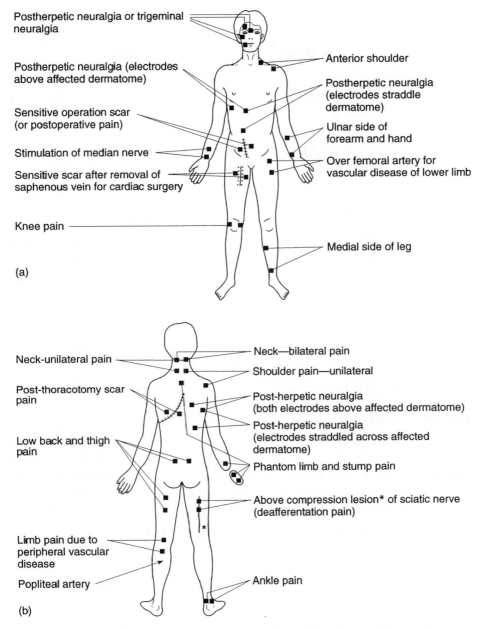

Postherpetic neuralgia or trigeminal neuralgia

Postherpetic neuralgia (electrodes above affected dermatome)

Sensitive operation scar (or postoperative pain)

Stimulation of median nerve

Sensitive scar after removal of saphenous vein for cardiac surgery

Knee pain

(a)

Anterior shoulder

Postherpetic neuralgia (electrodes straddle dermatome)

Ulnar side of forearm and hand

Over femoral artery for vascular disease of lower limb

Medial side of leg

Neck-unilateral pain

Post-thoracotomy scar pain

Low back and thigh pain

Limb pain due to peripheral vascular disease

Popliteal artery

(b)

Neck—bilateral pain

Shoulder pain—unilateral

Post-herpetic neuralgia (both electrodes above affected dermatome)

Post-herpetic neuralgia (electrodes straddled across affected dermatome)

Phantom limb and stump pain

Above compression lesion* of sciatic nerve (deafferentation pain)

Ankle pain

Fig. 13.4 Drawing of electrode positions commonly used for TENS. (a) Anterior aspect. (b) Posterior aspect.

Conducting rubber pads can be converted into self-adhesive electrodes by the use of Karaya pads (double sided sticky) and thereby eliminate the need for jelly and tape.

Some disposable electrodes are now available using a pregelled silver/silver chloride construction in order to avoid polarization. However, with stimulators of modern design the latter is not usually a problem. Other uncommon types of electrodes are available such as cotton pads and stainless steel but these are rarely used.

Treatment plan

As with all other forms of treatment it is essential to diagnose the cause of the pain before deciding to treat it. However it is not always possible to make a precise diagnosis, particularly with chronic pain. When using TENS for pain caused by a neoplasm, it is important to ensure that the condition does not require some form of urgent and/or more radical therapy. For some pain conditions (including those of neoplastic origin) it may take a considerable amount of time and patience on the part of both patient and therapist to establish effective electrode positions. It is also important to check that TENS does not aggravate the pain condition which occasionally occurs and usually indicates that this form of treatment is unsuitable for a particular patient.

Experience has shown that the best way to find out whether or not TENS will produce effective pain relief is to loan a stimulator to the patient for a trial period of, for example, one month. Then the treatment can be given an exhaustive test under normal everyday conditions of the patient's life. During the month's trial period, the patient is encouraged to contact the clinic to report progress. Initially each patient on TENS therapy should be reviewed at monthly intervals and thereafter according to need.

Indications for TENS therapy

Many different acute and chronic pains, including those associated with cancer, have been treated successfully with TENS (Table 13.3). Any pain that occurs in a patient suffering from cancer may well respond to TENS. As with all other pains, it is important to discover the cause of the pain; but treatment should not be withheld pending the completion of investigations. It is not possible to predict whether a particular pain problem in a particular patient will respond to TENS (Johnson *et al.* 1991). This situation also applies to the use of TENS for cancer-related pain. When embarking on a course of TENS, it is important not to raise excessive expectations but to indicate that 'a trial of TENS is well worthwhile and may result in useful and effective pain relief'. There are several pain conditions associated with cancer that may respond particularly well to TENS.

Predominantly nociceptive pains:

 (i) Pain from metastatic bone disease. The electrodes should be sited near the painful metastatic deposit or on healthy skin within the affected dermatome.

 (ii) Pain caused by initial compression of nerve roots following vertebral collapse. The electrodes should be placed in the affected dermatome or on an adjacent dermatome.

(iii) Pain in the abdomen including that due to an enlarged liver caused by secondary deposits. The electrodes should be placed over or near the painful area.

Predominantly neuropathic pains:

(i) Pain due to compression of a nerve by a neoplasm, for example, a lumbar nerve by a retroperitoneal tumour. The electrodes should be placed on skin innervated by the affected nerve but proximal to the site of compression and at a level where sensory function has been preserved.

(ii) Pain due to post herpetic neuralgia. Apply electrodes to skin of same or adjacent dermatome near (but not on) affected site.

(iii) Pain due to infiltration of nerves, for example, brachial plexus. Electrodes should be placed on skin of dermatome(s) that are adjacent (cephalad) to those affected.

(iv) Post chemotherapy neuropathy. Electrodes placed paravertebrally at or above the level of affected nerve roots and on affected limbs. Modulated mode can produce effective analgesia. Muscle power can also increase in hypotonic muscles with these peripheral placements.

(v) Mirror image (contralateral) TENS. When TENS therapy produces a poor response, it is worth trying mirror image or contralateral stimulation, that is applying stimulation to the corresponding normal site on the opposite side of the body. This may prove to be effective when ipsilateral TENS has produced little or no response. Sometimes the combination of ipsilateral and contralateral TENS produces a better response than ipsilateral TENS alone. If it is found that ipsilateral TENS cannot be tolerated when applied to the affected part (most likely to occur with a neuropathic pain), contralateral TENS to the mirror image site may be effective. This may be applied either alone or combined with ipsilateral TENS applied away from the affected area but within the same dermatome.

Without doubt, trial and error is the best method by which to discover the optimum form of TENS for treating a particular pain. Continuous (conventional) TENS may be better for those pains which are predominantly nociceptive, namely skeletal, paravertebral and joint pains and visceral referred pain. Pulsed and acupuncture-like TENS may be better for neuropathic pain especially where hyperaesthesia or dysaesthesia are prominent features (Table 13.4; Bowsher 1991).

Efficacy

There is now an extensive world literature on TENS and most of it supports the view that this is a useful form of analgesia, particularly for chronic pain (Mannheimer and Lampe 1984; Sjölund and Eriksson 1985; Woolf and Thompson 1994; Walsh 1997). Results of a number of controlled studies indicate that there is a significant and therapeutically useful analgesic response to TENS (Tulgar *et al.* 1991; Lander and Fowler-Kerry 1993; Marchand *et al.* 1993; Morgan *et al.* 1995) although others do not support this conclusion (Deyo *et al.* 1990). A recent study by Marchand *et al.* (1993) clearly differentiated the effect of TENS on pain intensity and pain unpleasantness. As with medication, there is a placebo response to TENS. This factor contributes to the initial but transient analgesic effect seen with some patients in response to electrical stimulation. Thus the response of a group of patients to TENS may be as high as 70–80% during the first week. Response falls to about 40% at the end of the first month and to about 35% at the end of the first year (Ray 1976; Bates and Nathan 1980; Johnson *et al.* 1991, 1993). In spite of this, there is a group of patients for whom TENS appears to offer significant and continued pain relief (Johnson *et al.* 1991) and where medication has often failed to help or where there are no alternatives with the possible exception of ablative procedures.

Evidence-based medicine and TENS

Currently the number of randomized controlled clinical trials on TENS is small. Therefore for both therapeutic and economic reasons there is an urgent need to confirm the efficacy of TENS for different chronic pain conditions. It must not be assumed that if TENS is shown to be effective for one type of chronic pain, is it necessarily effective for another type of chronic pain, even though the two pains may appear to be similar. A recent meta-analysis of thirty-eight randomized controlled trials on TENS has produced results from which several important conclusions have been drawn (McQuay and Moore 1998). These may be summarized:

1. In none of the trials was TENS judged to have been blinded. It is appreciated that blinding of TENS is much more difficult than blinding of drug studies.

2. An important aim is that the outcome measures should be a direct determination of pain intensity or pain relief. Thus it should not be an indirect measurement such as the need to use other analgesic interventions or a reduction of analgesic consumption.

3. The dose of TENS used to treat chronic pain conditions must be adequate. Those physicians who treat chronic pain regularly with TENS usually prescribe it for a *minimum* of 30 minutes twice daily continued for at least a month before significant benefit may be expected (Nash *et al.* 1990; Johnson *et al.* 1993). None of the trials included in the meta-analysis had used doses which came close to this amount.

4. The authors' conclude that the use of TENS in chronic pain may be justified. This remains to be proved with the aid of a multicentre randomized trial in which TENS is tested on a large number of patients. In spite of these conclusions, McQuay, Moore and their colleagues have confirmed that TENS has an analgesic effect in dysmenorrhoea (Leijon *et al.* 1997).

Practical issues in the use of TENS

When a patient is started on TENS and pain is relieved, it is not possible to distinguish whether this response is likely to be maintained or to wane. If the latter occurs it may be due either to a change in the severity of pain or in the response of the patient.

Changes in pain level

This may be due to an actual increase in the intensity of the pain for which TENS is being used or may be due to a change in the emotional response of the patient to his or her pain. Alternatively, the increase may be due to a change in the quality of pain, for example, the addition of a neuropathic component to an existing nociceptive pain. Alternatively, the increase may be due to the addition of one or more new pains to the original pain. This situation highlights the importance of continuously monitoring the site(s) and cause(s) of pain, especially in patients suffering from advanced cancer.

Changes in the patient response

There are three main causes that need to be considered.

The initially favourable response to TENS may have been due to a placebo response. The hallmark of a placebo response is that it is likely to fade rapidly, even abruptly, commonly within a week of starting treatment, although sometimes taking a little longer (Woolf and Thompson 1994).

The waning response may be due to the development of tolerance. This term conceals a considerable amount of ignorance as to its mechanism. Tolerance develops more slowly and insidiously than a placebo response. It may not occur for weeks or months after starting treatment. It appears to be akin to drug tolerance which may develop fairly quickly over the course of weeks (e.g. opioid tolerance) or very slowly over the course of months or years (e.g. insulin tolerance). Tolerance to TENS may include some or all of the following: dysfunction of pain-inhibitory neuronal pathways (e.g. waning neurotransmitter release or down-regulation of opioid, nor-adrenaline or 5-hydroxytryptamine receptors); interference by the production of increasing amounts of endogenous opioid antagonists e.g. the octapeptide form of cholecyst-okinin (CCK-8) (Wang *et al.* 1990). The neuropharmacology of the pain pathway and opioid mechanisms have been described elsewhere (Thompson 1990, 1994).

The effectiveness of these possible mechanisms whereby tolerance to TENS develops may depend upon the establishment of regular patterns of neuronal activity in the nerve pathways involved. This may be linked to the well-known phenomenon of habituation which the regular pulse patterns of TENS may help to establish. For this reason some stimulators are now constructed with the option of a random pulse output. This development has been carried to the furthest degree by the development of the Codetron stimulator. It applies randomly distributed pulses to a set of six electrodes (instead of the usual pair) and is claimed to be more effective than ordinary TENS (Librach and Rapson 1988). It is possible that random stimulation may help to delay or reverse tolerance. When it does so, it may achieve this via delaying or reversing the regular patterns of neuronal activity which may be an integral part of the tolerance mechanism.

The patient's response to TENS may be antagonized by concurrent medication. There is some equivocal clinical evidence to suggest that the concurrent use of opioids (more especially when opioid dependence is well developed), corticosteroids, or benzodiazepines may interfere with the efficacy of TENS (Mannheimer and Lampe 1984; Thompson 1989). However, these drugs are commonly prescribed to patients who obtain an excellent therapeutic response with TENS. It therefore seems unlikely that medication is a common cause of TENS failure. Nevertheless when the onset of failure with TENS therapy coincides with some change in medication, the possible occurrence of this mechanism should be considered and appropriate action taken.

In a survey on 179 patients, Johnson, Ashton and Thompson (1991) observed that the average length of use of TENS was 4 years (range 3 months to 9 years). During this time 47% of patients found TENS reduced their pain by more than half. Furthermore TENS analgesia was rapid both in onset (less than 30 minutes in 75%) and offset (less than 30 minutes in 75%). One-third of patients used this therapy for over 61 hours per week. It is known that in patients who suffer from more than one type of pain condition, TENS may be very effective for one pain and yet totally ineffective for another. All the foregoing evidence mitigates strongly against the view that TENS analgesia is a placebo response.

Unfortunately, tolerance to TENS occurs and may develop slowly or suddenly thus terminating what has previously been effective analgesia. The reasons for this are not fully understood but sometimes it is possible to overcome this problem by changing the type of stimulation. It is also important to note that some patients do not respond to TENS. The response to TENS may depend upon the level of cortical responsivity which is significantly lower in non-responders (Johnson *et al.* 1993).

The results of TENS for the treatment of malignant disease are summarized in Table 13.6. There is a wide range of efficacy for good (15–99%) or partial (2–44%) pain relief. This may be due to many variables including the small samples, severity of disease, the mode of application of TENS, and differences in methods of assessing pain relief. These results indicate the urgent need for further controlled trials of TENS in palliative medicine. This conclusion is supported by a search of the literature which failed to find any randomized controlled trials on this subject during the 20 years from 1979 to January 1999.

Complications and contraindications

Complications of TENS therapy may be related to the response of the patient or the performance of the equipment.

Serious complications due to TENS therapy are rare. Most problems are due to skin irritation, skin burn, or allergy (to the electrode, or associated conducting jelly, tape, or gum). Skin irritation can be minimized by ensuring that the skin area to which electrodes are applied is kept dry, clean, and free from grease (e.g. cosmetics). This keeps electrical resistance between the electrode and skin low and evenly distributed thus avoiding 'hot spots', caused by uneven current flow. This is important for electrodes requiring electrode jelly and those that are self-adhesive (pre-gelled). In a survey of nearly 200 patients using TENS regularly the only common problem was skin irritation (Johnson *et al.* 1991). This occurred in a third of cases probably due in part to drying out of electrode jelly (Mason and Mackay 1976; Yamamoto *et al.* 1986).

Equipment failure is uncommon. It may be due to faulty leads, stimulator, battery,

Table 13.6. TENS for the treatment of malignant disease

Author(s)	Good or complete pain relief	Partial pain relief or reduction of analgesics	No relief	Total patients
Long (1974)	3	—	2	5 malignancies in total series of 197 patients
Hardy (1975)	2	—	2	4: out of 53
Loeser *et al.* (1975)	—	3	4	7 out of 198
Campbell and Long (1976)	1	—	3	4
Ostrowski (1979)	4	4	1	9
Ventafridda (1979)	36 at 1–10 days	—	1	37
	4 at 30 days	—	33 at 30 days	37
Bates and Nathan (1980)	4 all longer than 1 week	—	1	5
Avellanosa and West (1982)				
2 weeks	17	22	21	60
3 months	9	11	40	60
Dil-din *et al.* (1985)	11	—	—	11 (abstract only available)
Rafter (1986) quoted by Librach and Rapson (1988)	34	1	4	49
Range (%)	15–99	2–44	3–75	Total 191 pts

or charger. When modern, well-designed and properly constructed equipment is used in accordance with the manufacturers instructions these problems are unusual. Disposable batteries have a finite life and rechargeable batteries cannot be recharged indefinitely.

Contraindications to TENS therapy are few.

• Do not place electrodes on inflamed, infected, or otherwise unhealthy skin.

• Do not stimulate over the anterior part of the neck. This is to avoid the possibility of stimulating the nerves of the larynx or the carotid sinus which could produce laryngeal spasm or hypotension.

• Do not stimulate over a pregnant uterus (except when TENS is being used for obstetric analgesia).

• Do not use the stimulator in the presence of a cardiac pacemaker. This restriction applies especially to an on-demand pacemaker. In order to err on the side of safety the manufacturers of TENS equipment apply this as a general restriction. In practice, it is not uncommon to operate fixed rate pacemakers in the presence of a TENS machine. This should only be done after consulting the cardiologist responsible for the patient and also, if necessary, the manufacturers of the pacemaker and the TENS equipment.

• Do not try to force the use of TENS onto a non-compliant patient. Patients with organic brain disease or limited understanding may have particular difficulty. In addition, some patients will be found to have a fear of, rooted objection to, or inability to use, electricity in any form for medical treatment, including TENS.

Neuroanatomy and neuropharmacology of TENS and acupuncture

During the past two decades considerable progress has been made with the study of the neuroanatomy and neuropharmacology of nociceptive systems including the possible mechanisms of both TENS and acupuncture (Han and Terenius 1982; Duggan and Foong 1985; Bowsher 1985; Garrison and Foreman 1994; Bowsher 1987).

The neuroanatomical and neuropharmacological basis of pain and the way in which this is modified by TENS and acupuncture is shown in Fig. 13.5. The diagram is based on the work of Duggan and Foong (1985), Bowsher (1985, 1987), Han and Terenius (1982), Le Bars *et al.* (1979), Fields and Basbaum (1994) and Jones *et al.* (1991). So-called 'first', 'rapid', or 'aversive' pain is due to the activation of small myelinated A delta fibres whereas 'second', 'slow' or 'tissue damage' pain is due to activation of mostly unmyelinated C fibres with activation of some A delta fibres (Bowsher 1987). There are four conditions to be considered:

Pathways for tissue damage pain: peripheral polymodal nociceptor afferents (C) are activated as the result of, for example, a painful scar (Fig. 13.5). The C fibre afferents terminate in the substantia gelatinosa (SG) (lamina II) where their axon terminals secrete Substance P (SP) or vasoactive intestinal peptide (VIP), according to whether these arise from skin or viscera, respectively. The substantia gelatinosa indirectly excites transmission cells (T) deep in the spinal grey matter whose axons form the spinoreticular tract. This forms one component of the crossed anterolateral funiculus which ascends to the brain. The spinoreticular tract sends collaterals to the hypothalamus (triggering autonomic responses to pain) and then synapses in the thalamus. Here it excites other neurones which are distributed widely over the cerebral cortex including the frontal area and the limbic system. These give rise to the conscious sensation and emotional experience of tissue-damage pain.

TENS: electrical stimulation excites A beta afferents connected to tactile receptors. After entering the spinal cord these afferents ultimately ascend in the dorsal columns. At spinal cord level the A beta fibres give collaterals which synapse with short interneurons, the endings of which terminate close to the C fibre terminals as the latter synapse with substantia gelatinosa cells. These interneurons probably release gamma-amino butyric acid (GABA) which causes presynaptic blockade of the C afferents. This

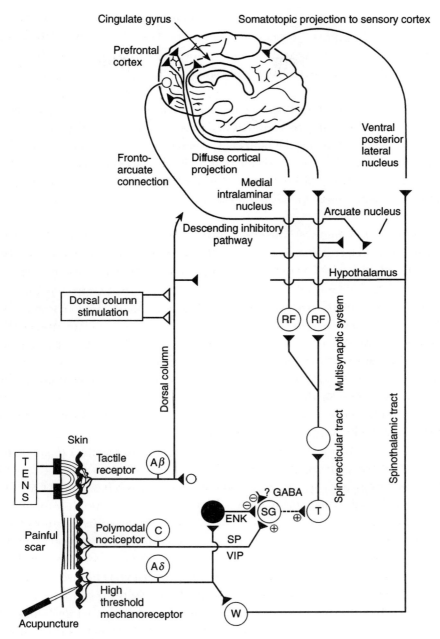

Fig. 13.5 Diagram to show neuronal circuits involved in TENS and acupuncture analgesia. The afferent pathways involved in transmitting nociceptive information from a painful scar to the higher centres via the dorsal horn, the ascending tracts and the thalamus are shown. The connections to the descending inhibitory pathways which descend in the dorsolateral funiculus are also shown. The connections to the hypothalamus are indicated. Abbreviations: Aβ, C and Aδ represent the posterior root ganglion cells of Aβ, C, and Aδ fibres, respectively; SP = substance P; VIP = vasoactive intestinal polypeptide; GABA = γ-amino-butyric acid; OP = opioid peptides; SG = cell in the substantia gelatinosa (lamina II); Enk = enkephalinergic neurone; T = transmission cell; W = Waldeyer cell; PAG = periaqueductal grey; mRG = cell in the nucleus raphe gigantocellularis; nRM = cell in the nucleus raphe magnus; Nad = noradrenaline; 5-HT = 5-hydroxytryptamine; + = stimulant effect; − = inhibitory effect.

prevents them from exciting the substantia gelatinosa cells and blocks the onward transmission of nociceptive information. The elegant demonstration by Garrison and Foreman (1994) that TENS decreases the activity of spontaneous and noxiously evoked dorsal horn cells is in accord with this explanation.

Segmental acupuncture: High threshold mechanoreceptors connected to small myelinated primary (A delta) afferents are activated by acupuncture. One central branch of the A delta afferent excites the inhibitory enkephalinergic interneuron (on the borders of laminae I and II), releasing enkephalin (Enk). This produces post-synaptic block of the substantia gelatinosa cell and prevents the onward transmission of noxiously generated information. This mechanism would explain segmental acupuncture.

Extra-segmental acupuncture: Waldeyer cells (W) in lamina I of the spinal grey matter are excited by acupuncture via another central branch of A delta primary afferents. The axons of the Waldeyer cells constitute another component (spinothalamic tract) of the crossed anterolateral funiculus. They convey pin-prick information to consciousness through the ventral posterolateral nucleus of the thalamus. This passes to the somatosensory cortex where there is somatotopic representation. Collaterals excite the periaqueductal grey (PAG) area, which in its turn projects to the nucleus Raphe Magnus (nRM) which is situated in the midline of the lower brainstem reticular formation.

Serotinergic (5HT) and adrenergic (Nad) axons of nRM cells descend through the dorsolateral funiculus of the spinal cord. These synapse eventually with the cells described above. Blocking the onward transmission of noxiously generated information in the same way as segmental acupuncture. However, this descending inhibitory pathway gives off connections at all levels of the spinal cord thereby explaining the extra-segmental effect of acupuncture.

A striking and puzzling difference between analgesia produced by TENS and acupuncture is the duration of pain relief. Whereas TENS usually produces analgesia for minutes or hours, acupuncture can, and often does, produce analgesia for weeks. The mechanisms discussed previously cannot account for the prolonged analgesia commonly seen after acupuncture. Some additional mechanisms must be involved. Acupuncture may set up a so-called meso-limbic loop of analgesia formed by the periaqueductal grey, the nucleus accumbens and the habenula (Han *et al.* 1986). Acupuncture may set in motion this particular loop of neuronal activity which, whilst it is in motion, blocks the upward transmission of nociceptive impulses from the spinal cord to the thalamus and cortex. In support of this hypothesis, acupuncture analgesia can be blocked by injecting naloxone into any one of the main neuronal stations on the loop (Zhou *et al.* 1984; Han *et al.* 1986). It seems unlikely that naloxone would have this effect unless these areas operate as a loop and are inter-dependent. Presumably, once the loop has been set in motion, it takes some time to slow down. It is during this time that analgesia occurs and so explains its prolonged effect. It is an exciting concept but it remains to be substantiated by further experiments. Changes an analgesic gene expression may also be responsible for the sustained effects of acupuncture (Zieglgansberger 1999, personal communication, Lee and Beitz 1993).

Acknowledgements

Much of the section on transcutaneous electrical nerve stimulation has been reproduced from the chapter entitled 'Transcutaneous electrical nerve stimulation (TENS) and acupuncture' in the *Oxford textbook of palliative medicine*, 2nd edition, 1998 (editors: D. Doyle, G.W.C. Hanks, and N. MacDonald) published by Oxford Medical Publications. We are most grateful to Oxford University Press for generously allowing reproduction of material. We also wish to record our thanks to Mrs Julia Jeffrey and to Mrs Jane Brooks for their secretarial help in the preparation of this chapter.

References

Aglietti, L., Roila, F., Tonato, M., Basurto, C., Bracarda, S., Picciafuoco., M., Ballatori, E., and Del-Favero, A. (1990). A pilot study of metoclopramide, dexamethasone, diphenhydramine and acupuncture in women treated with cisplatin. *Cancer Chemotherapy and Pharmacology*, **26**, 239–40.

Ahonen, E., Hakumaki, M., Mahlamaki, S., Partanen, J., Reikkinen, P., and Sivenius, J. (1983). Acupuncture and physiotherapy in the treatment of myogenic headache patients: Pain relief and EMG activity. *Advances in Pain Research and Therapy*, **5**, 571–6.

Avellanosa, A.M., and West, C.R. (1982). Experience with transcutaneous nerve stimulation for relief of intractable pain in cancer patients. *Journal of Medicine*, **13**, 203–13.

Baldry, P. (1998). Laser therapy. In *Medical acupuncture—a western scientific approach* (ed. J. Filshie and A. White) pp. 193–201. Churchill Livingstone, Edinburgh.

Baldry, P.E. (1993). Acupuncture, trigger points and musculo-skeletal pain (2nd edn). Churchill Livingstone, Edinburgh.

Bates, J.A.V., and Nathan, P.W. (1980). Transcutaneous electrical nerve stimulation for chronic pain. *Anaesthesia*, **35**, 817–22.

Baxter, D. (1989). Laser acupuncture analgesia: an overview. *Acupuncture in Medicine*, **6**, 57–60.

Belluomini, J., Litt, R.C., Lee, K.A., and Katz, M. (1994). Acupressure for nausea and vomiting of pregnancy: a randomized, blinded study. *Obstetrics and Gynecology*, **84**, 245–8.

Beyens, F. (1998). Reinterpretation of traditional concepts in acupuncture. In *Medical acupuncture—a western scientific approach* (ed. J. Filshie and A.W. White) pp. 391–407. Churchill Livingstone, Edinburgh.

Bianchi, M., Jotti, E., Sacerdote, P., and Panerai, A.E. (1991). Traditional acupuncture increases the content of beta-endorphin in immune cells and influences mitogen induced proliferation. *American Journal of Chinese Medicine*, **19**, 101–4.

Bliddal, H., Hellesen, C., Ditlevsen, P., Asselberghs, J., and Lyager, L. (1987). Soft laser therapy of rheumatoid arthritis. *Scandinavian Journal of Rheumatology*, **16**, 225–8.

Bowsher, D. (1985). Sensory mechanisms. In Frederiks JAM Ed. Clin. Neuropsychology, 45, 227–244. In Vinken, PJ, Bruyn, GW, Klawans, HL. *Handbook of Clinical Neurology* 1985, 1 (45). Publishers, Elsevier Science, Amsterdam.

Bowsher, D. (1987). The physiology of acupuncture. *Journal of the Intractable Pain Society of Great Britain and Ireland*, 5, 15–18.

Bowsher, D. (1991). Neurogenic Pain Syndromes and their management In *Pain mechanisms and Management* (ed. J.C.D. Wells and C.J. Woolf) *British Medical Bulletin*, 47, 644–66.

Bowsher, D. (1998). Mechanisms of acupuncture. In *Medical Acupuncture*—a Western scientific approach (ed. J. Filshie and A. White), pp. 69–82. Churchill Livingstone, Edinburgh.

Bowsher, D., Mumford, J., Lipton, S., and Miles, J. (1973). Treatment of intractable pain by acupuncture. *Lancet*, ii, 57–60.

Brockhaus, A., and Elger, C.E. (1990). Hypalgesic efficacy of acupuncture on experimental pain in man. Comparison of laser acupuncture and needle acupuncture. *Pain*, 43, 181–5.

Campbell, J.N., and Long, D.M. (1976). Peripheral nerve stimulation in the treatment of intractable pain. *Journal of Neurosurgery*, 45, 692–9.

Chapman, C.R., Wilson, M.E., and Gehrig, J.D. (1976). Comparative effects of acupuncture and transcutaneous stimulation on the perception of painful dental stimuli. *Pain*, 2, 265–83.

Christensen, B.V., Iuhl, I.U., Vilbek, H., Bulow, H., Dreijer, N.C., and Rasmussen, H.F. (1992). Acupuncture treatment of severe knee osteoarthrosis: A long-term study. *Acta Anaesthesiologica Scandinavia*, 36, 519–25.

Colov, H.C., Palmgren, N., Jansen, G.F., Kas, K., and Windelin, M. (1987). Convincing clinical improvement of rheumatoid arthritis by soft laser therapy. *Lasers in Surgery and Medicine*, 7, 77.

de Aloysio, D., and Penacchioni, P. (1992). Morning sickness control in early pregnancy by Neiguan point acupressure. *Obstetrics and Gynecology*, 80, 852–4.

Delaney, G.A., and McKee, A.C. (1993). Inter and intra-rater reliability of the pressure threshold meter in measurement of myofascial trigger point sensitivity. *American Journal of Physical Medicine and Rehabilitation*, 72, 136–9.

Deyo, R.A., Walsh, N.E., Martin, D.C., Schoenfeld, L.S., and Ramamurthy, S. (1990). A controlled trial of transcutaneous electrical nerve stimulation (TENS) and exercise for chronic low back pain. *New England Journal of Medicine*, 332, 1627–34.

Dil-din, A.S., Tikhonova, G.P., and Kozvov, S.V. (1985). Transcutaneous electrostimulation method leading to a permeation system of electroanalgesia in oncological practice. *Vopr-Onkologica*, 31, 33–6.

Dillon, M., and Lucas, C.F. (1999). Auricular stud acupuncture in palliative care patients: An initial report. *Palliative Medicine*, 13, 253–4.

Ding, V., Roath, S., and Lewith, G.T. (1983). Effect of acupuncture on lymphocyte behaviour. *American Journal of Acupuncture*, 11, 51–4.

Duggan, A.W., and Foong, F.W. (1985). Bicuculline and spinal inhibition produced by dorsal column stimulation in the cat. *Pain*, 22, 249–59.

Ernst, E., and Pittler, M.H. (1998). The effectiveness of acupuncture in treating acute dental pain: A systematic review. *British Dental Journal*, **184**, 443–7.

Ernst, E., and White, A.R. (1998). Acupuncture for back pain: a meta-analysis of randomized controlled trials. *Archives of Internal Medicine*, **158**, 2235–41.

Essentials of Chinese acupuncture (1980). Foreign Languages Press, Beijing.

Fields, H.L., and Basbaum, A.L. (1994). Central nervous system mechanisms of pain modulation. In *Textbook of pain* (3rd edn) (ed. P.D. Wall and R. Melzack) Ch. 12. Churchill Livingstone, Edinburgh.

Filshie, J. (1988). The non-drug treatment of neuralgic and neuropathic pain of malignancy. In *Cancer Surveys*, Vol. 7, No 1 (ed. G.W. Hanks) pp. 161–93. Oxford University Press.

Filshie, J. (1990). Acupuncture for malignant pain. *Acupuncture in Medicine*, **8**, 38–9.

Filshie, J., Penn, K., Ashley, S., and Davis, C.L. (1996). Acupuncture for the relief of cancer-related breathlessness. *Palliative Medicine*, **10**, 145–50.

Filshie, J., and Redman, D. (1985). Acupuncture and malignant pain problems. *European Journal of Surgical Oncology*, **11**, 389–94.

Filshie, J., Scase, A., Ashley, S., and Hood, J. (1997). A study of the effect of acupuncture on pain, anxiety and depression in patients with breast cancer. Abstract: *Pain Society Meeting*, Newcastle.

Filshie, J., and White, A. (1998). *Medical acupuncture. A western scientific approach*. Churchill Livingstone, Edinburgh.

Garrison, D.W., and Foreman, R.D. (1994). Decreased activity of spontaneous and noxiously evoked dorsal horn cells during transcutaneous electrical nerve stimulation (TENS). *Pain*, **58**, 309–15.

Gerwin, R.D., Shannon, S., Hong, C.Z., Hubbard, D., and Gevirtz, R. (1997). Inter-rater reliability in myofascial trigger point examination. *Pain*, **69** (1–2), 65–73.

Gunn, C.C., Milbrandt, W.E., Little, A.S., and Mason, K.E. (1980). Dry needling of muscle motor points for chronic low back pain: a randomised clinical trial with long term follow up. *Spine*, **5**, 279–91.

Halvorsen, T.B., Anda, S.S., Naess, A.B., and Levang, O.W. (1995). Fatal cardiac tamponade after acupuncture through congenital sternal foramen. *Lancet*, **345**, 1175.

Hammerschlag, R. (1998). Methodological and ethical issues in clinical trials of acupuncture. *Journal of Alternative and Complementary Medicine*, **4**, 159–71.

Han, J.S., Ding, X.Z., and Fang, S.G. (1986a). Cholecystokinin octapeptide (CCK-8): antagonism to electroacupuncture analgesia and a possible role in electroacupuncture tolerance. *Pain*, **27**, 101–15.

Han, J.S., and Terenius, L. (1982.) Neurochemical basis of acupuncture analgesia. *Annual Review of Pharmacology and Toxicology*, **22**, 193–220.

Han, J.S., Yu, L.C., and Shi, Y.A. (1986). A mesolimbic loop of analgesia. III. A neuronal pathway from nucleus accumbens to periaquaductal grey. *Asian Pacific Journal of Pharmacology*, **1**, 17–22.

Hansen, P.E., and Hansen, J.H. (1983). Acupuncture treatment of chronic facial pain: a controlled cross-over trial. *Headache*, **23**, 66–9.

Hardy, R.W. (1975). Current techniques in the management of pain. *Cleveland Clinical Quarterly*, **41**, 77–183.

Hester, J. (1998). Acupuncture in the pain clinic. In *Medical acupuncture. A western scientific approach* (ed. J. Filshie and A. White), pp. 319–40. Churchill Livingstone, Edinburgh.

Hubbard, D.R., and Berkoff, G.M. (1993). Myofascial trigger points show spontaneous needle EMG activity. *Spine*, **18**, 1803–7.

Hyodo, M. (1990). *Ryodoraku treatment*. Japanese Society of Ryodoraku Medicine, Osaka.

Jobst, K., Chen, J.H., McPherson, K., Arrowsmith, J., Brown, V., *et al.* (1986). Controlled trial of acupuncture for disabling breathlessness. *Lancet*, **ii**, 1416–19.

Johansson, K., Lindgren, I., Widner, H., Wiklund, I., and Johansson, B.B. (1993). Can sensory stimulation improve the functional outcome in stroke patients? *Neurology*, **43**, 2189–92.

Johnson, M.I., Ashton, C.H., and Thompson, J.W. (1991). An in-depth study of long term users of transcutaneous electrical nerve stimulation (TENS). Implications for clinical use of TENS. *Pain*, **44**, 221–9.

Johnson, M.I., Ashton, C.H., and Thompson, J.W. (1993). A prospective investigation into factors related to patient response to transcutaneous electrical nerve stimulation (TENS)—the importance of cortical responsivity. *European Journal of Pain*, **14**, 1–9.

Jones, A.K.P., Brown, W.D., Friston, K.T., Qi, Ly, and Frackowiak, R.S.J. (1991). Cortical and subcortical localisation of response to pain in man using positron emission tomography. *Proceedings of the Royal Society of London, Series B*, **244**, 29–44.

Jonsdottir, I.H. (1999). Physical exercise, acupuncture and immune function. *Acupuncture in Medicine*, **17**, 50–53.

Lander, J., and Fowler-Kerry, S. (1993). TENS for children's procedural pain. *Pain*, **52**, 209–16.

Lao, L., Bergman, S., Langenberg, P., Wong, R.H., and Berman, B. (1995). Efficacy of Chinese acupuncture on postoperative oral surgery pain. *Oral Surgery, Oral Medicine, Oral Pathology, Oral Radiology and Endodontics*, **79**, 423–8.

Lazarou, J., Pomeranz, B.H., and Corey, P.N. (1998). Incidence of adverse drug reactions in hospitalized patients: A meta-analysis of prospective studies. *Journal of the American Medical Association* **279**, 1200–5.

Le Bars, D., Dickenson, A.H., and Besson, J.M. (1979). Diffuse noxious inhibitory controls (DNIC). II Lack of effect on non-convergent neurons, supraspinal involvement and theoretical implications. *Pain*, **6**, 283–304.

Lee, J.H., and Beitz, A.J. (1993). The distribution of brain-stem and spinal cord nuclei associated with different frequencies of electroacupuncture analgesia. *Pain*, **52**, 11–28.

Leijon, G., Carroll, D., Gavaghan, D., Tramér, M., McQuay, H.J., and Moore, R.A. (1997). Transcutaneous electric nerve stimulation (TENS) in chronic pain; a qualitative systematic review. *Pain in Europe: II Congress of the European Federation of IASP chapters*, 23–27 September 1997. Proceedings, page 273.

Lewith, G.T., and Vincent, C.A. (1998). The clinical evaluation of acupuncture. In *Medical acupuncture. A western scientific approach* (ed. J. Filshie and A. White) pp. 205–24. Churchill Livingstone, Edinburgh.

Librach, S.I., and Rapson, L.M. (1988). The use of transcutaneous electrical nerve stimulation (TENS) for the relief of pain in palliative care. *Palliative Medicine*, **2**, 15–20.

Lim, J. (1989). Understanding acupuncture. Ph.D. Thesis, Cambridge University.

Loeser, J.D., Black, R.G., and Christman, A. (1975). Relief of pain by transcutaneous stimulation. *Journal of Neurosurgery*, **42**, 308–14.

Loh, L., Nathan, P.W., Schott, G.D., and Zilkha, K.J. (1984). Acupuncture versus medical treatment for migraine and muscle tension headaches. *Journal of Neurology, Neurosurgery and Psychiatry*, **47**, 333–7.

Long, D.M. (1973). Electrical stimulation for relief of pain from chronic nerve injury. *Journal of Neurosurgery*, **39**, 718–22.

Long, D.M. (1974). External electrical stimulation as a treatment of chronic pain. *Minnesota Medicine*, **57**, 195–8.

Lu, G.D., and Needham, J. (1980). *Celestial lancets. A history and rationale of acupuncture and moxa*. Cambridge University Press, Cambridge.

Lundeberg, T. (1999). Effects of sensory stimulation (acupuncture) on circulatory and immune systems. In *Acupuncture: a scientific appraisal*, pp. 93–106. Butterworth-Heinemann, Oxford.

Lundeberg, T., Hurtig, T., Lundeberg, S., and Thomas, M. (1988). Long-term results of acupuncture in chronic head and neck pain. *The Pain Clinic*, **2**, 15–31.

Ma, Kan-Wen (1992). The roots and development of Chinese acupuncture from prehistory to early 20th century. *Acupuncture in Medicine*, Vol X, suppl, pp. 92–9.

Macdonald, A.J., Macrae, K.D., Master, B.R., and Rubin, A.P. (1983). Superficial acupuncture in the relief of chronic low back pain. *Annals of Royal College Surgeons of England*, **65**, 44–6.

Macdonald, A.J. (1989). Acupuncture analgesia and therapy. In *Textbook of Pain* (ed. R. Melzack and P.D. Wall) (2nd edn), pp. 906–19. Churchill Livingstone, Edinburgh.

Macdonald, A.J.R., and Coates, T.W. (1995). The discovery of transcutaneous spinal electroanalgesia and its relief of chronic pain. *Physiotherapy*, **81**, 653–61.

Maciocia, G. (1997). *Tongue diagnosis in chinese medicine*, Eastland, Seattle, W.A.

Mann, F. (1992). *Reinventing acupuncture. A new concept of ancient medicine*. Butterworth-Heinemann, Oxford.

Mannheimer, J.S., and Lampe, G.N. (1984). *Clinical transcutaneous electrical nerve stimulation*. FA Davis Co., Philadelphia.

Marchand, S., Charest, J., Li, J., Chenard, J.-R., Lavignolle, B., and Laurencelle, L. (1993). Is TENS purely a placebo effect? A controlled study on chronic low back pain. *Pain*, **54**, 99–106.

Mason, J.L., and Mackay, N.A.M. (1976). Pain sensations associated with electrocutaneous stimulation. *IEEE Transactions on Biomedical Engineering*, **23**, 405–9.

McNulty, W.H., Gevirtz, R.N., Hubbard, D.R., and Berkoff, G.M. (1994). Needle electromyographic evaluation of trigger point response to a psychological stressor. *Psychophysiology*, **31**, 313–16.

McQuay, H., and Moore, A. (1998). Transcutaneous electrical nerve stimulation (TENS) in chronic pain. In *An evidence-based resource for pain relief*, pp. 207–11. Oxford University Press, Oxford.

Melzack, R. (1994). Folk medicine and the sensory modulation of pain. In *Textbook of pain* (3rd edn) (ed. R. Melzack and P.D. Wall), pp. 1209–17. Churchill Livingstone, Edinburgh.

Melzack, R., and Wall, P.D. (1965). Pain mechanisms: a new theory. *Science*, **150**, 971–9.

Moore, K.C., Hira, N., Kumar P.S., Jayakumar, C.S., and Ohshiro, T. (1988). A double-blind crossover trial of low-level laser therapy in the treatment of post herpetic neuralgia. *Laser Therapy*, **1**, 7–9.

Morgan, B., Jones, A.R., Mulcahy, K.A., Finlay, D.B., and Collett, B. (1995). Transcutaneous electric nerve stimulation (TENS) during distension shoulder arthrography: a controlled trial. *Pain*, **64**, 265–7.

Nakatani, Y., and Yamashita, K. (1977). *Ryodoraku acupuncture*. Ryodoraku Research Institute, Osaka.

Nash, T.P., Williams, J.D., and Machin, D. (1990). Does the type of stimulus really matter? *Pain Clinic*, **3**, 161–8.

Nogier, P.F.M. (1972). *Treatise on auriculotherapy*. Maisonneuve, France.

Oleson, T.D., Kroening, R.J., and Bresler, D.E. (1980). An experimental evaluation of auricular diagnosis: the somatotopic mapping of musculo skeletal pain at ear acupuncture points. *Pain*, **8**, 217–29.

Ostrowski, M.J. (1979). Pain control in advanced malignant disease using transcutaneous nerve stimulation. *British Journal of Clinical Practice*, **33**, 157–62.

Otsuka, N., Fukunaga, M., Morita, K., Ono., S., Nagai, K., Katagiri, M., Harada, T., and Morita, R. (1990). Iodine-131 uptake in a patient with thyroid cancer and rheumatoid arthritis during acupuncture treatment. *Clinical Nuclear Medicine*, **15**, 29–31.

Packham, R.J., and Chandler, C.S. (1992). A comparison of Likon and transcutaneous electrical nerve stimulation for the relief of pain in patients suffering from ankylosing spondylitis. *Clinical Rehabilitation*, **6** [supplement], 36–7.

Patel, M., Gutzwiller, F., Paccaud, F., and Marazzi, A. (1989). A meta-analysis of acupuncture for chronic pain. *International Journal of Epidemiology*, **18**, 900–6.

Rafter, J. (1986). *TENS and cancer pain*. Paper read to the Acupuncture Foundation of Canada Congress on Acupuncture and Related Techniques. Toronto, Canada, November 1986. Quoted by Librach and Rapson (1988).

Rampes, H., and James, R. (1995). Complications of acupuncture. *Acupuncture in Medicine*, **13**, 26–33.

Rampes, H. (1998). Adverse reactions to acupuncture. In *Medical acupuncture—a western scientific approach* (ed. J. Filshie and A. White), pp. 375–87. Churchill Livingstone, Edinburgh.

Ray, C.D. (1976). Electrical stimulation: new methods for therapy and rehabilitation. *Scandinavian Journal of Rehabilitation Medicine*, **10**, 65.

Reeves, J.L., Jaeger, B., and Graff-Radford, S.B. (1986). Reliability of the pressure algometer as a measure of myofascial trigger point sensitivity. *Pain*, **24**, 313–21.

Seichert, N. (1991). Controlled trials of laser treatment. In: *Physiotherapy; controlled trials and facts. Rheumatology*, vol 14 (ed. Sclapbach and Gerber) pp. 205–217. Karger, Basel.

Shealy, C.N., Mortimer, J.T., and Reswick, J.B. (1967). Electrical inhibition of pain by stimulation of the dorsal column: preliminary clinical reports. *Anaesthesia and Analgesia*, **46**, 488–91.

Sjölund, B., and Eriksson, M. (1985). *Relief of pain by TENS*. English translation. Chichester and New York: John Wiley and Sons 1985.

Sjölund, B.H., Eriksson, M., and Loeser, J.D. (1990). Transcutaneous and implanted electrical stimulation of peripheral nerves. In *The management of pain*, Vol II. (2nd edn) (ed. J.J. Bonica), pp. 1852–61. Lea and Febiger, Philadelphia.

Stacher, G., Wancura, I., Bauer, P., Lahoda, R., and Schulze, D. (1975). Effect of acupuncture on pain threshold and pain tolerance determined by electrical stimulation of the skin: a controlled study. *American Journal of Chinese Medicine*, **3**, 143–9.

Stamp, J.M., and Rose, B.A. (1984). *A comparative evaluation of transcutaneous electrical nerve stimulators* (TENS) Part II. *University and Area Health Authority (T)*, Sheffield.

Stamp, J.M., and Wood, D. (1981). *A comparative evaluation of transcutaneous electrical nerve stimulators*. University and Area Health Authority (T), Sheffield.

Streitberger, K., Kleinhenz, J. (1998). Introducing a placebo needle into acupuncture research. *Lancet*, **352**, 364–5.

ter Riet, G., de Craen, A.J., de Boer, A., and Kessels, A.G. (1998). Is placebo analgesia mediated by endogenous opioids? A systematic review. *Pain*, **76**, 273–5.

ter Riet, G., Kleijnen, J., and Knipschild, P. (1990). Acupuncture and chronic pain: a criteria-based meta-analysis. *Journal of Clinical Epidemiology*, **43**, 1191–9.

Thomas, M., Eriksson, S.V., and Lundeberg, T. (1991). A comparative study of diazepam and acupuncture in patients with osteoarthritis pain: a placebo controlled study. *American Journal of Chinese Medicine*, **19**, 95–100.

Thompson, J.W. (1987). The role of transcutaneous electrical nerve stimulation (TENS) for the control of pain. In *International Symposium on Pain Control* (ed. D. Doyle) 1986. Royal Society of Medicine Services International Congress and Symposium series.

Thompson, J.W. (1989). Pharmacology of transcutaneous electrical stimulation (TENS). *Journal of the Intractable Pain Society*, **7**, 33–40.

Thompson, J.W. (1990). Clinical pharmacology of opioid agonists and partial agonists. In *Opioids in the treatment of cancer pain* (ed. D. Doyle), pp. 17–38. Royal Society of Medicine Services International Congress and Symposium Series No. 146, Royal Society of Medicine Services Ltd, London.

Thompson, J.W. (1994). Neuropharmacology of the pain pathway. In *Pain management by physiotherapy* (2nd edn) (ed. P.E. Wells, V. Frampton, and D. Bowsher), Chapter 10. Butterworth Heinemann, Oxford.

Thompson, J.W., and Filshie, J. (1998). Transcutaneous Electrical Nerve Stimulation (TENS) and Acupuncture. In *Oxford textbook of palliative medicine* (2nd edn) (ed. D. Doyle, G. Hanks, and N. Macdonald), pp. 421–37. Oxford Medical Publications.

Travell, J.G., and Simons, D.G. (1983). *Myofascial pain and dysfunction. The trigger point manual*, Baltimore. Williams & Williams.

Tulgar, M., McGlone, F., Bowsher, D., and Miles, J.B. (1991). Comparative effectiveness of different stimulation modes in relieving pain. Part I. A pilot study. *Pain*, **47**, 151–5. Part II. A double-blind controlled long-term clinical trial. *Pain*, **47**, 157–62.

Veith, I. (1972). *The Yellow Emperor's Classic of Internal Medicine*. Berkeley: University of California Press.

Ventafridda, V. (1979). Transcutaneous nerve stimulation in cancer pain. In *Advances in pain research and therapy*. (ed. J.J. Bonica and V. Ventafridda), pp. 509–15. Raven Press, New York.

Vickers, A.J. (1996). Can acupuncture have specific effects on health? A systematic review of acupuncture antiemesis trials. *Journal of the Royal Society of Medicine*, **89**, 303–11.

Vincent, C.A. (1992). Acupuncture research: why do it? *Complementary Medical Research*, **6**, 21–24.

Vincent, C.A., Richardson, P.H., Black, J.J., and Pither, C. E. (1989). The significance of needle placement site in acupuncture. *Journal of Psychosomatic Research*, **33**, 489–96.

Von Roenn, J.H., Cleeland, C.S., Gonin, R., Hatfield, A.K., and Pandya, K.J. (1993). Physician attitudes and practice in cancer pain management. A survey from the eastern cooperative oncology group. *Annals Internal Medicine*, **119**, 121–6.

Walker, J.B., Akhanjee, L.K., Cooney, M.M., Goldstein, J., Tamayoshi, S. and Segal-Gidan, F. (1987). Laser therapy for pain of trigeminal neuralgia. *Clinical Journal of Pain*, **3**, 183–7.

Wall, P.D., and Sweet, W. (1967). Temporary abolition of pain in man. *Science*, **155**, 108–9.

Walsh, D.M. (1997). *TENS: clinical applications and related theory*. Churchill Livingstone, Edinburgh.

Wang, X.-J., Wang, X.-H., and Han, J. (1990). Cholecystokinin octapeptide antagonise opioid analgesia mediated by mu- and kappa- but not delta-receptors in the spinal cord of the rat. *Brain Research*, **523**, 5–10.

Ward, A. (1996). Spontaneous electrical activity at combined acupuncture and myofascial trigger point sites. *Acupuncture in Medicine*, **14**, 75–9.

Wen, H.L. (1977). Cancer pain treated with acupuncture and electrical stimulation. *Modern Medicine of Asia*, **13**, 12–15.

White, A. (1998). Electroacupuncture and acupuncture analgesia. In *Medical acupuncture—a western scientific approach* (ed. J. Filshie and A. White), pp. 153–75. Churchill Livingstone, Edinburgh.

White, A.R., Eddleston, C., Hardie, R., Resch, K.L., and Ernst, E. (1996). A pilot study of acupuncture for tension headache, using a novel placebo. *Acupuncture in Medicine*, **14**, 11–15.

White, A.R., Hayhoe, S., Ernst, E. (1997). Survey of adverse events following acupuncture. *Acupuncture in Medicine*, **15**, 67–70.

Woolf, C.J. (1989). Segmental afferent fibre-induced analgesia: transcutaneous electrical nerve stimulation (TENS) and vibration. In *Textbook of pain* (2nd edn) (ed. P.D. Wall and R. Melzack), pp. 884–96. Churchill Livingstone, Edinburgh.

Woolf, C.J., and Thompson, J.W. (1994). Stimulation-induced analgesia: transcutaneous electrical nerve stimulation (TENS) and vibration. In *Textbook of Pain*. (3rd edn) (ed. P.D. Wall and R. Melzack), pp. 1191–208. Churchill Livingstone, Edinburgh.

Xue, C.C. (1986). Acupuncture induced phantom limb and meridian phenomenon in acquired and congenital amputees. A suggestion of the use of acupuncture as a method for investigation of phantom limb. *Chinese Medical Journal*, **99**, 247–52.

Yamamoto, T., Yamamoto, Y., and Akiharu, Y. (1986). Formative mechanisms of current concentration and breakdown phenomena dependent on direct current flow through skin by a dry electrode. *IEEE Trans. Biomed. Eng.*, **33**, 396–404.

Yoshino, N., and Kumio, Y. (1977). *Ryodoraku acupuncture*. Research Institute Limited, Ryodoraku.

Zhou, Z.F., Xuan, Y.T., and Han, J.S. (1984). Analgesic effect of morphine injected into habenula, nucleus accumbens or amygdala of rabbits. *Acta Pharm. Sinica*, **5**, 1150–3.

FOURTEEN

Spinal cord stimulation

KEITH BUDD

The 'gate theory' of Melzack and Wall (1965) has had an astonishing effect upon research into pain and its treatment. The precision of its formulation enables scientists to design experiments to test its predictions and clinicians to devise new forms of pain relieving therapy. Many scientific experiments supported the concept of a spinal gate. Clinical work gave rise to transcutaneous neural and spinal cord stimulation and offered an intriguing scientific basis for some forms of acupuncture. The relationship of therapeutic spinal cord stimulation (SCS) to the gating mechanisms remains unclear at present even though it was the gate control theory that inspired its inception. The first patient to receive SCS was successfully treated for cancer-related pain. However, since that time, the response of nociceptive pain to SCS has not always been as successful.

Mode of action

Activation of large afferent axons by spinal cord stimulation causes only brief and mild effects on spinal segmental reflexes, but initiates a powerful and long lasting inhibition that descends from the brain. For many decades, electrical stimulation of the brain has been known to cause analgesia (Reynolds 1969). Much of this work studied the periaqueductal grey matter (PAG), stimulation of which has been shown to inhibit responses to noxious stimuli for periods of an hour or more. In man, pain relief following such stimulation has been reported for up to 24 hours (Hosobuchi 1980). Experimental evidence has shown that this inhibition is exerted on spinal neurones and that a polysynaptic pathway from the PAG projects to the cord via a relay in the ventromedial medulla with axons in the dorsolateral funiculus (DLF) (Fields and Basbaum 1984). Stimulation of brain areas other than PAG have also exhibited analgesia, but invariably accompanied by behavioural changes (Hilton and Redfern 1986). One area of the brain that, whilst giving strong analgesia at low stimulation intensity, did not evoke signs of aversion or stress is the anterior pretectal nucleus (APtN) (Prado and Roberts 1985). The effects of APtN stimulation can be attenuated by anticholinergic, opioid and α_2-adrenoceptor antagonist agents. There is evidence that analgesic, catecholamine cells project to the spinal dorsal horn (SDH) via the DLF (Rees et al. 1987). The APtN projects to these cells and it seems likely that they might be activated by APtN stimulation to release catecholamine in the spinal cord (Barbaro et al. 1985). There is no direct projection from APtN to the spinal cord and inhibitory effects of its stimulation must be relayed by a polysynaptic pathway. It seems that the PAG and APtN project to the spinal cord by different routes, hence 5-HT antagonists reduce the effect of PAG stimulation but not that of APtN. The analgesic effects of the latter are mediated via several lateral, mid, and hind brain structures projecting to the SDH to release adrenaline. This would account for the antagonistic action of α_2- adrenergic antagonists on APtN stimulation-produced analgesia (Roberts and Rees 1994).

Clinical approaches

Inspired by the gate control theory and the subsequent animal experimentation, Shealy and colleagues implanted the original spinal cord stimulator into man in 1967. This patient had pain from a chest wall cancer which was relieved with no impairment of vibration, position, touch or pinprick sensations, although deep pain sensation was felt as touch. Shealy and colleagues (1970) reported five further patients with various presenting pathologies including cancer. Good results were obtained in spite of four patients having perineal pain, normally a singularly difficult area to target.

Several early series included small numbers of patients with cancer-related pain showing variable results. The largest study included 10 good or excellent responses in 16 patients (Nielsen *et al.* 1975). A number of other series included only one or two cancer pain patients (Pineda 1975; Hunt *et al.* 1975; Urban and Nashold 1978; Richardson *et al.* 1979; Nashold and Friedman 1972), but two studies showed data containing important findings (Hoffenstein 1975; Larsen *et al.* 1975). These indicated that to obtain benefit from SCS cancer pain should have a neuropathic element.

Indications

In general, to obtain worthwhile benefit in the treatment of cancer-induced pain, the noxious sensation should have a burning quality with clinical evidence of neurological damage involving sensory and/or autonomic pathways. However, mid-line and facial pain together with pain generated within the central nervous system fare less well with SCS.

Success likely

- Complex regional pain syndrome Type 1.
- Nerve plexus involvement.
- Peripheral nerve damage or involvement.
- Cauda equina damage or involvement.
- Amputation stump pain.

Success reasonable

- Spinal cord involvement.
- Phantom pain.

Benefit unlikely

• Centrally placed pain e.g. rectum, vagina, perineum.

• Nociceptive pain especially incident pain.

Patient selection

In selecting patients who might benefit significantly from the use of SCS, a variety of factors must be taken into consideration. The decision-making process should involve the clinical management team rather than relying on a single person, however experienced.

Pathology

The more widespread the malignancy and the more rapid the spread or metastasis, the less likely is SCS to be of great and lasting value. The wider the area over which the pain is felt, the larger will be the area which stimulation will have to cover. This may increase the number of electrodes implanted and the complexity of the programming of the system. Ideally, there should be a well defined, dermatomally located pain pattern. This may be susceptible to stimulation by a single electrode which will cover the whole of the pain representation allowing some extension of the tumour.

Pain type

SCS is most likely to be successful in neuropathic and sympathogenic pain of a constant rather than an incidental nature. The distribution of the pain should be well defined in a dermatomal mode. In terms of descriptors, 'burning' and 'sharp' tend to be associated with a successful outcome whereas 'wretched', 'pounding', 'sickening', 'pressing', and 'terrifying' tend to be associated with a poor outcome (Nashold and Friedman 1972; North *et al.* 1993; North *et al.* 1991).

Life expectancy

Before exploring the use of expensive, 'high-tech' invasive procedures, all other agents, techniques, and procedures should have been considered and, possibly, implemented with inadequate success. Nevertheless, the patient must have an adequate life expectancy for the required device to be cost beneficial. Although prediction of a cancer patient's life span can be difficult, an estimate in terms of days, weeks, months or years is essential to guide the selection of the most appropriate system. Often the patient's condition will improve when adequate analgesia is provided, a possibility that must be considered. Although the cost of the SCS trial procedure is comparatively small when related to the whole care cost, the longer the complete system is in use the more cost-beneficial it becomes. Generally, cost-benefit can be achieved after a three to six month duration of treatment (Budd 1998).

Previous and current therapy

Generally, highly invasive procedures should be regarded as last stage techniques. This is so for SCS in cancer pain. Consequently, before considering SCS seriously, all other logical therapies should have been considered and, preferably, tried. SCS then becomes a 'last-ditch' effort. Current therapy should be considered carefully to make sure that its effects will not affect SCS or its institution e.g. anticoagulants.

Other pathology

Other pathology present in the patient may benefit from SCS; however, pathology or its treatment may interfere with SCS, for example spinal distortion affecting electrode placement or drug therapy affecting blood coagulation.

Planned therapy or investigations

Any planned treatment or investigation proposed should be known about in case SCS will interfere with it, for example MRI may be difficult with a spinal electrode in place, or CT results may be distorted by scatter from the SCS electrode. Consequently, liaison with colleagues prior to implantation is essential.

Psychological screen

In recent years, there has been a move away from the use of formal psychological and psychiatric screening for potential SCS patients. This may be partly a result of earlier experiences and partly because indications by diagnosis have become clearer. The situation is probably best summed up by quoting Nielsen who, in 1975, stated that 'accurate pre-operative psychological predictors are essential'. Unfortunately, they were not available then, nor are they now. Therefore, most implantation units rely on learned experience of patient response to evaluate the likelihood of possible psychological problems. The most difficult aspect is not only identifying the psychological factors but also identifying their importance (Sweet and Wespic 1974).

Response to transcutaneous electrical neural stimulation

Good correlation between the responses to TENS and to SCS have been reported (Miles and Lipton 1978; Mittal *et al.* 1987). More patients show a better response to SCS than to TENS and many nonresponders to TENS do respond to SCS (Dooley 1977; Spiegelmann and Friedman 1991). Thus TENS is not a useful predictor of outcome from SCS.

Patient's wishes

Last, but by no means least, is the response of the patient to the suggestion of using SCS. It is vitally important to explain not only the procedure, but also the possible problems, to the patient and carers in such a manner that understanding can be assured. Should the patient have any reservations about proceeding with SCS it is well to not press the point, but return again to the discussion at a later date. If the patient is still undecided then the procedure should be witheld. The patient must be well informed and in total agreement to proceed.

Technique

Specific details of implantation techniques can be gained from the many papers and monographs available. This section will deal only with principles. At this stage, detailed discussion with the patient will inform them about the trial procedure and how their necessary co-operation will be achieved. Where the type of pain may be difficult to determine precisely and the contribution of each component of the pain remains unclear, a trial of stimulation must be undertaken. This assesses whether the technique will achieve analgesia and also places the electrode (or electrodes) to obtain optimal stimulation patterns i.e. paraesthesiae covering the area of the pain.

To achieve correct placement, patient co-operation is necessary. The introduction of the electrode will, therefore, need to be under local anaesthesia. When the electrode is introduced into the epidural space and stimulation is engendered, the patient will be able to inform the operator whether the appropriate position has been achieved. Paraesthesiae need to be obtained in the area over which the pain is experienced or otherwise further manipulation of the electrode is necessary.

The electrode chosen should cover the widest dermatomal range so that if the cancer spreads, and the pain is felt over a wider area than originally, the stimulation pattern may be altered to cope with this. Should the area over which pain is experienced initially be greater than one electrode can cope with, a second electrode can be introduced to increase the total stimulation field. Electrodes are usually quadripolar with four available channels. However, to provide more sophisticated field planning, octopolar electrodes will provide up to sixteen channels (dual octopolar). Programming such a stimulator with several million possible electrode combinations requires patient-interactive computerized control systems (North *et al.* 1992). In terms of polarity, the most effective electrode configuration comprises narrowly separated longitudinal bipoles with the cathode rostral (Law 1983). More recently, it had been shown that with bipolar stimulation, a small contact separation gives a wider distribution of paraesthesiae than does a larger contact separation (Barolat *et al.* 1991).

In terms of placement of the electrode within the epidural space, the probability of successfully stimulating different anatomical areas varies with the rostrocaudal and lateral position of the electrodes. For example, to stimulate the shoulder, the cathode should be at C2–C4, for the hand at C5–C6 and for the thigh T7–T8. T8–T9 is usually satisfactory for legs and buttocks and the foot is easily stimulated at T9–T10 or even lower. Some areas remain very difficult to target selectively such as low back, perineum, and genitalia (Barolat *et al.* 1993).

For the setting of the trial stimulation parameters and subsequent ones, no clear pattern emerges of particular parameters being effective for different pain syndromes. There is a wide range of individual variation in use and the general trend is to vary the parameters to produce the most comfortable and effective stimulation for each individual patient (Simpson 1994). Discussion with the patient to determine their preference will indicate whether an internal or external stimulation generator is to be used. Both first and second stages of the procedure are undertaken using antibiotic cover during the procedure. It is usual to use a broad spectrum antibiotic, generally of the cephalosporin type.

Complications

The most serious complication of spinal cord stimulation (SCS) is infection. Should this occur in any part of the system, the complete unit must be removed, together with energetic antibacterial therapy. Fortunately, this is a rare occurrence considering that the implanted material could provide a convenient nidus around which bacteria could breed.

The most common occurrences that need attention are electrode migration, dislodgement, lead fracture, and current leakage. These may be corrected by the manipulation of the electrode into the correct location or the replacement of the broken part.

A troublesome complication of unexplained origin is that of prolonged or exaggerated postoperative pain, sometimes localized to the incisions or more diffusely over the back. Preemptive use of local anaesthetic in the wounds may help to prevent this and topical local anaesthetic cream postoperatively may help should it occur. Persistent sensitivity and discomfort over the site of the receiver may best be treated by the application of capsaicin cream (0.075%) four times daily for six to eight weeks.

Other complications recorded sporadically include excessive receiver mobility, receiver failure, subcutaneous wound haematoma, hypersensitivity to the implanted materials, skin ulceration, and erosion by the implanted components (Simpson 1994). It should also be observed that SCS systems should be removed from deceased patients who are going to be cremated otherwise they may explode when heated (K. Budd, personal observation).

Conclusion

When used in the correct indication and by experienced practitioners, spinal cord stimulation can be highly beneficial and cost-effective for patients with resistant cancer-induced pain. The apparently high capital cost of the system should be weighed against both the humanitarian benefit to patients, in whom no other therapy has relieved their pain, and also the cost-effectiveness when in use for a prolonged period of time. Cost alone should not deter this valuable technique from being considered and used.

References

Barbaro, N.M., Hammond, D., and Fields, H.L. (1985). Effects of intrathecally administered methysergide and yohimbine on microstimulation- produced antinocicetion in the rat. *Brain Research*, **336**, 133–42.

Barolat, G., Zeme, S., and Ketcik, B. (1991). Multifunctional analysis of epidural spinal cord stimulation. *Stereotactic and Functional Neurosurgery*, **56**, 77–107.

Barolat, G., Massaro, F., He, J., Zeme, S., and Ketcik, B. (1993). Mapping of sensory response to epidural stimulation of the intraspinal neural structures in man. *Journal of Neurosurgery*, **78**, 233–9.

Budd, K. (1998). Cost-benefit analysis of spinal cord stimulation. Abstracts of 2nd International Neuromodulation Society, Lucerne.

Dooley, D.M. (1977). Demyelinating, degenerative and vascular disease. *Neuro-surgery*, **1**, 220–4.

Fields, H.L., and Basbaum, A.J. (1984). Endogenous pain control mechanisms. In *Textbook of pain,* P.D. Wall and R. Melzack, ed. pp. 142–52. Churchill Livingstone, Edinburgh.

Hilton, S.M., and Redfern, W.S. (1986). A search for brainstem cell groups integrating the defence reaction in the rat. *Journal of Physiology*, **378**, 213–28.

Hoffenstein, R. (1975). Electrical stimulation of the ventral and dorsal columns of the spinal cord for relief of chronic intractable pain: preliminary report. *Surgical Neurology*, **4**, 187–94.

Hosobuchi, Y. (1980). The current status of electrical brain stimulation. *Acta Neurochirurgica*, **30**, 219–27.

Hunt, W.E., Goodman, J.H., and Bingham, W.G. (1975). Stimulation of the dorsal spinal cord for treatment of intractable pain: a preliminary report. *Surgical Neurology*, **4**, 153–6.

Larsen, S.J., Sances, A., Cusick, J.F. *et al.* (1975). A comparison between anterior and posterior spinal implant systems. *Surgical Neurology*, **4**, 180–6.

Law, J. (1983). Spinal stimulation: statistical superiority of monophasic stimulation of narrowly separated longitudinal bipoles having rostral cathodes. *Applied Neuro-physiology*, **46**, 129–37.

Melzack, R., and Wall, P.D. (1965). Pain mechanisms: a new theory. *Science*, **150**, 971–9.

Miles, J., and Lipton, S. (1978). Phantom limb pain treated by electrical stimulation. *Pain*, **5**, 373–82.

Mittal, B., Thomas, D.G.T., Walton, P., and Calder, I. (1987). Dorsal column Stimu-lation (DCS) in chronic pain: report of 31 cases. *Annals of the Royal College of Sur-geons of England*, **69**, 104–9.

Nashold, B.S., and Friedman, H. (1972). Dorsal column stimulation for control of pain: preliminary report on 30 patients. *Neurosurgery*, **36**, 590–7.

Nielsen, K.D., Adams, J.E., and Hosobuchi, Y. (1975). Experience with dorsal column stimulation for relief of chronic intractable pain: 1968–1973. *Surgical Neurology*, **4**, 148–52.

North, R.B., Ewend, M.G., Lawton, M.T. *et al.* (1991). Failed back surgery syndrome: 5-year follow-up after spinal cord stimulation. *Neurosurgery*, **28**, 692–99.

North, R.B., Fowler, K., Nigrim, D.J., and Szymanski, R. (1992). Patient interactive, computer controlled, neurological stimulator system: clinical efficacy in spinal cord stimulator adjustment. *Journal of Neurosurgery*, **76**, 967–72.

North, R.B., Kidd, D.H., Zahwak, M. *et al.* (1993). Spinal cord stimulation for chronic, intractable pain: experience over two decades. *Neurosurgery*, **32**, 384–95.

Pineda, A. (1975). Dorsal column stimulation and its prospects. *Surgical Neurology*, **4**, 157–63.

Prado, W.A., and Roberts, M.H.T. (1985). An assessment of the antinociceptive and aversive effects of stimulating identified sites in the rat brain. *Brain Research*, **340**, 219–28.

Rees, H., Prado, W.A., Rawlings, S., Roberts, M.H.T. (1987). The effects of intraperitoneal administraion of antagonists and development of morphine tolerance on the antinociception induced by stimulating the anterior pretectal nucleus of the rat. *British Journal of Pharmacol*, **92**, 769–79.

Reynolds, D.V. (1969). Surgery in the rat during electrical analgesia induced by focal stimualtion. *Science*, **164**, 444–5.

Richardson, R.R., Siqueira, E.B., and Cerullo, L.J. (1979). Spinal epidural neurostimulation for treatment of acute and chronic intractable pain. *Neurosurgery*, **5**, 344–8.

Roberts, M.H.T., and Rees, H. (1994). Physiological basis of spinal cord stimulation. *Pain Reviews*, **1**, 199–230.

Shealy, C.N., Mortimer, J.T., and Reswick, J.B. (1967). Electrical inhibition of pain by stimulation of the dorsal columns. Preliminary clinical report. *Anesthesia Analgesia*, **46**, 489–91.

Shealy, C.N., Mortimer, J.T., and Hagfors, N.R. (1970). Dorsal column electroanalgesia. *Journal of Neurosurgery*, **323**, 560–4.

Simpson, B.A. (1994). Spinal cord stimulation. *Pain Reviews*, **1**, 199–230.

Spiegelmann, R., and Friedman, W.A. (1991). Spinal cord stimulation: a contemporary series. *Neurosurgery*, **28**, 65–71.

Sweet, W.H., and Wespic, J.G. (1974). Stimulation of the posterior columns of the spinal cord for pain control: indications, technique and results. *Clinical Neurosurgery*, **21**, 278–310.

Urban, B.J., and Nashold, B.S. (1978). Percutaneous epidural stimulation of the spinal cord for relief of pain. *Journal of Neurosurgery*, **48**, 323–8.

FIFTEEN

Radiotherapy

WENDY P. MAKIN

Radiotherapy can achieve pain relief by directly influencing the disease process. Intensive or 'radical' treatment may be given with the intention of eradicating cancer completely and thereby curing the patient. If successful, there is resolution of pain and other symptoms associated with the presence of tumour. Radiotherapy also has an important role in palliation, especially for metastatic disease. Although the patient cannot be cured, treatment to symptomatic tumour sites may contribute considerably to quality of life without necessarily influencing survival. Such palliative treatments account for up to half of the workload of a radiotherapy department, and many of these are given to help pain. The aim of this chapter is to provide the non-radiotherapist with an understanding of the principles of treatment, what can be achieved and what it entails for the patient, to help clinical decisions concerning pain management.

Principles

Radiotherapy uses ionizing radiation, which is directed in a carefully controlled way to a target volume of tissue containing tumour. The principal treatment machines in radiotherapy departments are called linear accelerators (Fig. 15.1) and produce high energy beams of X-rays and electrons. These machines have largely replaced lower energy orthovoltage X-ray equipment and telecobalt units. Radioactive sources are also used, implanted or placed in close proximity to the tumour (for example, in treatment of gynaecological cancers) and can deliver a high dose to a very localized area. Sometimes unsealed radioisotopes are administered such as radioiodine, which is taken up preferentially by thyroid cancers.

Radiation causes DNA damage in both normal and malignant cells. Although some damage can be repaired, a critical amount leads to a failure of subsequent cell division and thereby the extinction of that cell line. If enough cancer cells are affected, there will be shrinkage and possibly eradication of the tumour. The therapeutic benefit of radiotherapy depends upon the exploitation of a number of factors which maximize the effects upon cancer cells and spare the normal tissues as far as possible. These include careful treatment planning to deliver a high dose to the tumour volume and as little normal tissue as possible; care is taken to keep critical normal structures out of the irradiated volume or to limit the dose to these, sometimes by shielding. Intrinsic differences between normal and cancer cell populations can be enhanced by fractionation, which refers to the delivery of the total dose in a course of small exposures. This is usually

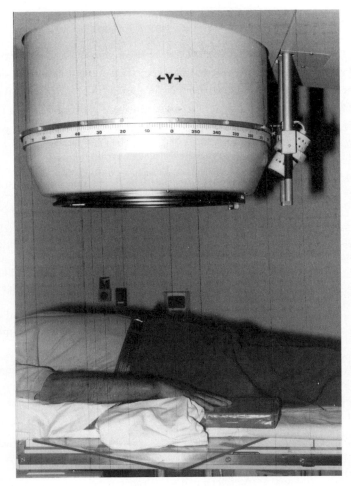

Fig. 15.1 Patient set up under linear accelerator for palliative radiotherapy to bone metastases in forearm.

given once daily on weekdays but in some circumstances may be two or three times daily (hyperfractionation) or three times or less each week (hypofractionation). Palliative radiotherapy is generally given in short courses and sometimes in a single session. This is acceptable where the aim is no longer cure. It enables treatment to be given quickly with minimum visits or duration of stay at the oncology centre. Usually a lower dose is prescribed for palliative treatments, as the aim is to achieve a useful symptomatic response without troublesome side-effects.

Radiotherapy dose is a measure of ionising radiation delivered to the tumour volume. It is possible to calculate accurately the dose received on the surface of the patient, at depth, within the tumour, and adjacent normal tissues. The old unit of the Rad has now been superceded by the Gray (Gy)—sometimes given in centigrays (cGy). There is a complex relationship between the dose, number, and size of fractions and overall time; thus a dose is only meaningful when related to a specified schedule. These bewildering figures are therefore of limited use to those in other disciplines!

Side-effects of radiotherapy

The side-effects of radiotherapy arise from the normal tissues that have been exposed to radiation. While most patients do experience some side-effects during and after treatment, these are often well tolerated, particularly with palliative radiotherapy. Side-effects are related to the site treated and the dose received, but the severity also varies between individuals; those encountered following palliative radiotherapy are summarized in Table 15.1.

Table 15.1. Common side-effects following palliative radiotherapy

Side-effect	Onset	Site or treatment	Management	Duration
Nausea and vomiting	Early (hours)	Abdomen; lumbar spine; hemibody irradiation; brain	Anti-emetics before and during treatment (5HT3 antagonists, cyclizine)	Limited to treatment period; settles in 24 hours after single fractions
Skin erythema/soreness	Early	Superficial tissues; otherwise minimal	Avoid soap; keep dry and open; 1% hydrocortisone cream	Heal within 4 weeks of completion
Skin pigmentation/telangectasia	Late	As above; rarely significant in palliation	None	Permanent
Hair loss	Early	Any hair-bearing site; whole brain	Warn patient and order wig if needed	Usually temporary
Mucositis	Early	Thorax; cervical/dorsal spine	Soft diet; soluble analgesics; Mucaine suspension	Settles within 4 weeks of completion
Diarrhoea	Early	Abdomen/pelvis (small bowel in treated volume)	Loperamide; adequate fluid intake	As above
Cystitis/proctitis	Early	Central pelvis	Analgesics; avoid constipation	As above
Marrow Suppression	Early	Large fields; hemibody irradiation; previous chemotherapy	Check blood count and avoid treatment if already compromised	As above
Systemic: lethargy, tiredness	Early	Whole brain; often attributed to any X-ray treatment	None except limit activities	As above

Acute radiation effects are experienced during the first 1–2 weeks after starting radiotherapy. These are the result of radiation upon active cell populations such as those in epithelial tissues or bone marrow. They will usually resolve completely within a few weeks. Patients are warned about these symptoms and given advice on how to cope with them. Nausea and vomiting is often expected by patients but is unusual unless treatment is given to the upper abdominal area or when large volumes of the body are treated. It can develop within hours of exposure to radiation, but is now effectively prevented or minimized with antiemetics such as ondansetron.

Late effects may be encountered 6 months to several years following radiotherapy. They may be evidence of radiation damage to normal tissues within a high dose zone, or to tissues that are particularly vulnerable, such as kidney, lung, or spinal cord. Over a long period of time, irradiated tissues develop fibrosis with changes in the small blood vessels leading to a relatively poorer blood supply. In rare cases this may lead to breakdown of the tissues or radionecrosis; sometimes this occurs after trauma. Late effects upon the spinal cord lead to progressive myelitis and ischaemia with paraplegia or quadriplegia. It must be emphasized that serious problems are uncommon, even with radical treatments. They are very unusual following palliative radiotherapy; not only are relatively lower doses used, many patients do not survive long enough to develop them. Nevertheless, care is always taken to minimize the risk of serious damage and this may also preclude re-treatment of an irradiated area.

Pain associated with cancer: how and when can radiotherapy help?

Cancer pain is the result of invasion, distension, or compression of pain-sensitive somatic and visceral structures by the tumour. It is easy to imagine how the simple mechanism of tumour shrinkage can directly relieve pain due to nerve compression. Eradication of tumour will enable healing of ulcerated epithelium. Repair of bone is a longer process and radiological evidence of this may take up to 4 months. Mechanisms for pain and the response to radiation are less well understood at a cellular level. Tumour invasion is often associated with an inflammatory response. Erythema, soreness, and itch may accompany infiltration of superficial tissues, for example recurrent breast cancer extending over the chest wall. Symptomatic response to non-steroidal anti-inflammatory drugs suggests that this is partly mediated by prostaglandin activity. These and other mediators can be produced by a host immune response to tumour and this may have a part to play in bone pain. This is supported by the rapid response to regional radiotherapy in patients with extensive bone metastases. It has been suggested that this is the result of rapid lymphocyte depletion and a fall in cytokine production (Ross Garrett 1993).

The published data on the results of radiotherapy tend to highlight easily measured end-points, such as tumour response or survival. Pain is rarely well documented although it is reasonable to expect some correlation between pain relief and tumour response. Further growth of the tumour is accompanied by return or worsening of pain. However in many patients, pain may be caused by new sites of metastatic spread.

In a prospective study of palliative radiotherapy in pain relief (Rutten *et al.* 1997), an attempt was made to identify factors which would predict a complete response. The closest correlation was with a relatively low pain score prior to treatment and the presence of radiating pain. Although there was distinction between nociceptive and neuropathic pain, it is not clear how many of the latter responded completely. Pain syndromes are often complex and radiotherapy can only achieve partial improvement.

It may deal successfully with pain from bone involvement of a vertebral body or an epidural soft tissue mass encroaching on the cord itself, but the patient may still be left with incident pain as a result of structural spinal instability. Although often successful in relieving pain due to nerve compression of recent onset, radiotherapy does not modify established neuropathic pain that is the consequence of nerve destruction.

Applications of radiotherapy in pain relief

Skin and superficial tissues

Indications: Cutaneous nodules may be painful, especially if arising on pressure areas; they may ulcerate. These lesions may be metastases from a number of different types of cancer particularly lung, breast, adenocarcinomas of the upper gastrointestinal tract, and malignant melanoma. Kaposi's sarcoma in association with HIV infection produces painful skin and mucosal lesions. Isolated tumour deposits and small areas are easily treated by radiotherapy, especially if painful or disfiguring and where fungation is likely. The larger the area, the lower the dose that can be given, so radiotherapy may not be practicable. Widespread cutaneous involvement by breast cancer is best treated with hormone therapy or chemotherapy, although radiotherapy might still be used for individual troublesome lesions. Enlargement of superficial lymph nodes by tumour can cause pain by pressure from the mass or fixation to skin and underlying tissues.

Techniques: Planning is usually simple as the area to be treated is easy to define. Electron beams are used which give a high dose to skin and superficial tissues, sparing deeper structures. Palliative treatments to small lesions are often given a single treatment while fractionated courses are used for larger areas.

Side-effects: A skin reaction is inevitable and is treated with topical 1% hydrocortisone cream. 1% silver sulphadiazine (Flamazine) cream can be applied to sore areas, but only after radiotherapy has been completed. Hair loss occurs within the treated area, which may be permanent depending upon the dose. This can be conspicuous if scalp nodules are irradiated. Other side-effects are unlikely, although radiotherapy can produce severe mucosal reactions in immunocompromised patients and low doses are used to treat Kaposi's sarcomas. Small cutaneous deposits and localized metastatic nodes are expected to resolve completely. Although melanoma may respond less well than metastatic carcinomas, troublesome deposits are worth treating (Jenrette 1996). Most locoregional recurrences of breast cancer respond well and many achieve complete response.

Head and neck

Indications: Radiotherapy is important in the management of many patients with head and neck cancers. The use of palliative regimens for advanced disease is more contentious. Pain is among a number of problems experienced, due to bone invasion, nerve infiltration, and an expanding mass within a confined space. Radical regimens might still used for localized but inoperable disease. Some would argue that palliative treatment that achieves only a partial response, and still produces side-effects, is of no advantage to the patient. However it is possible to offer palliation to carefully selected patients, for example those with tumours of the nasal sinuses involving orbit, ethmoids, and maxilla; these are commonly associated with pain. Treatment is also given to locally advanced or metastatic tumours involving the base of skull and causing pain and cranial nerve palsies.

Brain tumours present with a wide range of situations from curative treatment to palliation of primary and secondary tumours. The main aim of treatment is to reduce and control the tumour and so improve neurological function and survival. Pain relief can be important for patients with meningiomas and large pituitary tumours. Reduction in cerebral swelling and intracranial pressure will help to reduce headache. For patients with cerebral metastases, radiotherapy enables a reduction in the dose of steroid needed to control headache and other symptoms (Priestman *et al.* 1996).

Techniques: Radical treatments for head and neck cancer involve complex technical plans. Shells are used to immobilize the patient during sessions to ensure accurate delivery of the dose. Some palliative treatments to whole brain, base of skull, and neck nodes can be planned simply using a simulator. High energy X-rays are used, plus electrons if disease is more superficial.

Side-effects: The worst acute reaction for many is the painful mucositis that develops if some of the oral cavity and pharynx is included within the treatment volume. Dry mouth follows irradiation to salivary glands. Whole brain radiotherapy is likely to cause initial headache and nausea especially if some cerebral oedema is present (this will respond to steroids); complete but temporary alopecia will develop in the following month.

Thorax

Indications: Patients with cancer of lung and oesophagus; mesothelioma; breast cancer; Hodgkin's disease, and lymphoma involving the mediastinum. Radiotherapy is the primary treatment for inoperable non-small cell lung cancer. It is usually the more peripheral tumours which cause pain by invasion of the chest wall. Tumours that arise in the superior sulcus of the lung apex (Pancoast's tumours) invade the adjacent pleura, lower brachial plexus, upper ribs often the vertebral body. Many patients have difficult pain by the time the diagnosis is made. Radiotherapy may relieve somatic pain in the upper chest, but there may be little effect upon neuropathic ipsilateral arm pain. Mesothelioma does respond to radiotherapy although improvements in pain may be of short duration (Bisset *et al.* 1991). The whole hemithorax can be treated if there is no useful lung function on that side; sometimes it is possible to target smaller areas where pain is the result of rib or vertebral erosion. Poorly-localized back and chest pain is a feature of mediastinal node involvement or paravertebral invasion in association with oesophageal and lung cancers. It implies incurable disease but may respond to a course of palliative radiotherapy.

Techniques: Radical regimens may be used for early oesophageal cancer and lung cancer, sometimes if the patient is unfit for surgery. This includes some patients with apical tumours, in whom more prolonged treatment and a higher dose is given to improve the likelihood of local control and pain relief. Most patients with lung cancer receive palliative regimens.

Side-effects: In general radiotherapy to the thorax is well tolerated. It is unlikely to cause nausea. Skin reactions are insignificant. A transient radiation oesophagitis is an acute side-effect of treatment to the central chest. The spinal cord is within the held so the dose must be limited to reduce the risk of late radiation myelitis. Lung tissue is sensitive to radiation; fibrosis develops within the treated fields but these changes in relatively small volumes are not usually clinically significant.

The MRC trial of palliative radiotherapy in non-small cell lung cancer (Rees *et al.* 1997) compared the symptomatic responses to 17 Gy in 2 fractions or 22.5 Gy in 5 fractions. 216 patients entered this trial and 88% reported improvement in chest wall pain with similar results in both arms. 61% (47/77) had complete relief of pain within 4 weeks.

Abdomen and pelvis

Indications: Cancer of the bladder, prostate, cervix, and rectum may all be treated with radical radiotherapy. This may also be used for recurrent pelvic disease following surgery, for example in rectal cancer where pain is often associated with invasion of the sacrum or perineal soft tissues. Long term control and even cure may be achieved by prolonged treatments over 4 to 6 weeks. These may be justified to achieve good palliation in locally advanced pelvic cancer. Shorter schedules of palliative radiotherapy are used to treat advanced primary tumours or involved pelvic lymph nodes.

Many abdominal tissues, especially liver, kidney, and the gastrointestinal tract, have low tolerance to radiotherapy. This limits the dose that can be given safely and therefore the likelihood of a beneficial response. Radiotherapy is seldom used to treat painful hepatomegaly in solid tumours such as breast cancer. It can provide palliation of liver and splenic distension due to infiltration by lymphomas, which are more radiosensitive. Palliative radiotherapy may be given to patients with inoperable cancer of the pancreas or kidney, or with metastatic involvement of para-aortic and pelvic lymph nodes. Such patients develop pain syndromes which include: somatic pain due to infiltration of abdominal wall, retroperitoneum and spine; neuropathic pain from damage to the lumbosacral plexus, spinal roots and cord itself; and visceral pain. Radiotherapy will only be of benefit if the disease can be encompassed in a reasonable treatment volume; it will not help in cases with extensive disease from abdomen to pelvis. Chemotherapy may be a better means of palliation for these individuals, although radiotherapy can be directed at a localized site which is causing troublesome symptoms.

Techniques: Information from surgical operations and CT or MRI scanning is needed to define extent of disease and the feasibility of useful treatment. Careful planning may be needed to minimize the volume and avoid sensitive structures. Simple techniques are used in palliative radiotherapy to para-aortic nodes or occasionally to localized, painful tumour infiltration of the abdominal wall.

Side-effects: Skin reactions are not troublesome unless superficial areas such as the perineum are treated. Nausea and vomiting is related to the volume treated and the dose; it is reduced by fractionated treatments. This can usually be controlled effectively by oral antiemetics and resolves when treatment is completed. The radiation effects on small bowel induce diarrhoea from the second week onwards and are managed with loperamide. Smaller volume but high dose pelvic treatments can cause troublesome radiation cystitis and proctitis. Although these effects are self-limiting, radical treatments can lead to serious late radiation problems in these tissues. This is unlikely with palliative schedules.

Control of local recurrence of rectal cancer in 159 patients with rectal cancer produced pain relief in 63%, although both surgery and radiotherapy were used (Frykholm *et al.* 1995). A review of radiotherapy for recurrent rectal cancer found pain relief achieved in 70–90% of patients with a median duration of 3 months (Wong *et al.* 1996). A review of the results in cancer of the pancreas described pain relief in half of the patients who had a median survival of 10 months (Roth *et al.* 1985).

In a series of 30 patients with lumbosacral plexopathy, 48% were shown to have an objective tumour response at 6 weeks, two-thirds of which were complete; 89% had some subjective pain improvement (Ampil 1986). Perhaps even a relatively small amount of tumour regression can help pain, but this is very unlikely to be of any duration in those who do not achieve a complete response. Russi *et al.* (1993) reported complete pain relief following radiotherapy in 13 patients with lumbosacral carcinomatous plexopathy. Radiotherapy achieved reasonable palliation, in 33 patients with ovarian cancer, in whom chemotherapy had failed to control pelvic and abdominal tumour; pain relief was reported in 83% and the duration of response was 4 months (Corn *et al.* 1994). Symptomatic improvement in liver capsule pain and also adrenal metastases has been described after radiotherapy (Borgelt *et al.* 1981; Short *et al.* 1996).

Bone

Bone pain is caused by local invasion by tumour at many sites and is a presenting symptom of primary cancers arising in bone or marrow, such as myeloma. The most common cause of bone pain is metastatic disease, especially in patients with cancers arising from prostate, breast, and lung, who often require palliative radiotherapy. Bone pain is a feature of hypertrophic pulmonary osteopathy, which is also amenable to radiotherapy (Yeo *et al.* 1996). Although many patients have widespread skeletal involvement, radiotherapy is primarily used to treat the symptomatic sites that cause pain from bone invasion and from nerve and spinal compression by tumour. There is no evidence that treatment to other, asymptomatic deposits will improve survival, so most patients are managed by a watch and wait approach. Systemic treatment by chemotherapy or hormonal manipulation is possible in same cases, and palliative radiotherapy can still be used in conjunction with these as necessary. Prophylactic radiotherapy may be given to obvious areas of lytic disease where further progression could lead to pathological fracture, particularly in weight-bearing bones. It is used postoperatively following fixation to enable healing of normal bone without further damage by tumour.

The diagnosis of metastatic bone disease must be carefully established, especially if this is the first site of relapse or a long time has elapsed since the primary treatment. Usually this is made radiologically, although occasionally a bone biopsy may be needed. Investigations will determine the precise cause of symptoms and the area to be irradiated. This may be obvious from plain X-rays but a more sensitive isotope bone scan may be needed to localize the metastatic deposit. If there is persistent pain with no obvious cause, a CT or MRI scan can demonstrate bone involvement as well as soft tissue disease even if the bone scan appeared to be normal. Different radiotherapy techniques are available depending upon whether there are relatively few symptomatic sites, or multiple areas with more diffuse bone pain.

Radiotherapy to localized sites

Most patients are simply treated with a small field that encompasses the obvious disease with a margin; this is planned using X-rays and bone scans, with a treatment simulator. Careful clinical assessment is needed to define the actual source of the pain, which may be referred from another site, for example when metastatic disease involves both the spine and pelvic bones. Large lytic lesions (3 cm or more) with evidence of cortical destruction warrant surgery first, especially if in a weight-bearing bone, as fracture will not be prevented by radiotherapy. Patients with vertebral metastases in whom there is suspicion of impending cord compression should have MRI scanning as there may be more than one level of disease encroaching upon the spinal canal.

Patients are treated using linear accelerators, usually with high energy X-rays; sometimes electrons may be used to treat ribs or sternum. The treatment area will encompass the obvious symptomatic disease with a margin. Other fields may be matched on in the future, avoiding overlap of irradiated sites if possible.

Palliative radiotherapy to bone metastases is often given as single treatments at a number of UK centres although this is not accepted practice in some other countries, notably North America. Short courses may be used, especially for larger volumes, for example whole pelvis, or if a substantial section of the spine requires treatment. Re-treatment to the same site may be considered, depending on the previous dose that was given and the presence of any dose-limiting normal tissues within the field, especially the spinal cord. There is little point in repeating treatment if that given earlier had no beneficial effect. If local radiotherapy was effective there is some evidence that re-treatment can produce similar response rates (Mithal *et al.* 1994). Side-effects are related to the site (Table 15.1).

While there is more published on radiotherapy for metastatic bone pain than for relief of other symptoms, attempts to quantify this are often poor. Radiological evidence of bone healing may take up to 4 months and is an indirect indication of response (Neilson *et al.* 1991). Furthermore the wide range of dose and fractionation schedules in use, heterogeneity of extent and types of malignant disease and the poor survival of many patients compound the difficulties in accurate evaluation.

Recent interest in the use of single treatments versus short fractionation schedules has provided valuable data from studies which have attempted to analyse pain ratings and other parameters. A comparison between 8 Gy as single fraction and 30 Gy in 10 sessions demonstrated a response in over 80% of patients at 4 weeks in both arms; 45% of the patients given a single treatment had complete relief of pain (Price *et al.* 1986). There was no difference in the time to response, its duration, or overall survival in the two groups, which supported the use of a single radiotherapy sessions for palliation of bone pain. A separate study found that a drop in dose to 4 Gy compared with 6 Gy led to more re-treatments for further bone pain (20% compared with 9%) at the same site (Price *et al.* 1986). Other UK studies have supported the use of single, large fractions (Cole 1989).

A systematic review of radiotherapy for painful bone metastases has been completed: this rigorous analysis of thirteen trials showed lower figures for pain relief than are usually quoted by radiotherapists and others (McQuay *et al.* 1997). However, at least 49% of patients achieved 50% pain relief (range 28–81%) and 30% had a complete response at one month following radiotherapy. The median duration of complete pain relief was 12 weeks.

One large retrospective analysis of 463 treatments demonstrated a relationship between dose and pain response (Arcangeli *et al.* 1989). A complete response was independent of the underlying primary tumour type, except for a poor response with adenocarcinoma of kidney and non-small cell lung cancers. Others have documented the relative radioresistance of renal cancer (Onufrey and Mohiuddin 1985). In contrast, myeloma and bone involvement with lymphoma is treated very effectively with relatively low doses. Leigh *et al.* (1993) reviewed the results of over 3000 radiotherapy treatments in 101 patients with myeloma. The overall response was 97%, of which 26% were complete pain responses and re-treatment was necessary in only 6%.

Radiotherapy for widespread bone metastases

Extensive bone disease associated can be treated by large radiotherapy fields which encompass up to half the body (hemibody irradiation or HBI), or by administration of bone-seeking radioisotopes. Both techniques treat multiple deposits and as well as effectively relieving diffuse bone pain may also delay onset of symptoms from silent deposits. They are used most often in patients with breast, lung, prostate cancer, and also myeloma (but not if marrow function is already compromised by previous chemotherapy or infiltration by tumour). Caution is needed if the white cell count is below 3.0×10^6 or platelets under 100×10^9.

Hemibody irradiation is given to the upper or lower half body by a large parallel pair of beams in a single session; 6 Gy is prescribed for upper half treatments and 8 Gy to the lower. There is usually a rapid and high response rate, with over 70% experiencing some improvement in pain within 24–48 hours (Qasim 1981). Large volumes are irradiated, so more side-effects are produced. Critical dose-limiting tissues in this technique are the lungs and bone marrow. If treatment to both halves of the body is contemplated, there must be an interval of 4–6 weeks between them to allow the remaining stem cells to repopulate the entire marrow. Patients are usually admitted to hospital for this treatment. They are given prophylactic 5HT3 antiemetics and dexamethasone. Although this considerably reduces side-effects, some experience nausea and vomiting in the first 24 hours. Those who receive lower hemibody irradiation are warned to expect diarrhoea. Upper half treatments may be planned from below the eyes to avoid hair loss.

Radioisotopes which are preferentially taken up by bone can be used to irradiate sites of metastatic tumour throughout the skeleton. Radiophosphorus (P-32) is an established treatment in myeloproliferative disorders, but in cancer patients has the disadvantage of causing significant myelosuppression. Strontium-89 (Sr-89) is more widely used for palliation of metastatic bone disease associated with osteoblastic activity. It is used in patients with prostate cancer that has escaped from control by hormonal manipulation and has also been used in breast cancer (Robinson 1993).

Sr-89 is administered as a single intravenous injection. It is a pure beta-emitter and can be given safely to outpatients without special precautions provided the patient is continent (it is excreted in the urine). Patients are warned that there can be a flare in bone pain within 2–4 days following the injection. There are no other significant side-effects, importantly no nausea, vomiting, or hair loss. As analogue of calcium, it remains within bone and in effect delivers radiotherapy throughout the skeleton, but especially at disease sites, for some weeks. Improvement in symptoms is seen within a month and may continue for up to 3 months. Compared with P-32 there is relatively little effect upon marrow function, which may be evident from a dip in platelet count by 6 weeks following administration. If there has been a beneficial response, further Sr-89 may be repeated at 6-monthly intervals. A controlled trial comparing local radiotherapy alone or combined with 400 MBq Sr-89 in metastatic prostate cancer demonstrated improved pain control, with reduction in further radiotherapy treatments in the patients given the radioisotope, but without significant haematological toxicity (Porter and McEwan 1993). A retrospective comparison of 200 MBq Sr-89 with hemibody irradiation in patients with prostate cancer showed similar benefits; at 3 months, 63% of the HBI group had improvement in pain compared with 52% given Sr-89 (Dearnley *et al.* 1992). Transfusion requirements and treatment side-effects were greater in those given external radiotherapy and the time to response was slower for those treated with the radioisotope. Although a valuable treatment for diffuse bone pain, the wider use of Sr-89 may be limited by its high cost.

Radiotherapy offers valuable means of achieving pain relief for both localized and more diffuse sites of bone pain. In general the techniques used are simple and well tolerated by patients. However there may be a delay of some weeks between referral, treatment, and achieving a response, during which it is important to relieve pain by appropriate use of drugs and other means. It is also important to identify patients with

complex pain syndromes including incident pain or neuropathic pain; while radiotherapy may be indicated to prevent further damage associated with tumour progression, it cannot provide the complete solution to pain for these individuals.

Radiotherapy—the patient's experience

The first stage on arrival at the radiotherapy department will be to plan the treatment,
using investigations that have localized the tumour responsible for symptoms and
defined the extent of disease. Treatment of bone metastases may require only plain
X-rays and a bone scan; in other situations CT and MRI scans may be needed. Radical
treatment of deep-seated tumours may be planned from the scan images using a computer. Most palliative treatments are planned using clinical assessment and a treatment
simulator, a diagnostic X-ray machine that exactly reproduces the set-up of the linear
accelerator. Treatment fields are marked on the patient in ink in relation to bone and
other landmarks. Discreet permanent dots are tattooed to indicate the corner or centre
of a field, except on the face. Measurements are taken and calculations made to produce the treatment prescription. The radiotherapy will be started as soon as possible
after this. Single fraction palliative treatments will probably be done on the same visit,
when it may be possible to treat more than one painful site.

During radiotherapy treatment, the patient holds a still position close to the machine
itself. Usually the individual lies supine on quite a hard couch; sometimes prone
and occasionally on one side or sitting up if these are the only positions that can be
tolerated because of pain or breathlessness. It is important to provide effective pain
relief to enable radiotherapy to be given. An additional dose of analgesia by mouth or
injection may be sufficient. If there is severe pain on movement, a strategy must be
planned to deal with this. In difficult situations, regional infusion of local anaesthetic,
for example via an epidural catheter, may be necessary in the short term. Unless
orthovoltage X-rays or electrons are used, the machine does not come into contact with
the patient. Care is taken over the patient's position to ensure comfort, accurate
delivery of radiation in every session, and also to enable accurate matching of treatments to adjacent areas in the future; the tattoos provide a 'landmark' for subsequent
radiotherapy.

As it is not desirable to expose professional staff to ionizing radiation, the patient
remains alone during treatment which takes only a few minutes each session. A
television monitor is used throughout. Treatment is stopped immediately if the patient
moves or shows any sign of distress; in practice this is rarely necessary. The room
is quite large and not claustrophobic; some people bring tapes of favourite music to
play and the supportive radiographers plus camaraderie among patients help considerably. Above all, the delivery of radiotherapy is painless (unless the position is
uncomfortable). This is one of its advantages in palliation, even for children and ill
patients.

To treat or not to treat?

These points should be considered when palliative radiotherapy is contemplated for pain relief. Decisions about treatment interventions in advanced disease can be difficult. It is always worth discussing the patient with a clinical oncologist at the radiotherapy department. Judgement about the likely prognosis of each individual is important in this process; even when a single treatment to a bone metastasis is contemplated, the expected survival should be at least 6 weeks or more to make this worthwhile. However in distressing situations such as incipient spinal cord compression, radiotherapists would be prepared to treat immediately unless the patient was already confined to bed.

Disease related factors

- Is the cause and type of pain clearly defined?
- Is it possible to localize the site of disease responsible for the symptoms?
- Are further investigations needed?
- Is urgent treatment needed?

Treatment factors

- Can an effective dose of radiotherapy be given to the symptomatic site?
- Has the area been irradiated in the past?
- Are the likely side-effects outweighed by potential benefits from pain relief?
- Are there other options such as surgery to be considered?

Patient factors

- Does this patient want further treatment?
- Is the prognosis long enough for them to benefit?
- Is the patient fit enough to travel to the radiotherapy department, lie still, and co-operate with treatment?
- What can be done immediately to relieve pain while awaiting radiotherapy and its outcome?

References

Ampil, F.L. (1986). Palliative irradiation of carcinomatous lumbosacral plexus neuropathy. *International Journal of Radiation Oncology*, **12**, 1681–6.

Arcangeli, G., Micheli, A., Arcangeli, G., Giannarelli, D., La Pasta, O., Tollis, A., Vitullo, A., Ghera, S., and Benassi, M. (1989). The responsiveness of bone metastases to radiotherapy: the effect of site, histology and radiation dose on pain relief. *Radiotherapy and Oncology*, **14**, 95–101.

Bisset, D., Macbeth, F.R., and Cram, I. (1991). The role of palliative radiotherapy in malignant mesothelioma. *Clinical Oncology*, **3**, 315–17.

Bogelt, B.B., Gelber, R., Brady, L.W., Griffin, T., and Hendrickson, F.R. (1981). The palliation of hepatic metastases: the results of the Radiation Therapy Oncology Group pilot study. *International Journal of Radiation Oncology, Biology and Physics*, **7**, 587–91.

Cole, D. (1989). A randomised trial of a single treatment versus conventional fractionation in the palliative radiotherapy of painful bone metastases. *Clinical Oncology*, **1**, 59–62.

Corn, B.W., Lanciano, R., Boente, M., Hunter, W.M., Ladazack, B.S., and Ozols, R.F. (1994). Recurrent ovarian cancer. Effective radiotherapeutic palliation after chemotherapy failure. *Cancer*, **74**, 2979–83.

Dearnley, D.P., Bayly, R.J., Hern, R.P., Gadd, J., Zivanovic, M.M., and Lewington, V.J. (1992). Palliation of bone metastases in prostate cancer. Hemibody irradiation or Strontium-89? *Clinical Oncology*, **4**, 101–7.

Frykholm, G.J., Pahlman, L., and Glimelius, G. (1995). Treatment of local recurrences of rectal carcinoma. *Radiotherapy and Oncology*, **34**, 185–94.

Jenrette, J.M. (1996). Malignant melanoma: the role of radiation therapy revisited. *Seminars in Oncology*, **6**, 759–62.

Leigh, B.R., Kurtts, T.A., Mach, C.F., Matzener, M.B., and Schim, D.S. (1993). Radiation therapy for palliation of multiple myeloma. *International Journal of Radiation Oncology, Biology and Physics*, **5**, 801–4.

McQuay, H.J., Carroll, D., and Moore, R.A. (1997). Radiotherapy for bone metastases: a systematic review. *Clinical Oncology*, **9**, 150–4.

Mithal, N.P., Needham, P.R., and Hoskin, P.J. (1994). Retreatment with radiotherapy for painful bone metastases. *International Journal of Radiation Oncology, Biology and Physics*, **29**, 1011–14.

Nielson, O.S., Munro, A.J., and Tannock, I.F. (1991). Bone metastases: pathophysiology and management policy. *Journal of Clinical Oncology*, **9**, 509–24.

Onufrey, V., and Mohiuddin, M. (1985). Radiation therapy in the treatment of metastatic renal cell carcinoma. *International Journal of Radiation Oncology, Biology and Physics*, **11**, 2007–9.

Porter, A.T., and McEwan, A.J.B. (1993). Strontium-89 as an adjuvant to external beam radiation improves pain relief and delays disease progression in advanced prostate cancer: results of a randomised, controlled trial. *Seminars in Oncology*, **20**, 38–43.

Price, P., Hoskin, P.J., and Easton, D. (1986). A prospective randomised trial of single and multifraction radiotherapy schedules in the treatment of painful bony metastases. *Radiotherapy and Oncology*, **6**, 247–55.

Priestman, T.J., Dunn, J., Brada, M., Rampling, R., and Baker, P.G. (1996). Final results of the Royal College of Radiologists' trial comparing two different radiotherapy schedules in the treatment of cerebral metastases. *Clinical Oncology*, **8**, 308–15.

Qasim, M.M. (1981). Half body irradiation (HBI) in metastatic carcinomas. *Clinical Radiology*, **32**, 215–19.

Rees, G.J.G., Devrell, C.E., Barley, V.L., and Newman, H.F.V. (1997). Palliative radiotherapy for lung cancers: two versus five fractions. *Clinical Oncology*, **9**, 90–5.

Robinson, R.G. (1993). Strontium-89—Precursor targeted therapy for pain relief of blastic metastatic disease. *Cancer*, **72**, 3433–5.

Ross Garrett, I. (1993). Bone destruction in cancer. *Seminars in Oncology*, **20**, 4–9.

Roth, S., Sach, H., Thesen, N., and Modder, U. (1985). Radiotherapy of pancreas cancer. *Radiologie*, **1**, 41–7.

Russi, E.G., Pergolizzi, S., Gaeta, M., Mesiti, M., D'Aquino, A., and Delia, P. (1993). Palliative radiotherapy in lumbosacral carcinomatous neuropathy. *Radiotherapy and Oncology*, **26**, 172–3.

Rutten, I.H.J.M., Crul, B., van der Toorn, P.P.G., Otten, A.W., and Dirksen, R. (1997). Pain characteristics help to predict the analgesic efficacy of radiotherapy for the treatment of cancer pain. *Pain*, **69**, 131–5.

Short, S., Chaturvedi, A., and Leslie, M.D. (1996). Palliation of symptomatic adrenal gland metastases by radiotherapy. *Clinical Oncology*, **8**, 387–9.

Wong, R., Thomas, G., Cummings, B., Froud, P., Shelley, W., Withers, R.H., and Williams, J. (1996). The role of radiotherapy in the management of pelvic recurrence of rectal cancer. *Canadian Journal of Oncology*, **1**, 39–47.

Yeo, W., Leung, S.F., Chan, A.T.C., and Chiu, K.W. (1996). Radiotherapy for extreme hypertrophic pulmonary osteoarthropathy associated with malignancy. *Clinical Oncology*, **8**, 195–7.

SIXTEEN

Chemotherapy and hormonal manipulation

DAWN L. ALISON

Chemotherapy

Chemotherapy can play an important part in the control of pain and other symptoms in cancer patients. Its use in the context of curable disease is not disputed but as part of a palliative approach to cancer care, chemotherapy has an unacceptable image in the eyes of many non-oncology health-care workers. It is often cited as a cause of significant symptoms due to the associated toxicities and side-effects. As a result the positive outcome for some patients may be overlooked. Lack of knowledge and of experience in caring for patients undergoing cytotoxic chemotherapy are both reasons why some clinicians fail to consider using chemotherapy as a method of symptom relief.

When to refer

Important aims of the recent re-organization of cancer services in Britain are to increase speed of referral and to improve access to specialists in cancer care throughout the country (Calman and Hine 1995). Optimal care requires that the opinion of surgical and non-surgical oncologists should be sought about the most appropriate treatment for patients with cancer as soon as possible after a diagnosis of cancer has been made or when such a diagnosis is suspected. It is also recommended that specialist palliative care services are integrated with cancer services to allow early involvement of relevant professionals to help address the complex needs of cancer patients and their families. The key to translating these laudable aims into effective practice is by regular open communication between referring clinicians, oncologists, and palliative care specialists. Failure to recognize what can be achieved in terms of disease control and palliation of symptoms by specific anticancer treatment even for patients presenting with fairly advanced metastatic disease still occurs for want of appropriate referral. Collaborative working can avoid this pitfall as illustrated by the following case history.

A 43-year-old woman was admitted acutely via the accident and emergency department of a teaching hospital under the care of a general surgeon. She was confused, a little drowsy and complained of abdominal pain. There was a 5-week history of weight loss and nausea. Clinical examination revealed marked abdominal distension, ascites, and hepatomegaly. Abdominal ultrasound showed multiple liver metastases which were biopsied and a CT scan showed extensive abdominal and pelvic ascites, massive hepatomegaly, and widespread peritoneal metastases. The patient was commenced on a subcutaneous infusion of diamorphine for pain relief by the admitting team and referral was made to the hospital palliative care team. The patient was very drowsy, confused, and agitated when first seen. The histology from the liver biopsy had been reported as a poorly differentiated adenocarcinoma of unknown primary origin and the admitting team felt there was no treatment available to reverse the patient's rapid deterioration. At the request of the palliative care team the patient's serum calcium was assessed and urgent referral made to the oncology team. The patient was found to be hypercalcaemic and after review by the oncologist and discussion with the patient's relatives the hypercalcaemia was treated by hydration and bisphosphonate infusion. The patient became increasingly lucid and less agitated and it was possible to reduce the opioid dose. When her clinical condition became more stable options for palliative chemotherapy were discussed with the patient and her husband. She agreed to undergo a trial of combination chemotherapy with a regimen containing cisplatinum which has a 20–30% response rate in the context of unknown primary tumours (Sporn and Greenberg 1990). She tolerated this well experiencing only transient mild nausea. Pyrexia at the time of her neutropenia was treated with broad spectrum antibiotics. No infective source was found and she recovered quickly. She was discharged home approximately 3 weeks after admission. Opioid analgesia was no longer needed. She completed 5 cycles of chemotherapy at 3 weekly intervals with excellent symptomatic improvement. She relapsed approximately 5 months after finishing chemotherapy and died 11 months after her original presentation. The chemotherapy had undoubtedly allowed her to survive nearly 1 year longer than she would have done without it and provided a period of good symptom relief which she was able to spend at home.

This case highlights several important points about use of chemotherapy as palliation which are considered in more detail later.

- Early referral to an oncologist is essential to allow choices to be considered even when a patient appears very ill.

- Many factors influence the decision to offer chemotherapy including tumour type and responsiveness to chemotherapy, performance status of the patient, co-morbidity, presence of significant organ dysfunction and toxicity of the drugs which are active against individual cancer types (Rubens *et al*. 1992).

- Patients are prepared to accept much higher levels of toxicity from chemotherapy for a smaller chance of likely benefit than doctors or nurses believe (Slevin *et al*. 1990). The role of the oncologist is to provide as clear information as possible about the risks and benefits of chemotherapy in individual situations to enable the patient to choose whether or not they wish to undergo the treatment.

- Regular review of toxicities and benefits is necessary to decide on whether continuing with treatment is appropriate (Maher *et al*. 1994).

- Good supportive care is crucial to patient safety whilst undergoing toxic treatments. Patients, their carers, and involved health-care professionals should all be aware of the need for vigilance regarding life-threatening complications such as neutropenic sepsis.

Tumour responses

Tumour types

There is a spectrum of responsiveness of different cancer types to the chemotherapy drugs currently available as indicated in Table 16.1. Cancer pain occurs in many sites due to local growth and invasion by the primary and metastatic disease. There are some pain syndromes which prove particularly difficult to control with conventional analgesics which can be relieved by cytotoxic therapy. An example of this is the superficial soreness and itching of skin infiltration caused by locally advanced breast cancer.

Table 16.1. Results with cytotoxic chemotherapy

Cure of advanced disease >50% of cases	Cure of advanced disease <50% of cases
Hodgkin's disease	Non-Hodgkin's lymphoma
Testicular cancer	Ovarian cancer
Paediatric cancers	Small cell lung cancer
Acute lymphoblastic leukaemia	Neuroblastoma
Choriocarcinoma	

Increased cure rate in high risk locoregional disease

Breast cancer
Colorectal cancer
Small cell lung cancer

Remissions in most patients

Curable tumours (see above)
Breast cancer
Small cell lung cancer
Ovarian cancer

Prolonged survival but few cures in advanced disease

Non-small cell lung cancer
Colorectal cancer
Gastric cancer
Breast cancer

Palliation of symptoms only

Renal cancer
Bladder cancer
Melanoma
Head and neck cancer

The likelihood of chemotherapy or hormone therapy contributing to pain relief is directly related to the predicted response rate of the cancer to the drugs used. There are no specific pain types which respond better than others. Pain relief occurs due to shrinkage of tumour masses or by influencing biological effects caused by tumours. It is therefore helpful to have accurate histological information whenever possible. This will ensure that cancer patients who have the potential to be cured or whose survival can be prolonged significantly are offered appropriate treatment. It will also help to indicate the chances of symptomatic benefit being achieved by chemotherapy for patients with less chemosensitive disease. For those patients found to have cancers with poor response rates to chemotherapy this information can be a crucial part in the decision making process. The balance between anticipated benefits and burdens of chemotherapy when aiming for symptom relief with no hope of improving overall survival is a difficult one to achieve. The situation is analogous to that when offering other drugs with unpleasant side-effects such as those used for neuropathic pain (e.g. amitriptyline, carbamazepine). The response rates may be low, the time for demonstrable improvement can take several weeks and side-effects are potentially debilitating in a frail group of patients.

It is not always possible to make a definitive diagnosis even with the use of increasingly sophisticated laboratory and radiological techniques. The oncologist then needs to make an assessment of the treatment options most likely to help based on the mode of presentation, pattern of metastases identified, serum tumour markers, and available histological data (Bradley and Selby 1992).

Measurement of response

Oncologists have traditionally focused on objective measurements of response to chemotherapy and for purposes of clinical trials these are categorized as complete, partial, no change, or progression. Objective responses are determined by clinical, radiological, biochemical, or surgicopathological staging. Where measurable disease exists bidimensional or unidimensional measurements are taken for marker lesions and these are repeated at agreed intervals during a course of treatment, (usually after 2–3 of a potential 6 treatments). At the end of treatment a 'complete response' is defined as the disappearance of all known disease, determined by observations not less than 4 weeks apart. A 'partial response' is a 50% or more decrease in total tumour size of the lesions that have been measured to determine the effect of therapy by two observations not less than 4 weeks apart. In addition there can be no appearance of new lesions or progression of any lesion. 'No change' is recorded when there is a less than 50% decrease in size of lesions and no lesion has increased in size by 25%. 'Progressive disease' is recorded when there is a 25% or more increase in the size of one or more measurable lesions or appearance of new lesions. Some disease cannot be measured accurately, for example pleural effusions, lymphangitic pulmonary metastases, skin involvement in breast cancer, palpable but unmeasurable abdominal masses. In these cases an estimate is made and responses are recorded using similar criteria as for measurable disease. Bone metastases require separate response criteria and the time allowed for response is longer in keeping with the slower observed changes.

Objective response rates are necessary to make comparisons between different treatments, but of more importance to patients, especially in the context of palliative therapy, is their subjective response. Some patients report benefit symptomatically even when the overall objective response rate is of 'no change' (Gough *et al*. 1981). Quality of life measurement has gained recognition as a necessary part of assessment in recent years (Slevin 1992). An increasing number of clinical trials incorporate some means of evaluating this. There are many different quality of life measurement tools, sometimes tumour site specific, which include several domains of function: (physical function, physical symptoms, psychological function, social function) (Maguire and Selby 1989; Aaronson *et al*. 1988).

If chemotherapy treatment is intended to improve unpleasant symptoms such as pain, symptoms must be recorded at the start and regularly thereafter using either a simple verbal or numerical scale as a routine part of clinical practice. A body chart to indicate sites of pain will help remind clinicians of the focus of the treatment.

Toxic effects of chemotherapy must also be assessed and recorded at frequent intervals usually before each treatment is due and at least once in between each treatment. There are recognized scales for this (World Health Organization 1979). The impact of drug related toxic effects, the inconvenience of hospital visits, and possible in-patient stays can only be judged against the perceived subjective improvement by the patient. A study of the benefits and deleterious effects of chemotherapy in advanced breast cancer has highlighted this issue (Ramirez *et al.* 1998).

Techniques for chemotherapy administration

Oral

The route of cytotoxic chemotherapy administration is dependent on the individual drug being used. A few drugs have sufficiently good oral bioavailability to allow for tablet treatment, for example chlorambucil, cyclophosphamide. Oral chemotherapy is not necessarily easier for patients some of whom may already experience nausea. Additional tablets for patients who are frequently subject to polypharmacy can be difficult especially if they exacerbate existing nausea.

Peripheral venous infusions

The majority of treatments rely on intravenous injections or infusions, many of which can be given by trained specialist nurses in outpatient departments. Care must be taken with peripheral venous cannulation as some drugs are irritant and some damaging if extravasated. Dilution in free-flowing intravenous fluids can reduce damage to the endothelial lining. If extravasation occurs specific measures need to be taken immediately to minimize the destruction of tissues. Occasionally surgical debridement and skin grafting are needed when damage has been severe (Clamon 1992).

Some cytotoxic chemotherapy regimens require in-patient stay because of the supportive measures needed to minimize toxicity. An example of these drugs is cisplatinum which has activity against several different tumour types including germ cell tumours, ovarian cancer, breast cancer, and gastrointestinal tumours. One of the most dangerous toxic effects of cisplatinum is its renal toxicity which can be reduced by intravenous pre-hydration and post-hydration with careful attention to fluid balance.

Central venous cannulae

Some situations require central venous cannulae placement to deliver chemotherapy. Cannulae can remain in place for the duration of treatment provided there are no complications. In suitable patients these may be inserted peripherally and should be considered at the start of treatment for patients who wish to avoid multiple peripheral venous cannulations or in whom the smaller peripheral veins appear problematic. Additionally there are a variety of subcutaneous ports which can be used for administration of chemotherapy. Central venous cannulation has other advantages for those patients who choose to receive chemotherapy this way. Blood samples can be taken from the cannula and transfusions of blood or platelets, if needed, can also be given via this route.

Some cytotoxic drugs work best by slow continuous infusion and this necessitates use of a tunnelled long-term central venous cannula for example Hickman or Groshong line. Lightweight small battery operated pumps into which bags of cytotoxic drugs are inserted and connected to the central venous catheter to allow ambulatory infusions. This is not suitable for all cytotoxic drugs and is not acceptable to all patients some of whom find the constant presence of infusion equipment a constant reminder of their condition.

The risks and potential complications associated with use of long-term indwelling central venous cannulae include a pneumothorax at insertion (in up to 5%), thrombosis, and sepsis. Some clinicians favour anticoagulation of all patients who have long-term central venous cannulae inserted. All patients receiving cytotoxic therapy are at risk of infection during periods of neutropenia, and cannulae as a possible source of sepsis must not be overlooked (Lopez 1992).

Other routes of chemotherapy administration

Whilst most chemotherapy is given via a systemic intravenous route there are some situations where regional perfusion is used to deliver a higher drug level to a particular organ or anatomic site than is achieved elsewhere in the body. Such approaches involve intra-arterial, intra-ventricular, intraperitoneal, intrapleural, or intravesical routes. These are specialist techniques with limited applicability. The intrathecal route is also sometimes used particularly in the treatment of leukaemia, lymphoma, and for meningeal metastases from breast cancer. This may seem intrusive in the context of disease palliation, but it offers the best chance of delivering chemotherapy into a fluid compartment not generally well reached by cytotoxic drugs. Only a few drugs can be used safely intrathecally and special preparations are required. The improvement in headache and other neurological symptoms and signs when disease response is achieved can be dramatic. Omaya reservoirs can be inserted into the ventricles to ensure ease of access and reduce patient discomfort by avoiding multiple lumbar punctures.

Cytotoxic schedules and duration

Cancer chemotherapy drugs work by interfering with normal cell replication in a variety of different ways. Some drugs require cells to be in a specific phase of the cell cycle to have their effect. The drugs currently available are rarely selective for cancer cells and as a result their use causes damage to normal healthy body tissues. Normal tissues will tolerate or recover from the effects of cytotoxic drugs within quite narrow dose limits. The scheduling of chemotherapy regimens is dictated by the need for recovery of normal tissues. Commonly treatments are given every 3–4 weeks. It is usual for 2–3 treatments to be given before evaluating whether a useful response is being achieved. Individual circumstances may require modification of this strategy particularly if the cancer is clearly progressing very quickly. When benefit is observed treatments generally continue for a total of 6 cycles lasting 4½–6 months depending on the scheduling.

Many cancer treatments use combinations of cytotoxic drugs. The drugs in a particular regimen will each have a modest activity against the cancer being treated and a different site of effect. Although there may be some overlap in toxicities they also usually have differing toxicities. This allows the cancer to be exposed to several different mechanisms of attack whilst minimizing the toxicity to any one organ or tissue. It is likely that use of combination regimens also helps reduce development of resistance by the cancer to cytotoxic treatment.

In some situations, if a drug has a high activity against a specific cancer this drug may be used alone allowing the dose to be maximized because there will be no contribution to its main toxicity from other drugs. Carboplatin is an example of a drug used frequently as a single agent for treatment of ovarian cancer, a disease most likely to arise in elderly women who may have poor tolerance of cytotoxic drugs.

Cytotoxic chemotherapy toxicities

Cytotoxic chemotherapy can damage most normal tissues as a result of its effect on cell replication. In addition some drugs have toxicities related to their specific chemical properties or their interference with other biochemical functions. Knowledge of the range of predicted toxicities and individual risk factors which potentiate them is necessary in order to inform patients as fully as possible about what a chemotherapy regimen will involve.

Bone marrow toxicity

All cytotoxic drugs can affect the bone marrow. A few do so only minimally whereas others may cause significant myelosuppression with the associated risks of neutropenic sepsis, thrombocytopenic bleeding, and anaemia. It is common practice to assess a patient's nadir blood count after a cycle of chemotherapy. This will occur 10–14 days after treatment with many regimens, although some drugs affect the marrow more quickly and a few have a more delayed action. Doses are sometimes adjusted to reduce the impact of treatment on the marrow particularly in the context of palliative treatments. Growth factors such as growth colony stimulating factor can be used to minimize the period of neutropenia. In recent years it has become possible to salvage marrow function by use of peripheral blood stem cell transplants following high dose chemotherapy.

Gastrointestinal and oral toxicity

Gastrointestinal mucosa is sensitive to many chemotherapy drugs. The oral, oesophageal, and bowel mucosa can all become inflamed and even ulcerated giving rise to sore mouths, diarrhoea, and malabsorption. In severe cases supportive care with analgesics and fluid replacement is required.

Nausea and vomiting

Many cytotoxic drugs cause nausea and vomiting which is often worst within a few hours of receiving treatment, but sometimes extends over several days. $5HT_3$ receptor antagonist drugs used in conjunction with steroids have significantly reduced this side-effect for the most emetogenic drugs such as cisplatinum and dacarbazine but some patients still have problems. Occasionally nausea and vomiting can become anticipatory, hence, there is a need to try to optimize emesis control from the time of the first treatment.

Renal

Several drugs are toxic to the kidneys and this may be minimized by hydration schedules before and after treatment. Even with careful hydration there can be a cumulative damaging effect on tubular function. Creatinine clearance should be checked routinely before each cycle of treatment and doses adjusted or treatment stopped if significant reductions occur. In the case of patients with pelvic disease causing ureteric obstruction in whom treatment with renal toxic chemotherapy is indicated it may be appropriate to optimize renal function first by use of ureteric stents or occasionally nephrostomies.

Neurological

Central and peripheral neurotoxicities can be seen with some chemotherapy agents. Best known are the peripheral and autonomic neuropathies caused by vinca alkaloids (vincristine, vinblastine) and cisplatinum. In addition to impaired sensory and motor function patients may experience unpleasant sensations which may resolve only slowly and partially. These effects are generally worse in elderly patients.

Alopecia

Not all cytotoxic drugs cause hair thinning or loss but this is a distressing symptom when it occurs. For some drugs it is possible to reduce hair loss by use of cold caps to cool the scalp (and thereby reduce blood flow locally) before and during the time of drug infusion. Not all patients can tolerate this and it is impractical for drugs with long infusion times. Hair re-grows after finishing treatment but may be altered in texture.

Other toxicities

There are several organ related toxicities specific to a few frequently used drugs or classes of drugs. Anthracyclines (doxorubicin, epirubicin) cause cardiac toxicity with cumulative effect. Other drugs damage lung tissue e.g. bleomycin and some can damage bladder mucosa e.g. cyclophosphamide, ifosfamide. There are many other rare toxicities. Careful monitoring is, therefore, essential at all stages of treatment. Tiredness and non-specific malaise are frequently described by patients undergoing chemotherapy and whilst difficult to quantify this may have a significant impact on perceived quality of life.

Choice of drug regimen and dose adjustments

Dose intensity (dose size and frequency) is thought to correlate with improved survival in the treatment of some cancers (Henderson *et al.* 1988; Hryniuk and Bush 1984) although this is not proven in all situations. More intensive treatment may result in better palliation despite more side-effects, due to better overall response rates and disease control (Glimelius *et al.* 1989). Although it is tempting to reduce doses to minimize toxicities or to select less toxic (and possibly less effective) regimens this may not serve the patient best. Dose reductions are clearly important in specific situations where reduced organ function will alter drug pharmacokinetics. The elderly are more at risk for some toxicities and sensible adjustments should be made. Whatever regimen is chosen there is a need for robust support for patients to optimize control of treatment related side-effects.

Care of patients receiving cytotoxic chemotherapy

General

The complexity of chemotherapy treatments demands that they be supervized and delivered by specialist multi-disciplinary oncology teams. Guidelines for the prescribing and administration of chemotherapy have been published by the Joint Council for Clinical Oncology and these make explicit the standards required (Joint Council for Clinical Oncology 1994). Patient education and psychological support are both required along with specialist skills in giving treatments either on wards or in outpatient departments. Written information about treatments and side-effects to supplement the verbal information given by doctors and nurses can be helpful. These may be of value to community health-care workers who may have limited knowledge of anti-cancer treatments.

Some patients may benefit from a short period of in-patient care aimed at rehabilitation and convalescence after receiving the first one or two chemotherapy treatments, especially if they have advanced disease and multiple symptoms. Close co-operation between oncology and hospice units may allow patients to benefit from in-patient hospice care in a more pleasant less clinical environment whilst their progress is reviewed. This demonstrates the best of shared care for patients receiving palliative treatments. It may also allow patients to reflect on their experience of chemotherapy and explore with health professionals not directly responsible for this aspect of treatment, the overall benefits to their symptom control. Patients may have difficulty opting out of treatments perhaps because they do not wish to disappoint those who have supplied them.

Neutropenic sepsis

There is no room for complacency in the management of patients with neutropenic sepsis. This is a reversible complication and failure to treat it appropriately and promptly can cause untimely death. For this reason clear guidance on how to deal with worrying symptoms developing after cytotoxic treatment should be given to everyone concerned with a patient's care including the primary health care team and community specialist palliative care services. In particular it should be stressed that the development of a fever during a period of potential neutropenia should be managed as a medical emergency with prompt referral to the oncology team. It is negligent to attempt management of the patient at home with oral antibiotics. Patients with neutropenic pyrexia require immediate hospital admission and commencement of broad spectrum intravenous antibiotics whilst awaiting the results of investigations which should routinely include blood cultures, urine culture, throat swabs, chest X-ray, and swabs of any infective lesions. If a long-term intravenous cannula is in place the exit sites should be observed for signs of infection and cultures taken from blood withdrawn from all lumens. Additional antibiotics are required when cannula infection is suspected. Sometimes cannula removal is necessary to eradicate infection.

Oncology units have clear antibiotic guidelines for use in patients with neutropenic sepsis. If a patient's symptoms and clinical condition fails to improve with first line treatment other antibiotics are introduced and sometimes antifungal treatment is required. Close liaison with microbiology colleagues is of great benefit.

Prolonged nausea and vomiting

Occasionally patients experience severe and prolonged nausea and or vomiting after chemotherapy. This is particularly worrying if patients are unable to maintain adequate oral hydration and especially so if they are taking other nephrotoxic medication such as non-steroidal anti-inflammatory drugs. Admission to hospital for intravenous hydration and adjustment of antiemetic medication can often improve the situation quickly.

Hormone therapy

The growth of some cancers is influenced by hormone levels and interference with these hormones can cause tumour regression or growth arrest. This is a useful strategy not only in adjuvant first line treatment of certain cancers but also when attempting to palliate advanced metastatic disease. Hormonal manipulation is generally less toxic than chemotherapy and should be considered as a means of attempting pain relief in patients with potentially responsive cancer. As with chemotherapy, hormone treatments should be initiated and supervised by oncologists, but less frequent monitoring is required as complications are rare.

Tumour responses

Cancers arising in tissues which are themselves under hormonal control of normal cellular proliferation or survival are commonly hormone sensitive (Table 16.2). Other cancers may exhibit less hormone dependency and for these, hormone treatments are used only occasionally and are the subject of research. In breast cancer there is a spectrum of responsiveness to endocrine therapy dependent on the oestrogen and progesterone receptor status of the tumour. Overall the response rate in advanced breast cancer is 30% (Veronesi *et al*. 1995). Prostate cancer is extremely sensitive to hormonal manipulation with an 80% subjective and 50% objective response rate (Horwich *et al*. 1995).

Techniques of hormone manipulation

Removing the source of growth promoting hormones

Surgical methods such as bilateral oophorectomy in pre-menopausal women and bilateral orchidectomy in men have been superseded generally by medical techniques. Radiotherapy induced ovarian ablation is another technique used in pre-menopausal women with breast cancer. Alternatively 'medical castration' can be achieved by use of long acting luteinizing hormone release hormone (LHRH) analogues for example goserelin and leuprorelin which cause receptor down regulation in the pituitary, block

Table 16.2. Hormone treatment responsiveness of human cancers

Tumour type	Hormones involved	Treatment
Breast	Sex hormones	Hormone treatment established
Prostate	Sex hormones	
Endometrium	Sex hormones	
Lymphoma	Corticosteroids	Hormone treatment established
Leukaemia	Corticosteroids	
Myeloma	Corticosteroids	
Neuroendocrine	}	
Pancreatic	}	Limited value
Renal	} Various	Subject of research
Hepatocellular	}	
Ovarian	}	
Lung	}	

luteinizing hormone (LH) and follicle stimulating hormone (FSH) production and in turn gonadal hormone output.

In post-menopausal women sex hormone production is mainly extragonadal, therefore, other techniques are needed. Inhibitors of the peripheral aromatase enzymes, which are used in the conversion of adrenally secreted androstenedione to oestrogens, are an option. Aminoglutethimide was the first such drug but newer drugs such as anastrazole and exemestane, are more specific and have less toxicity.

Hormone inhibitors

In breast cancer treatment tamoxifen acts in part by blocking the binding of oestrogens to their receptors in tumour cells. It also has some pro-oestrogenic effects and some non-oestrogen receptor mediated actions. Tamoxifen is well established in the management of early and advanced breast cancer. New more potent specific antioestrogens are being developed.

Anti-androgen drugs are available with a steroidal and non-steroidal structure which give rise to variations in effect. Steroidal anti-androgens such as cyproterone acetate inhibit the androgen receptor in tumour cells and mimic testosterone in the hypothalamus so causing negative feedback inhibition of LHRH release. Nonsteroidal anti-androgens such as flutamide inhibit testosterone in both tumour cells and the hypothalamus so feedback inhibition is lost and serum testosterone levels rise. Commonly an LHRH analogue and anti-androgen are used simultaneously for a short period. This avoids the testosterone 'flare' which can arise when LHRH analogues are first used as they cause initial pituitary stimulation before inhibition of gonadotrophin release (Waxman *et al.* 1988). Total androgen blockade over a prolonged period is favoured by some clinicians.

Increasing hormones

Increased levels of some sex hormones can induce negative feedback loops. Stilboestrol, a synthetic oestrogen, can thus down-regulate hypothalamic LHRH in prostate cancer but is now less frequently used than other hormonal manipulations due to its worse side-effect profile. Tachyphylaxis or down regulation of receptors in breast cancer can be caused by high dose oestrogens but again is not commonly used.

Synthetic analogues of progesterone (medroxyprogesterone acetate and megesterol acetate) are both used in breast and endometrial cancer. Their modes of action are unclear but direct inhibition of tumour growth via the progesterone receptor and negative feedback on the pituitary/gonadal axis are both possibilities.

Glucocorticoids in high concentration induce apoptosis in some malignant lymphoid cells and hence their use in the treatment regimens for lymphoma, lymphoid leukaemias, Hodgkins disease, and myeloma. High dose pulses of treatment are usually used for 7–14 days.

Beneficial effects of hormonal treatment

The two most common cancers where hormone therapy has a clear therapeutic role are breast cancer and prostate cancer. Bone metastases are a frequent source of morbidity in both cancers and skeletal pain exacerbated by movement is a problem. This can be relieved by hormone treatment which may have a gradual effect. Occasionally drugs such as tamoxifen can initially cause increased bone pain due to tumour flare (Henderson and Harris 1991). A similar effect when using LHRH analogues alone in prostate cancer is seen. Therefore prophylactic peripheral androgen blockade is given as well.

Rapidly progressive visceral metastases in breast cancer patients rarely respond to hormone treatment and more indolent bone metastases appear to respond better. Sometimes sequential hormone manipulations are of benefit in patients who have responded well to the initial hormone treatment.

Side-effects of hormonal treatment

Hormonal manipulations are fairly well tolerated. Drug treatments are often tablets or sometimes depot injections (goserelin). The predictable side-effects vary with the drug used and can be troublesome to some patients. In women with breast cancer these may include flushing, nausea, weight gain, fluid retention, menstrual irregularity, mood disturbance, headaches, rashes, and other rarer ones.

In prostate cancer the unwanted effects of hormone treatments also vary, older drugs such as stilboestrol causing an increased risk of cardiovascular complications and impotence. Gynaecomastia, disturbances of hepatic function, and gastrointestinal toxicity are well described with the newer anti-androgens although potency may be preserved depending on drug choice.

Corticosteroids, even in short term use, can cause mood disturbance, insomnia, dyspepsia, fluid retention, and weight gain. Progestagens can give rise to improved appetite and weight gain which may be of benefit in a palliative care setting.

Summary

Cytotoxic chemotherapy and hormonal therapies should be included in the range of treatments considered for symptom relief including pain relief in cancer patients. Other methods of pain control can continue along with these treatments. The drugs used can have toxic effects but for some patients these may be offset by the benefits sustained. Different tumour types and stages of disease have different treatment options available. Early referral to an oncologist enables discussion of the possible advantages and disadvantages of treatment in individual situations. Patients should play the most important part in the decision to start chemotherapy and regular careful review of patient quality of life and symptoms is required as treatment proceeds. Excellent supportive care is essential to minimize risks and toxicities with close liaison between the specialist oncology and primary health care teams and, when indicated, specialist palliative care workers.

References

Aaronson, N.K., Bullinger, M., and Ahmedzai, S. (1988). A modular approach to quality of life assessment in cancer clinical trials. *Recent Results in Cancer Research*, **111**, 231–49.

Bradley, C., and Selby, P. (1992). In search of the unknown primary. *British Medical Journal*, **304**, 1065–6.

Calman, K., and Hine, D. (1995). *A policy framework for commissioning cancer services*. A report by the expert advisory group on cancer to the chief medical officers of England and Wales—Guidance for purchasers and providers of cancer services. EL(95)51.

Clamon, G.H. (1992). Extravasation. In *The chemotherapy source book* (ed. M. Perry), pp. 548–52. Williams and Wilkins, Baltimore.

Glimelius, B., Hoffman, K., Olafsdottir, M., Pahlaman, L., Sjoden, P., and Wennberg, A. (1989). Quality of life during cytostatic therapy for advanced symptomatic colorectal carcinoma: a randomized comparison of two regimens. *European Journal of Cancer and Clinical Oncology*, **25**, 829–35.

Gough, I.R., Furnival, G.M., and Burnett, W. (1981). Patient attitudes to chemotherapy for advanced gastrointestinal cancer. *Clinical Oncology*, **7**, 5–11.

Henderson, Y.C., Hayes, D.F., and Gelman, R. (1988). Dose response in the treatment of breast cancer: a critical review. *Journal of Clinical Oncology*, **6**, 1501–15.

Henderson, I.C., and Harris, J.R. (1991). Principles in the management of metastatic disease. In *Breast diseases* (2nd edn), (ed. J.R. Harris, S. Hellman, I.C. Henderson and D.W. Kinne) pp. 547–677. J.B. Lippincott, Philadelphia.

Horwich, A., Waxman, J., and Schroder, F.H. (1995). Tumours of the prostate. In *The Oxford textbook of oncology* (ed. M. Peckham, H.M. Pinedo, and U. Veronesi), pp. 1498–530. Oxford Medical Publications, Oxford.

Hryniuk, W., and Bush, H. (1984). The importance of dose intensity in chemotherapy of metastatic breast cancer. *Journal of Clinical Oncology*, **2**, 1281–8.

Joint Council for Clinical Oncology. (1994). Quality control in cancer chemotherapy: Management and procedural aspects. London, JCCO.

Lopez, M.J. (1992). Central venous access for chemotherapy. In *The chemotherapy source book* (ed. M. Perry), pp. 780–98. Williams and Wilkins, Baltimore.

Maguire, P., and Selby, P. (1989). Assessing quality of life in cancer patients. *British Journal of Cancer*, **60**, 437–40.

Maher, E.J., Hopwood, P., Girling, J., Macbeth, F.R., and Mansi, J.L. (1994). Measurement of outcome in palliative oncology. *Journal of Cancer Care*, **3**, 94–102.

Ramirez, A.J., Towlson, K.E., Leaning, M.S., Richards, M.A., and Rubens, R.D. (1998). Do patients with advanced breast cancer benefit from chemotherapy? *British Journal of Cancer*, **78**, 1488–94.

Rubens, R.D., Towlson, K.E., Ramirez, A.J., Coltart, S., Slevin, M.L., Terrell, C., and Timothy, A.R. (1992). Appropriate chemotherapy for palliating advanced cancer. *British Medical Journal*, **304**, 35–40.

Slevin, M. (1992). Quality of life: philosophical question or clinical reality? *British Medical Journal*, **305**, 466–9.

Slevin, M., Stubbs, L., Plant, H., Wilson, P., Gregory, W., Armes, P., and Downer, S. (1990). Attitudes to chemotherapy: comparing views of patients with cancer with those of doctors, nurses and general public. *British Medical Journal*, **300**, 1458–60.

Sporn, J.R., and Greenberg, B.R. (1990). Empiric chemotherapy in patients with carcinoma of unknown primary site. *American Journal of Medicine*, **88**, 49–55.

Veronesi, U., Goldhirsch, A., and Yarnold, J. (1995). Breast Cancer. In *The Oxford textbook of oncology* (ed. M. Peckham, H.M. Pinedo, and U. Veronesi), pp. 1243–89. Oxford Medical Publications, Oxford.

Waxman, J., Williams, G., and Sandow, J. (1998). The clinical and endocrine assessment of three different antiandrogen regimens combined with a very long acting gonadotrophin-releasing hormone analogue. *American Journal of Clinical Oncology*, **11**, 152–5.

World Health Organization (1979). *Handbook for reporting results of cancer treatment*. WHO, Geneva.

SEVENTEEN

Homeopathic medicine

ELIZABETH A. THOMPSON

Much has been achieved in the management of cancer pain with the range of effective pain relieving drugs now available. However these drugs do not necessarily impinge on the emotional, psychological, and existential aspects of human suffering. There is clearly a need for modalities of care that can, when used alongside orthodox treatments, address these areas of hurt. The homeopathic approach to pain is one such modality that does not attempt to separate the psyche from the soma, but offers a truly holistic perspective. The person in pain is encouraged to tell their story in their own language, placing weight on those issues that are uppermost in their mind. An individual picture is thereby built up which embraces the many influences that have come to bear on that person.

Anecdotal reports in the homeopathic literature suggest that pain may be diminished or conventional drug requirements reduced using this approach (Payrhuber 1994). Research into the role of homeopathy in cancer pain can be difficult. It is essential to tease out the truth of what homeopathy can offer particularly when combined with conventional approaches of pain management. This chapter seeks to provide an overview of homeopathy and it's application in cancer pain.

Homeopathy and its historical context

It was Samuel Hahnemann (1755–1843), a German physician and scientist, who first began to uncover the central tenets of homeopathic philosophy. Whereas Descartes had reduced the human body to a machine, Hahnemann believed in the vital force, that which animates and regulates the human form and directs growth, healing, and repair. He postulated that the homeopathic remedy acted through the vital force stimulating a healing response.

The law of similars

Hahnemann began to draw out patterns of symptoms in relationship to homeopathic medicines, in a process called a 'proving'. The first proving (*prüfung* meaning a trial of a substance) used Cinchona, the Peruvian yew bark, known for its beneficial action in malaria and from which we eventually derived quinine. When given to a healthy person Hahnemann found that a pattern of symptoms developed similar to those found in the malaria sufferer. He went on to build up a catalogue of these symptom pictures with a variety of substances including belladonna (deadly nightshade) and arsenic. These symptom pictures particular to a medicine, could be matched to the symptoms in the sick person before him. Having discovered that medicines given in this way could be curative in acute diseases, he stated the fundamental law of similars, 'let like be treated with like'. Some psychotherapeutic techniques might be said to share this homeopathic approach, focusing, clarifying, and reflecting back the same story with the hope of stimulating a healing response. Conventional drugs may create the symptoms they are used to treat, thereby demonstrating the homeopathic principle; amphetamine which induces hyperactivity, and is used in hyperactivity disorder; aspirin, used in fever has, as a side-effect, hyperthermia; chemotherapy used to treat malignancy can induce malignant change. Provings are performed to this day as there are infinite substances, plant, mineral, and animal whose symptom pictures could be ascertained.

The minimum dose

Hahnemann pursued the minimum dose—the smallest amount of a substance that could be given to avoid side-effects and yet would still bring about a healing response. Much to his surprise, at some of the lower doses, the curative action of certain preparations seemed to be stronger, particularly when shaken vigorously (a process known as succussion). The preparation of a homeopathic medicine using serial dilution and succussion, he termed potentization. Drugs such as digitalis, which were known to be harmful in large doses, at the very low doses appeared to have a marked beneficial action without side-effects. The biological phenomenon of hormesis may explain some of these effects.

The homeopathic remedy as an ultramolecular dilution—scientific and clinical evidence for a therapeutic action

Hormesis

Hahnemann had chanced upon the observation that very low doses of a substance appeared to stimulate a healing response. Modern pharmacology has traditionally taught that very low concentrations of medicines have little or no effect on living mechanisms. As early as the 1940s, in radiation and toxicology research, it was observed that certain toxins in high doses were inhibiting metabolism and ultimately causing death, but at low doses they produced a stimulatory effect. As evidence accumulated, the phenomenon became known as hormesis. This refers to a bi-phasic dose–response relationship in which higher doses cause an inhibitory, and lower doses cause a stimulatory effect.

Clinical research

The role of a powerful consultation effect has been put forward as a key factor in initiating the positive changes associated with the administration of the homeopathic remedy. However clinical responses to ultramolecular preparations have been shown in randomized placebo controlled trials (Reilly *et al*. 1986, 1994). Using the test model of homeopathic immunotherapy in hay fever and subsequently asthma, Reilly and his co-workers showed that the homeopathically treated patients had a significant reduction in patient and doctor assessed symptom scores. No evidence emerged to support the idea that placebo action fully explains the clinical responses to homeopathic drugs. In a meta-analysis of 100 trials using homeopathy, over 77% were positive and the authors suggested further research was warranted (Kliejnen *et al.* 1991). A more recent meta-analysis of placebo controlled trials of homeopathy were not compatible with the hypothesis that the clinical effects of homeopathy are completely due to placebo (Linde *et al.* 1997).

Clinical evidence for homeopathy's role in cancer care

Downer (1994) and colleagues using a questionnaire-based study, showed that homeopathy is one of the eight most popular complementary therapies used by cancer patients. In an uncontrolled study from the London Homeopathic Hospital 50 patients were followed up over 6 months, 75% of whom had metastatic disease (Clover *et al.* 1995). A package of care, including homeopathy in every case, improved hospital anxiety and depression (HAD) scores and stabilized physical symptoms, including pain. A recent observational study, investigating 100 patients with cancer attending the Glasgow Homeopathic Hospital, showed that pain was the commonest problem symptom. In those patients completing the study, 75% found the homeopathic approach helpful for their symptoms assessed 4–5 visits later (Thompson 1999). In a Russian study, 37 patients with prostatic adenoma were treated with homeopathy over a 6–9 month period (Vozianov and Simeonova 1990). Surgical therapy was contra-indicated because of severe accompanying diseases. In the 19 patients complaining of pain as their main symptom, 18 reported improvement in perineal, groin, and loin pain over the course of homeopathic treatment.

Practical application in cancer pain

Decisions are needed about which, out of the 3000 homeopathic remedies currently available, might be most useful for cancer pain. The initial consultation can take up to 90 minutes. The first part can resemble a detailed conventional assessment. At the same time the homeopath may be taking in details of the language of the patient, physical characteristics, and demeanour—building up a framework as to the nature of the person, how they relate to the world and where they see the centre of their distress to lie. The diagnosis is important as a means to integrate the information as a whole, but what the patient says and the language that they use is paramount in deciding what remedy may be beneficial. Sometimes the present picture of pain connects with previous experiences of pain whether they be physical, psychological, or emotional. It is as if unresolved painful experiences in our lives can become awakened by the present experience of pain. Encouraging the person to speak of past and present hurt can allow a fuller picture of their suffering to become apparent. Themes within the person's story can then be matched to the themes of specific remedies. This can be illustrated with a clinical example.

72-year-old retired heavy metal worker.

Diagnosis renal cell carcinoma with bony secondaries. Symptom of painful muscle spasms due to spinal cord compression from metastatic disease. Past medical history: whooping cough as a child with painful spasmodic coughing.

He chooses first to talk about the violence he had experienced at the hands of fellow navy personnel during the war. This theme of violence was then repeated in the nature of the muscle spasms, which in the acute phase would throw him to the floor and which he described 'like preparing yourself for a punch in a fight'. On admission to the hospice he was in a violent confusional state. Intrathecal baclofen helped the spasms but a meningitis necessitated the removal of the catheter. A midazolam pump was started and the patient began to deteriorate.

After taking a 90 minute homeopathic case history, the remedy cuprum was chosen, a homeopathic preparation of copper. It has themes of violence, spasms, and cramps. It is used for the spasms of whooping cough. The cuprum was administered in liquid form three times daily. After 48 hours of taking this remedy his spasms were worse (a possible homeopathic aggravation) and then improved steadily over a ten day period, as did his general well-being. During this time the midazolam was gradually stopped (Thompson and Hicks 1998).

Choosing symptoms which most reflect the central themes and then finding the relevant remedies is known as repertorization. This process is aided by the use of the *Repertory* and *Materia medica*. Both of these are now available as computerized software.

The Repertory   lists thousands of symptoms arranged in sections according to their anatomical site of origin. Alongside each symptom are recorded all the remedies that include this symptom in their picture.

Materia Medica   complements the repertory by listing remedies along with their characteristic symptoms. Information from toxicology, provings, and clinical experience are collected together to create a comprehensive picture for each remedy (Table 17.1).

Table 17.1   Repestorization of case history above.

Case of Cuprum Metallicum	ARS	CUPR MET	BELL	CALC	COLOC	PHOS	HYOS	SIL
CARA Chart, Printed:5/11/98 9:37:42 PM Analysis type : Totality **Remedy filters** **Rubric filters** Polychrest: Yes Rubric weightings: No Frequent: Yes Stress significance: No Small: Yes Emphasise SRP: No Nosodes: Yes Emphasise small: No Remedy Class: All Remedy Family: All Miasms: All								
Total (weighted) score	11	11	9	8	8	7	7	7
Total rubrics covered	5	5	4	4	3	5	4	4
Total grades scored	11	11	9	8	8	7	7	7
1 Combined Synthetic Mentals DELIRIUM, VIOLENT	3	2	3			1	3	
1 Combined Kent Extremities CRAMPS	2	3	3	2	3	1	2	2
1 Combined Kent Extremities CRAMPS, LOWER LIMBS	1	3		2	3	1	1	1
1 Combined Synthetic Mentals LAMENTING, (BEMOANING, WAILING)	2	1	2	2	2	1	1	1
1 Combined Synthetic Generals (TIME) NIGHT MIDNIGHT, AFTER	3	2	1	2		3		3

Focusing on an unresolved emotional component to the pain

Certain groups of remedies are known for their use in anxiety states or depression. Below is an example of combining orthodox and complementary approaches to enhance pain relief using a remedy known to be useful in grief.

76-year-old gentleman referred to the pain clinic with intractable pain.

Diagnosis of squamous cell carcinoma of the left ear. Local recurrence despite radiotherapy. Using MST 100 mg twice daily. Pain excrutiating, 10/10 at all times, shooting in nature, extending around the ear. Assessment: post-auricular nerve involvement—treatment sodium valproate. Rates the death of his wife six months ago as more distressing than the physical pain and weeps with the mention of it. Had nursed her through the night sitting at her bedside. He would hold her hand, his left ear pressed against the armchair. Assessment: overwhelming grief reaction contributing to the pain. One month later says pain is still there but shooting component has gone. Still weeping with mention of wife.

Prescribed causticum, a remedy associated with grief in the affectionate and sympathetic person, particularly after nursing the sick. Pains are worse for cold wind and tend to be left sided, shooting in nature. Two months later reports 'pain is away' and wants to decrease morphine.

Focusing on the existential component

In some circumstances even with skilled communication, patients can get stuck in their journey towards the acceptance of disease progression, and death. Fear and anxiety can heighten the experience of pain and as carers we can be at a loss to know how to approach this block. Sometimes relief of distress without sedation is not possible. However having a range of non-drug approaches widens the potential to break through into a calmer space whilst the person remains as alert as they might wish.

69-year-old retired vicar

Diagnosis of mesothelioma. Referred because of difficulties with open communication, increasing anxiety and continuing chest pain. He had found the acceptance of women clergy into the church devastating. He remarked on my lack of punctuality, being two minutes later than the appointed hour. The noise of passing ambulances at some distance was a great irritation to him. His chest pain was left sided. In general the pain was better since admission with an increase in morphine and the addition of sodium valproate. However it was still wakening him at 4–5 a.m. and he was then distressed by thoughts going around in his head. He denied anxiety but mentioned his godson whom he worried about.

Prescribed Kali carbonicum. This is a remedy useful for those who desire order and punctuality. Symptoms tend to be worse around 4.00 a.m. and there is a marked irritation to noise. On review 5 days later he reported that the pain at night had gone. The consultation was more open and he spoke of John as his partner and his hope for acceptance of their relationship in the hospice. Pain was never an issue although very difficult night sweats were treated successfully with the homeopathic remedy arsenicum. He died peacefully five months later with John by his side.

Focusing on the physical component

Further research is needed to clarify which types of cancer pain may benefit most from the homeopathic approach. Two examples of the use of homeopathic medicines are

Visceral pain

42-year-old pianist
Diagnosis of ovarian carcinoma with extensive peritoneal spread and liver metastases. Six laparotomies with many adhesions. Symptom of abdominal colic. Very severe pain, comes on suddenly. Feels bloated. Uses the homeopathic remedy carbo vegetablis instead of buscopan to abort an attack.

Key notes of carbo vegetablis include excessive flatus with abdominal distension especially upper part. Griping pain in the abdomen below the naval extending from the left to the right side.

Postoperative incisional neuropathic pain

62-year-old lady with pain in scar post-mastectomy. This is a severe aching pain with the sensation of a ball in armpit. Prescription: 3 doses of arnica—a useful remedy in neuralgic pains post trauma or surgery.
Pain helped—within one week of powders the ball sensation had gone. Effect lasted 4 months before returning. Remedy repeated.

Problems encountered using homeopathy

Much of the homeopathic philosophy is based around the ideal of health and the expectation of full recovery. What is not yet clear is what outcome can be hoped for using the homeopathic approach for advanced disease. Cancer sufferers are a vulnerable group and fostering unrealistic expectations may engender denial or false hopes of recovery. Offering homeopathy as another approach to symptom control, rather than suggesting that remedies may have an impact on the disease itself, is more realistic. Occasionally a transient worsening of symptoms can occur after starting a homeopathic remedy. This is known as a homeopathic aggravation and can lead to confusion if there are other causes for an apparent deterioration. The homeopathic medicine should be stopped and the aggravation should settle quickly. The remedy can then be restarted at a lesser frequency of administration to avoid a further aggravation. Regular reviews are essential.

References

Clover, A., Last, P., Fisher, P., Wright, S., and Boyle, H. (1995). Complementary therapy: a pilot study of patients, therapies and quality of life. *Complementary Therapies in Medicine*, **3**, 129–33.

Downer, S.M., Cody, M.M. *et al.* (1994). Pursuit and practice of complementary therapies by cancer patients receiving conventional treatment. *British Medical Journal*, **309**, 86–9.

Kleijnen, J., Knipscild, P., Ter Riet, G. (1991). Clinical trials of homoeopathy. *British Medical Journal*, **302**, 316–23.

Linde, K., Clausius, N., Ramirez, G., Meichart, D., Eitel, F., Hedges, L., Jonas, W. (1997). Are the clinical effects of homoeopathy placebo effects? A meta-analysis of placebo-controlled trials. *Lancet*, **350**, 834–43.

Payrhuber, D. (1994). Treatment in cancer. *Homoeopath Links*, **7**(4), 17–19.

Reilly, D., Taylor, M.A., McSharry, C., and Beattie, N. (1986). Is homoeopathy a placebo response? Controlled trials of homoeopathic potency with pollen in hayfever as a model. *Lancet*, **ii**, 881–6.

Reilly, D., Taylor, M.A., Beattie, N.G.M., Campbell, J.M., McSharry, C., and Aitchison, T.C. (1994). Is the evidence for homoeopathy reproducible? *Lancet*, **344**, 1601–6.

Thompson, E., and Hicks, F. (1998). Intrathecal baclofen and homoeopathy for the treatment of painful muscle spasms associated with malignant spinal cord compression. *Palliative Medicine*, **12**, 119–21.

Thompson, E. (1999). The homeopathic approach to symptom control in the cancer patient—an observational study, oral presentation. European Association of Palliative Care Congress, Geneva.

Vozianov, A.F., and Simeonova, N.K. (1990). Homoeopathic treatment of patients with adenomas of the prostate. *British Homoeopathic Journal*, **79**, 148–51.

Index